Surgery
of the Veins of the Leg
and Pelvis

Other monographs in the series / Major Problems in Clinical Surgery:

Child: *The Liver and Portal Hypertension*
Welch: *Polypoid Lesions of the Gastrointestinal Tract,* 2nd edition
Madding and Kennedy: *Trauma to the Liver*
Barker: *Peripheral Arterial Disease,* 2nd edition
Spratt and Donegan: *Cancer of the Breast*
Haller: *Deep Thrombophlebitis*
Colcock and Braasch: *Surgery of the Small Intestine in the Adult*
Jackman and Beahrs: *Tumors of the Large Bowel*
Ellis and Olsen: *Achalasia of the Esophagus*
Botsford and Wilson: *The Acute Abdomen*
Colcock: *Diverticular Disease of the Colon*
Spratt, Butcher and Bricker: *Exenterative Surgery of the Pelvis*
Shires, Carrico and Canizaro: *Shock*
Child: *Portal Hypertension as Seen by 16 Authorities*
Sedgwick: *Surgery of the Thyroid Gland*
Thorbjarnarson: *Surgery of the Biliary Tract*
Greenfield: *Surgery in the Aged*
Menguy: *Surgery of Peptic Ulcer*
Salisbury and Pruitt: *Burns of the Upper Extremity*
Bushkin and Woodward: *Postgastrectomy Syndromes*
Blaisdell and Lewis: *Respiratory Distress Syndrome of Shock and Trauma*

SURGERY OF THE VEINS OF THE LEG AND PELVIS

by

Dr. med. Robert May

Surgeon, F. I. C. A.
Innsbruck, Austria

Translated by

Hans J. Hirsch, M. D.
London, Great Britain

Volume XXIII in the Series
MAJOR PROBLEMS IN CLINICAL SURGERY

PAUL A. EBERT, M. D.
Consulting Editor

W. B. Saunders Company, Philadelphia, London, Toronto
and Georg Thieme Publishers Stuttgart 1979

Authorized English edition co-published 1979
by W. B. Saunders Company, Philadelphia, London, Toronto
and Georg Thieme Publishers, Stuttgart

Original German edition: Chirurgie der Bein- und Beckenvenen

Typeset by William Clowes, Colchester, UK. Printed in Germany by Karl Grammlich, Pliezhausen
ISBN 3-13-545901-2 (Thieme)
ISBN 0-7216-6200-5 (Saunders)
LCCCN 76-028942 (Saunders)

Editor

Univ.-Doz. Dr. med. ROBERT MAY, F.I.C.A., Facharzt für Chirurgie, Privatkrankenhaus der Kreuzschwestern, Boznerplatz 6, A-6020 Innsbruck, Austria

Authors

BLÜMEL, G., Prof. Dr. med., Direktor des Instituts für experimentelle Chirurgie der Technischen Universität, Ismaninger Straße 22, D-8000 Munich 80, Germany

BRUNNER, U., Prof. Dr. med., Leiter der Abteilung für periphere vaskuläre Chirurgie an der Chirurgischen Universitätsklinik B, Kantonsspital, CH-8006 Zürich, Switzerland

COCKETT, F. B., M.S., F.R.C.S., Surgeon, St. Thomas's Hospital, London, Great Britain

GOTTLOB, R., Prof. Dr. med., Leiter der Abteilung für experimentelle Chirurgie, I. Chirurgische Universitätsklinik, A-1014 Vienna, Austria

KUNLIN, A., Dr. med., Chef de chirurgie-assistant, Hôpitaux de Paris, Paris, France

KUNLIN, J., Dr. med., 95, rue de Sèvres F-92100 Boulogne, France

MAY, R., Univ.-Dozent Dr. med., F.I.C.A., Facharzt für Chirurgie, Privatkrankenhaus der Kreuzschwestern, Boznerplatz 6, A-6020 Innsbruck, Austria

NISSL, R., Univ.-Doz. Dr. med., Facharzt für Röntgenologie, Neuhauserstraße 2, A-6020 Innsbruck, Austria

PURTSCHELLER, W., Dr. med., Facharzt für Anaesthesiologie, Neugasse 6a, A-6064 Rum/Innsbruck, Austria

SCHLOSSER, V., Prof. Dr. med., Leiter der Abteilung für Herz- und Gefäßchirurgie, Chirurgische Universitätsklinik, Hugstetter Straße 55, D-7800 Freiburg i. Breisgau, Germany

SCHWARZ, H., Prof. Dr. med., Chefarzt der Chirurgischen Abteilung des Spitals Limmattal, Urdorferstraße 100, CH-8952 Schlieren, Switzerland

VOLLMAR, J. F., Prof. Dr. med., Leiter der Abteilung Chirurgie II im Chirurgie-Zentrum der Universität, Steinhövelstraße 9, D-7900 Ulm, Germany

DEWEESE, J. A., M.D., Prof. of Surgery, Division of Cardiothoracic Surgery, University of Rochester, Medical Center, 601 Elmwood Avenue, Rochester, New York 14642, USA

Translator

HIRSCH, HANS J., M.B., B.Ch., F.R.C.Path., 6, Graham Lodge, Graham Road, London NW4, 3DG, Great Britain

Thomas Mann, from *Joseph and His Brothers,* Prelude: Descent into Hell: "Appropriately . . . the unfathomable plays a mocking game with our research urges; it offers apparent stops and goals behind which, when attained, new reaches open—just as before the beachcomber who never finds an ending, since beyond each headland of muddy dune he set off for, new expanses lure toward farther foothills."

George Bernard Shaw: In October 1930 a dinner was given in honor of Albert Einstein at the Savoy Hotel in London. Bernard Shaw was the speaker. His secretary of many years, Blanche Patch, reports on it: "Shaw, who was then 74, considered this speech to be so important that I had to type it beforehand—an extraordinary request, for usually he spoke without notes. He said, 'Of these great natural philosophers, only three created a whole universe: Ptolemy, Newton, and Einstein. The others only patched it. These great Three became the leaders of a movement of humanity, which had an effect in two directions. One is called religion, the other science.' He continued, 'Religion solves all problems, thus eliminating the problems of the universe. It gives us certainty, peace, and absolute concepts. *Science is the direct opposite. It is always wrong. It never solves a problem without exposing new ones.*' "

Preface

In the last few years, surgery of the arteries has made such vital progress that special departments have had to be established in most hospitals.

Venous surgery long remained in the background. Widmer's studies on the working population in industry in Basel showed that roughly 30 percent of men and 34 percent of women had diseased veins. The surgical approach to veins has changed in important ways for treatment of varices, ulcers, venous malformations and so forth. Surgical removal of thrombi has become a routine procedure. Only one problem still needs solution — the post-thrombotic syndrome. Three percent of the workers in the Basel study had severe insufficiency of the veins. This means that in Switzerland and Austria at least 100,000 people and in Germany more than a million people suffer from lifelong, slowly deteriorating, deep vein disease that only inadequately can be overcome by conservative means. This reveals the magnitude of the problem. First steps have been taken, however. Experimental surgery played an important role in the solution of this problem; for this reason, we have devoted a large chapter to it. At the same time, precise roentgenologic and venous pressure studies are essential, and these too have been dealt with.

The publishers considered the time propitious for a comprehensive presentation of our experience. It seemed important to us to illuminate the whole problem from many aspects and to offer the views of not only the author. We therefore chose the multi-author approach with its divergent opinions.

Recently I saw the most beautiful mosaics in the world in Istanbul. The Byzantine artists intentionally placed the chips at different angles in order to achieve greater brilliance. I intended in the same way to present a book about present-day venous surgery—a mosaic, not a monotonous picture.

I also asked my coauthors to provide a brief bibliography emphasizing essentials. Repetitions from chapter to chapter were unavoidable if completeness was to be preserved.

I thank all my coauthors and personal assistants, especially my radiologist Dr. Raimund Nissl, the artist Rudolf Schulz, and my sister Heidi Rudolph.

For reasons unknown to me, it is the practice to thank the publisher last. Dr. med. h.c. Günther Hauff ought to be mentioned first in this book as in many others. Without his courage and patient advice and without the technically excellent reproduction of the illustrations, this book would never have been accomplished.

Innsbruck, August 1978

Robert May

Contents

9. Venous Trauma

10. Malformations of Leg and Pelvic Veins

1 Anatomy

R. May

What the vascular surgeon requires first is exact roentgenologic illustrations. Interpretation of the findings is sometimes not easy.
For this reason, the chapter on the *anatomy of the veins of the leg and pelvis* has deliberately been treated as x-ray anatomy. Surgically important features are discussed under individual procedures.
Knowledge of normal anatomic relations is essential for description and interpretation of x-ray pictures.

Veins of the Foot

Although they are insignificant from a pathologic point of view, the veins of the foot are important because contrast media are injected into them. They are divided into four systems, according to Winckler (1923).

Superficial Veins of the Sole of the Foot

The superficial veins of the sole of the foot form such a dense plexus that the French justly speak of a "semelle veineuse plantaire," an insole of veins, which forms a large venous arcade at the distal end of the foot. This plexus is widely connected with the superficial venous plexus of the dorsum of the foot by the interdigital and the dorsal collateral veins of each toe. It fans out into 12 to 15 branches to the medial and lateral margins of the foot. These veins can be seen medially on a standing, overtired foot. They form broad connections with the external and internal marginal veins, which course along the outer and inner margins of the foot. Despite their thin walls they are used for injection when the dorsal veins cannot be seen.

Superficial Veins of the Dorsum of the Foot

The superficial venous system of the dorsum of the foot, which is usually used for injection, is clearly visible through the skin. Despite their apparent variety the governing veins are constant. Beginning at the distal third of the dorsum of the foot there runs the wide, distally convex arch of the superficial dorsal venous arcade, whose terminations extend as the internal and external marginal veins; these in turn continue in the leg as the great and lesser saphenous vein (Fig. 1.1).
The widely curved arch of the superficial dorsal venous arcade collects the venous blood from the toes and transports it via the dorsal collateral veins into the median veins. These continue into the superficial dorsal interosseous veins. The internal collateral vein, which is particularly well developed, continues into the internal marginal vein after having collected blood from superficial connecting veins, not only from the dorsal but also from the plantar aspect of the big toe, and from the medial plantar margin of the foot.
The internal collateral vein and the median vein of the big toe, called also the unguinal vein, are therefore well suited to use for injection in phlebography, because of their size and drainage. By analogy, the external collateral vein of the fifth toe continues as the external marginal vein, having received the outer portion of the dorsal venous arch. Furthermore, at the base of each toe, the superficial interdigital veins flow into the internal collateral vein of its corresponding toe, thus connecting the superficial plantar with the superficial dorsal plexus. This connection is further safeguarded by the fact that the dorsal superficial interdigital veins are connected by the perforating interosseous veins with the corresponding plantar interosseous veins distally. As already mentioned, the internal malleolar vein continues as the *great saphenous vein*. It communicates with the posterior tibial vein by a large internal marginal vein just below the internal malleolus. Thus the contrast medium, which is usually injected into the trunk or ramifications of the internal marginal vein, certainly also reaches the deep veins of the leg (Fig. 1.2).
The considerably smaller external marginal vein runs below the external malleolus, thence becoming the *lesser saphenous vein*. During its entire

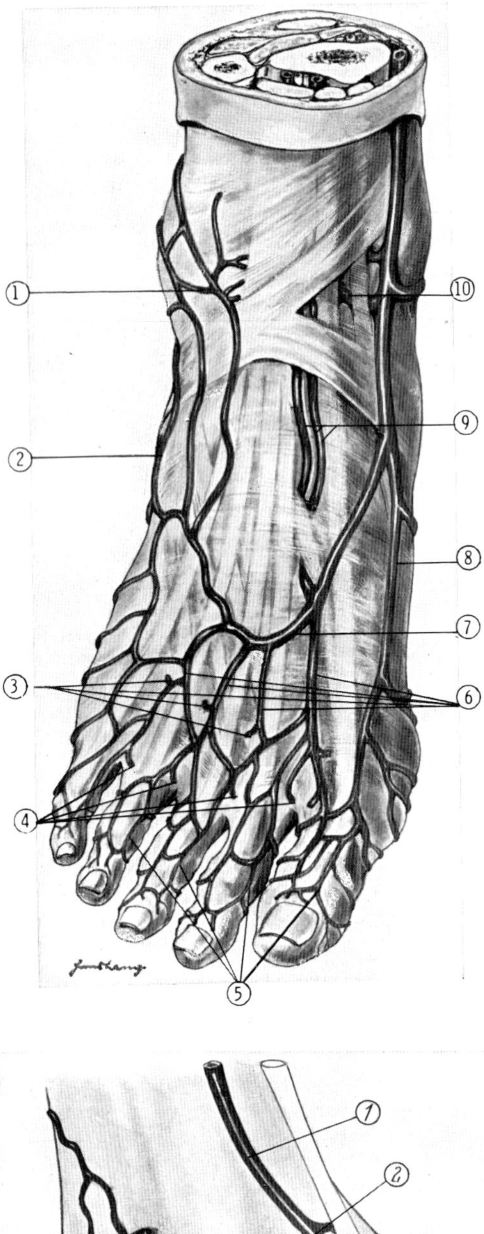

Fig. 1.1. Superficial veins of the dorsum of the foot.
1 V. malleolaris anteroexterna
2 V. marginalis externa
3 Arcus venosus dorsalis pedis
4 Vv. interosseae perforantes
5 Vv. interdigitales
6 Vv. digitales pedis dorsales
7 Vv. digitales communes pedis
8 V. marginalis interna
9 Vv. dorsales pedis
10 V. malleolaris anterointerna
(Figs. 1.1–1.4, 1.11, 1.44, 1.45, 1.47–1.54, 1.56–1.58 from May, R., and R. Nissl: Die Phlebographie der unteren Extremität. Thieme, Stuttgart 1959.)

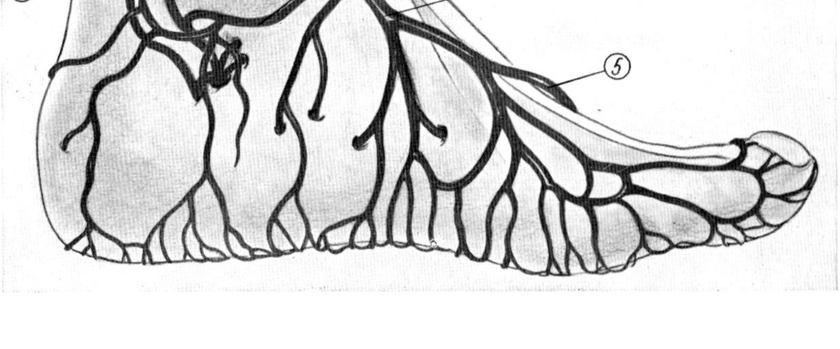

Fig. 1.2. Veins at the internal malleolus.
1 V. saphena magna
2 V. malleolaris interna
3 V. tibialis posterior
4 V. marginalis interna
5 Arcus venosus dorsalis pedis

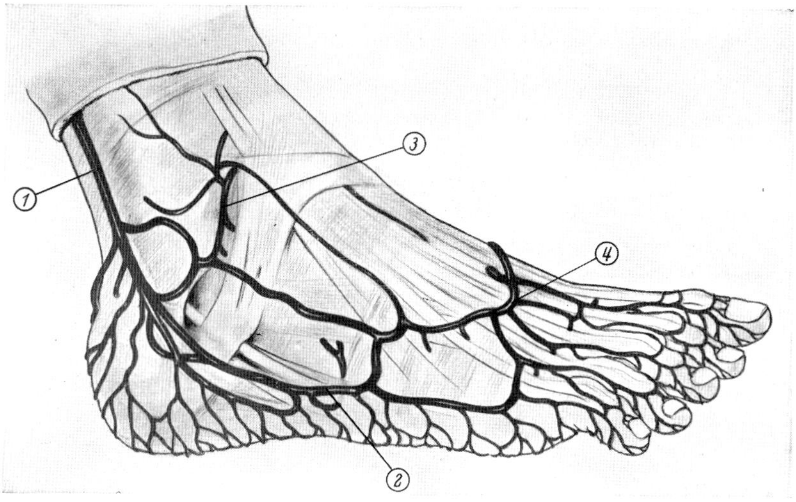

Fig. 1.3. Veins at the external malleolus.
1 V. saphena parva
2 V. marginalis externa
3 V. malleolaris antero-externa
4 Arcus venosus dorsalis pedis

course it, like the internal marginal vein, receives at regular intervals branches from the superficial plantar plexus which lie around the outer margin of the foot. Running over the instep, a strong constant anteroexternal malleolar vein connects the anterior tibial with the small saphenous vein (Fig. 1.3).

Deep Veins of the Sole of the Foot

The deep plantar veins usually accompany homonymous arteries (Fig. 1.4). Thus a single or twin external plantar vein accompanies the artery, sweeping in a wide arch from the first metatarsal interspace to the calcaneus canal, where it becomes the *posterior tibial vein*. Its connection with the superficial dorsal venous plexus is secured by a strong communicating vein in the first interosseous space, as well as by the plantar interosseous veins, which receive all communicating veins.

The much smaller internal plantar vein, also communicating with a neighboring plexus, accompanies the homonymous artery without special features. Dos Santos (1947) pointed out that, unlike those in the leg, the deep veins of the foot play an entirely subordinate part. The same is true of the deep dorsal veins.

Communicating Veins

The communicating veins of the foot interconnect the three venous systems described so far. They are numerous and variable. Van Limborgh (1961, 1963) divided them into plantar communicating veins, lateral marginal communicating veins and dorsal communicating veins of the foot.

It was thus clearly shown why all plexuses are filled on injection of any vein within reach and,

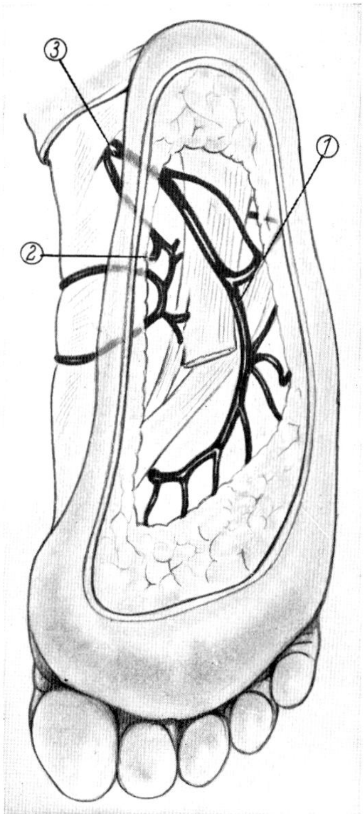

Fig. 1.4. Deep veins of the sole of the foot.
1 V. plantaris externa
2 V. plantaris interna
3 V. tibialis posterior

more important, why the distribution of the contrast medium to all deep leg veins is guaranteed.

Veins of the Lower Extremity

For functional reasons, four types of veins are distinguished in phlebography of the lower extremity (Figs. 1.5 and 1.6):

—deep leg veins;
—subcutaneous superficial veins;
—muscle veins; and
—communicating and perforating veins.

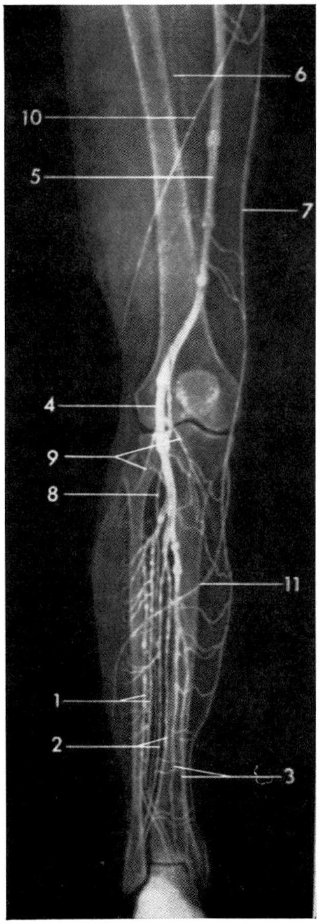

Fig. 1.5. Ascending phlebogram of the veins of the lower extremity.
1 Vv. tibiales anteriores
2 Vv. peroneae
3 Vv. tibiales posteriores
4 V. poplitea
5 V. femoralis superficialis
6 V. femoralis profunda (punctate line, only exceptionally demonstrable on ascending phlebography)
7 V. saphena magna
8 V. saphena parva
9 Vv. gastrocnemicae
10 V. saphena accessoria
11 R. anterior of V. saphena magna
(Figs. 1.5, 1.7–1.10, 1.18, 1.23, 1.24, 1.33–1.35 from May, R. and R. Nissl: Fortschr. Röntgenstr. 104 (1966) 172–180.)

Knowledge of normal anatomic relations and their variants is essential for description and interpretation of roentgenograms. The percentage figures quoted for normal anatomic variants are based on roughly 6000 phlebographic procedures performed by us.

Deep Veins of the Lower Limb

Deep Veins of the Leg

The three arteries of the leg are accompanied by three corresponding pairs of deep veins: the anterior tibial veins, the posterior tibial veins and the peroneal veins. They occur in pairs but occasionally ramify distally into three or four branches and, anastomosing among themselves, embrace the arteries. Proximally the paired branches fuse to single trunks.
These again unite at different levels to form the popliteal vein.
In 47.5 per cent of the population, the confluence of the deep leg veins lies distal to the popliteal space (Fig. 1.7*a*); in 8.35 per cent, level with the popliteal space (Fig. 1.7*b*); and in 44.15 per cent, above the popliteal space (Fig. 1.7*c*), which is equivalent to a double-barreled popliteal vein.
The local relations of the deep veins of the leg to each other and to the small saphenous vein on radiographs in different projections were studied in detail by Netzer (1958) (Fig. 1.8). On the anteroposterior view, the peroneal veins lie lateral to the anterior tibial veins at the level of the malleolus. They curve slightly medially, cross the tibial veins anteriorly approximately a thumb's thickness above the malleolus, and, in radiographs of all planes, are seen to lie between the anterior and posterior tibial veins. On radiographs made with slight internal rotation of the leg, in which the deep leg veins are best demonstrated because the greater part of them projects into the interosseous space, the crossing point of the anterior tibial with the peroneal veins moves proximally.

Popliteal Vein

Most textbooks of anatomy show only artificially normalized pictures of the vessel that are not consistent with the facts. Recent anatomic studies were made by Kobak and Lev (1954) and by Williams (1953).
Generally two points are important: (1) Irregularity is the rule. (2) Textbook descriptions notwithstanding, the popliteal vein does not occur as a single vessel; usually there are two veins in the popliteal space, and sometimes three.

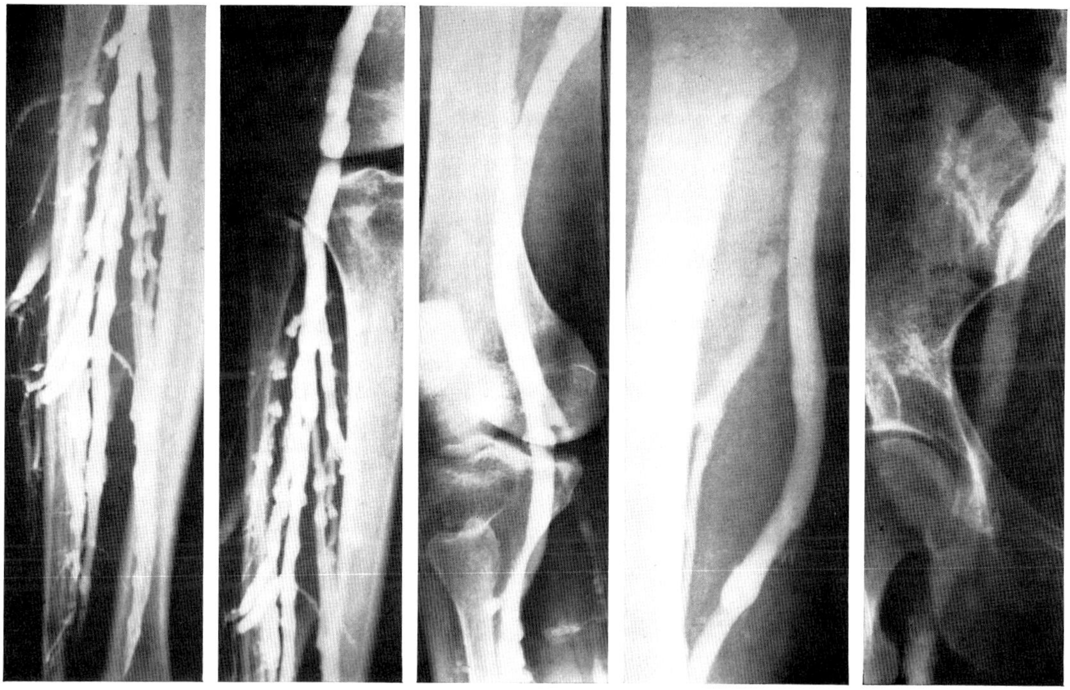

Fig. 1.6. Phleboscopic details of an ascending phlebogram of the lower extremity. Veins from the malleolus up to the cava showing the typical details of the normal deep and superficial venous systems.

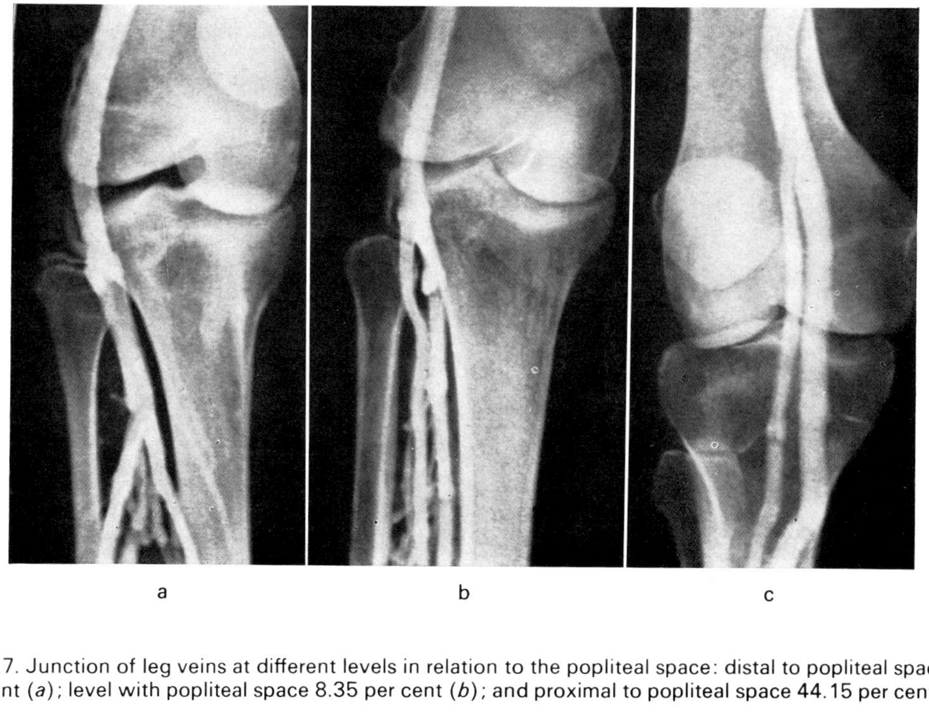

a b c

Fig. 1.7. Junction of leg veins at different levels in relation to the popliteal space: distal to popliteal space 47.5 per cent (*a*); level with popliteal space 8.35 per cent (*b*); and proximal to popliteal space 44.15 per cent (*c*).

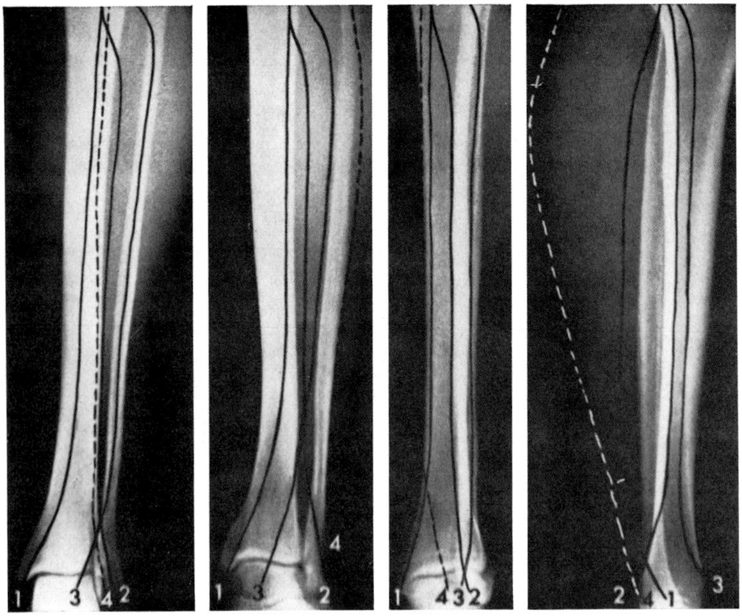

a b c d

Fig. 1.8. Relation of leg veins and small saphenous vein to each other in different planes (after Netzer). Antero-posterior ray path (*a*); 25-degree internal rotation (*b*); 30-degree external rotation (*c*); and lateral view (*d*).

1 Vv. tibiales posteriores
2 Vv. peroneae
3 Vv. tibiales anteriores
4 V. saphena parva

As already mentioned, this depends on the level of confluence of the deep veins of the leg.

In our material there was a single popliteal vein at the level of the popliteal space in 55.85 per cent of those studied (Fig. 1.9*a*). In 39.15 per cent there were two branches, which united just above the popliteal space to form a femoral vein (Fig. 1.9*b*). In 2.78 per cent confluence of the two branches was lacking and they continued as double-barreled femoral vein (Fig. 1.9*c*). In 2.22

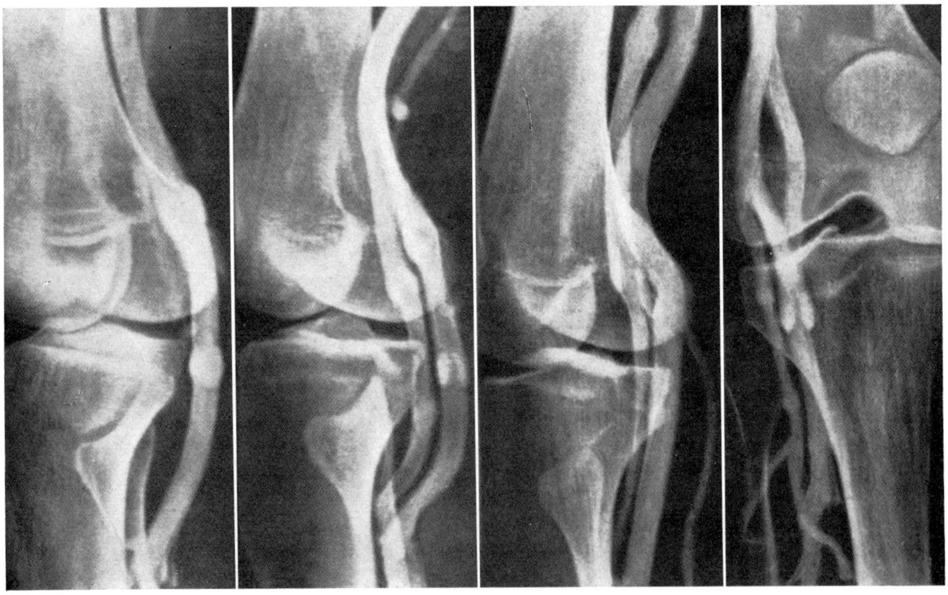

a b c d

Fig. 1.9. Variants of the popliteal vein. Single popliteal (55.85 per cent) (*a*); double popliteal (33.15 per cent) flowing into femoral vein (*b*); double popliteal (2.78 per cent) flowing into double femoral (*c*); and triple popliteal (2.22 per cent) (*d*).

per cent there was a triple-barreled popliteal vein at the level of the popliteal space (Fig. 1.9*d*).

Femoral Vein

Continuing the popliteal vein, the superficial femoral vein slants toward the inguinal region. At an average distance of 9 cm below the inguinal ligament, it receives the stout branch of the deep femoral vein, which is only exceptionally demonstrable on ascending phlebography; it is now named the common femoral vein. Anatomic studies of Cockett (1955) showed, however, that these textbook demonstrations applied in only approximately 16 per cent of cases. According to Cockett, there is frequently duplication of the main branch, which receives a large number of communicating veins at the level of the adductor canal, or the deep femoral vein anastomoses with the distal portion of the femoral vein or even the popliteal, so that two marked thigh veins are seen on radiography.

The material we examined revealed the single-barreled type of Cockett in 62.34 per cent of cases (Fig. 1.10*a*). In 21.16 per cent, the popliteal vein branches into two main femoral trunks, which reunite beneath the inguinal ligament (Fig. 1.10*b*). In 13.72 per cent there is multiple branching of the main trunk (Fig. 1.10*c*), and in 2.78 per cent a double-barreled popliteal vein changes into a double-barreled femoral vein, which does not join until it reaches the level of the inguinal ligament (Fig. 1.10*d*). The caliber of the two veins may vary markedly.

Superficial Veins of the Lower Limb and Muscle Veins

The superficial veins of the lower extremity and the veins in the gastrocnemius and soleus muscles are considered together since the termination of the small saphenous vein coincides with that of the gastrocnemius veins; here there are variations that have practical significance. All superficial lower limb veins vary in course and are linked by multiple anastomoses. Phlebography should demonstrate these unpredictable individual deviations.

Great Saphenous Vein

The great saphenous vein (Fig. 1.11), mostly deeply embedded in subcutaneous fat of the thigh, was aptly named "saphena," the hidden, by the Hebrews and later by the Arabs, in the early Middle Ages. The great saphenous vein is

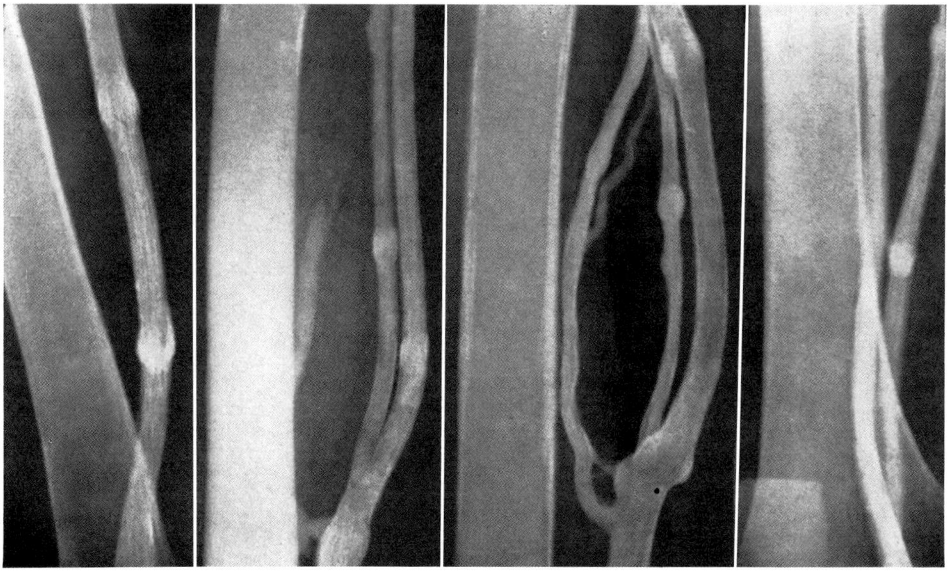

a b c d

Fig. 1.10. Variants of the femoral vein. Single femoral (62.34 per cent) (*a*); two main trunks of the femoral which join again distal to inguinal ligament (21.16 per cent) (*b*); multiple division of the main femoral trunk (13.72 per cent) (*c*); and double popliteal draining into double femoral (2.78 per cent) (*d*).

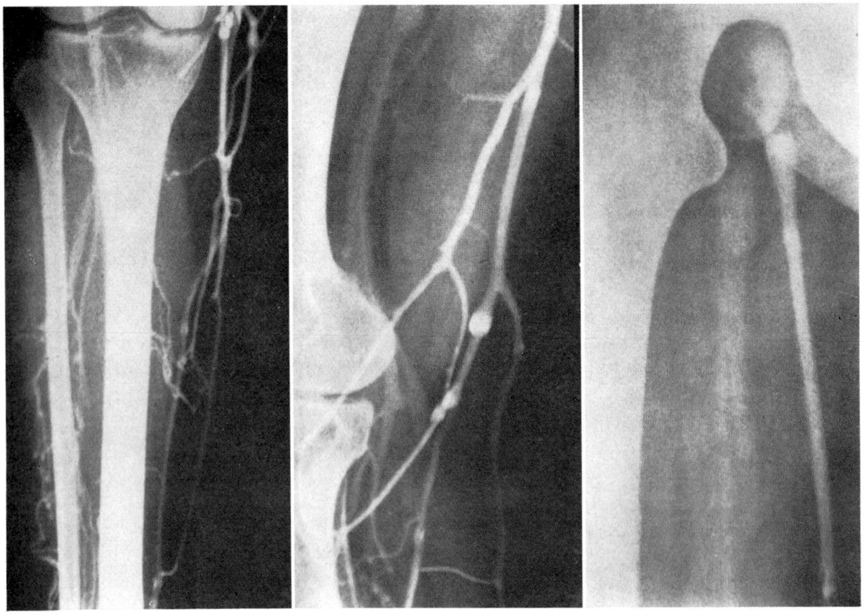

Fig. 1.11. Roentgenograms of a normal great saphenous vein.

the continuation of the medial marginal vein, which runs along the medial margin of the foot and ascends on the inner aspect of the leg in front of the internal malleolus, where it is always easily visible and palpable. At the posterior margin of the sartorius muscle it reaches the medial surface of the thigh and flows through the saphenous opening into the common femoral vein. In 73 per cent of cases the saphenous vein is single in the thigh; in 27 per cent it is double-barreled and the two trunks unite just beneath the fossa ovalis or in the fossa ovalis at the confluence with the common femoral vein. Subinguinally, in the region where the great saphenous unites with the femoral vein, level with the saphenous hiatus, several accessory veins join (Fig. 1.12).
These are

—both accessory saphenous veins—the medial or tibial and the lateral or fibular—whose termination in the great saphenous vein varies between the middle of the thigh and the hiatus saphenus;
—the superficial epigastric vein, whose termination is fairly constant;
—the superficial external pudendal vein, whose union is very variable and which may flow directly into the trunk of the femoral vein;
—the superficial medial and lateral circumflex veins of the femur, which are inconstant; and
—the superficial circumflex vein of the ilium.

The vascular variability in this region is so marked, however, that Hilty (1955) described it in a monograph of 148 pages. There are also very

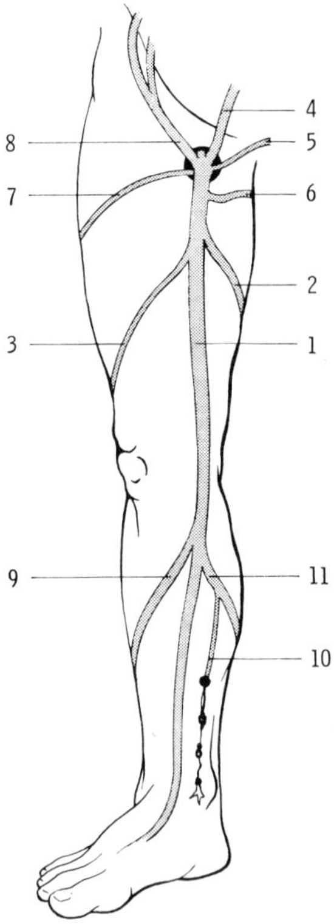

Fig. 1.12. Drawing of the great saphenous vein with the superficial subinguinal veins of the lower extremity.
1 V. saphena magna
2 V. saphena accessoria medialis
3 V. saphena accessoria lateralis
4 V. epigastrica superficialis
5 V. pudenda externa
6 V. circumflexa femoris medialis
7 V. circumflexa femoris lateralis
8 V. circumflexa ilium superficialis
9 Anterior ramus of great saphenous
10 Posterior ramus of great saphenous
11 Anastomosis with small saphenous

extensive studies by Cockett and Dodd (1956). It seems hopeless to attempt to classify these variants into groups. We can only advance an idealized scheme and emphasize that there are no typical and atypical cases, that any conceivable deviation is possible. This variation includes the external pudendal artery which, while always running obliquely across the union, lies at times above and at times below the great saphenous vein and occasionally even under the femoral vein.

As will be explained on page 85, the variable course and relations of the femoral artery and its branches to the venous system must also be considered. Bevan et al. (1956) described a rare variant of *low termination* of the great saphenous, in which the latter does not unite in the groin but a few fingerbreadths to a handbreadth distally, forming a special order of termination of the accessory vein which, however, is also inconstant (Fig. 1.13).

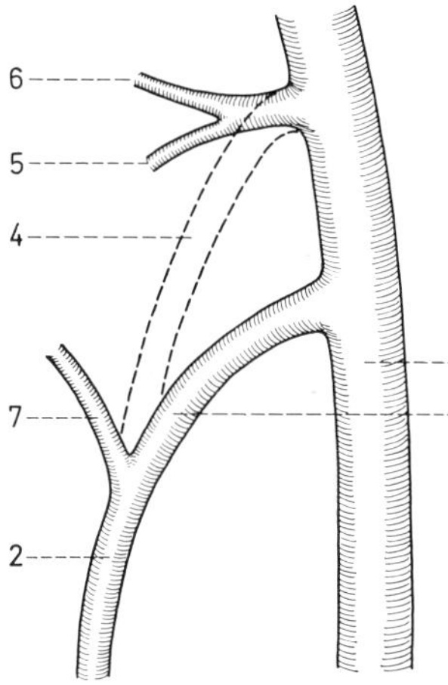

Fig. 1.13. Drawing of the junction of accessory veins with low termination of the great saphenous. (After Bevan, Green and Stammers.)
1. V. femoralis
2 V. saphena magna
3 Perforating vein developed to main trunk of great saphenous
4 Obliterated portion of great saphenous
5 V. pudenda externa
6 V. epigastrica superficialis
7 V. circumflexa ilium superficialis

The great saphenous vein further receives a number of accessory branches throughout its course which cannot be classified. The most important ones of the leg are the anterior and the posterior branches. Among the great number of anomalous junctions of the great saphenous vein, two types may be emphasized:

—*Low termination* of the great saphenous vein described by Bevan et al. (1956), in which the external pudendal and the superficial epigastric vein indeed terminate at the normal termination of the saphenous just below the inguinal ligament, but the great saphenous joins the femoral vein 3 to 5 cm below this point. The lower termination occurs when the next lower perforating vein develops as the great saphenous trunk and the most proximal portion of the saphenous is obliterated.

—The great saphenous vein does not flow into the femoral vein in the hiatus saphenus, as is normal, but crosses this vessel in the proximal part of the thigh, runs lateral to the femoral vein over the inguinal ligament and terminates in a subcutaneous abdominal vein. Siegelbauer (1944) pointed out that this drainage is the phylogenetically older path of the great saphenous vein and is atavistic.

Small Saphenous Vein, Femoropopliteal Vein and Veins of the Muscles

The following veins flow into the popliteal vein at the level of the popliteal fossa (Figs. 1.14 and 1.15):

—*Small saphenous vein*;
—*gastrocnemial veins*; and
—*communicating veins around the knee*.

Figure 1.16 shows that these junctions may be complex. Nevertheless, the anatomic order is normally relatively constant.

The small saphenous vein (Fig. 1.17) originates from the lateral marginal vein of the dorsum of the foot, runs below and behind the external malleolus up to the middle of the calf, disappears at varying levels through the fascia, and enters the popliteal vein between the heads of the gastrocnemius. Figure 1.18 shows a diagram Moosmann and Hartwell (1964) devised to demonstrate the relation of the small saphenous vein to the fascia. The level of entry of the small saphenous vein under the fascia is of importance if this vein is varicosed, for frequently the small saphenous vein contains varicosities distal to the point of entry through the fascia, but is sufficient proximal to it. Probably the fascia plays a part in supporting the vein, like an elastic stocking. The small saphenous enters the popliteal vein at various levels.

According to the surgical material of Haeger (1962), the small saphenous vein flows into the popliteal 1 to 3 cm above the popliteal space in 60 per cent of cases, and in the majority, 3 cm proximal to it. In approximately 8 per cent the site of entry is dorsal to the knee joint and in 32 per cent it is higher than 3 cm above the popliteal space. Our phlebographic examinations of 1000 patients yielded the following distribution of the inflow of the small saphenous vein, which approximates the surgical findings of Haeger (1962). If the small saphenous vein enters the popliteal in the popliteal space and does not continue into a femoropopliteal vein, the junction takes place between 3 and 5 cm above the popliteal fossa in 78.73 per cent of cases. Infrequently (1.46 per cent

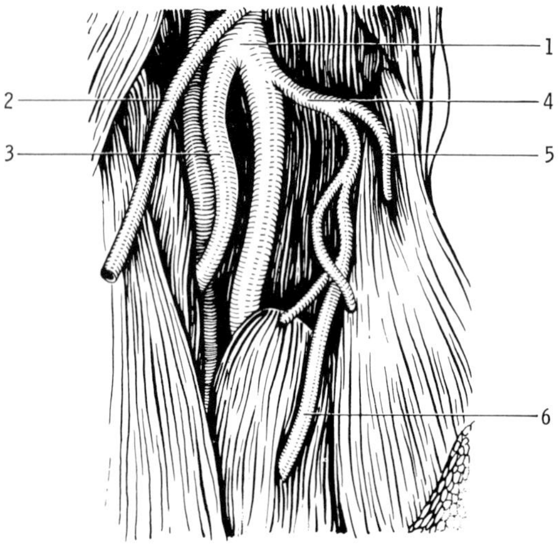

Fig. 1.14. Veins of the popliteal fossa. (From May, R., and R. Nissl: Fortschr. Röntgenstr. 109 (1968) 614.)
1 V. poplitea
2 V. saphena parva
3 V. gastrocnemia medialis
4 V. gastrocnemia lateralis with
5 branches from the head of gastrocnemius and
6 from soleus

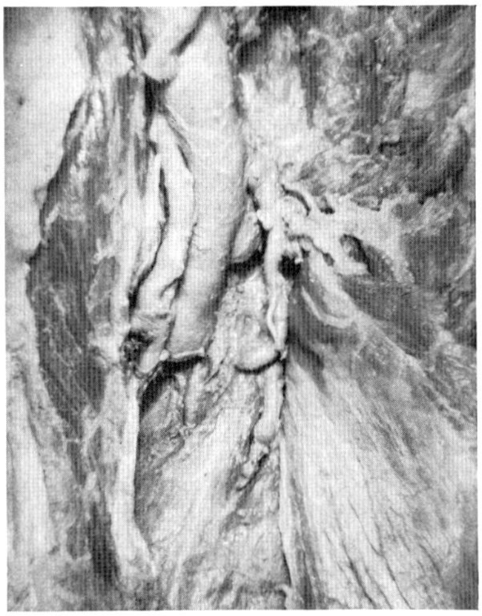

Fig. 1.15. Anatomic preparation of the veins in the popliteal fossa, corresponding with Figure 1.14.

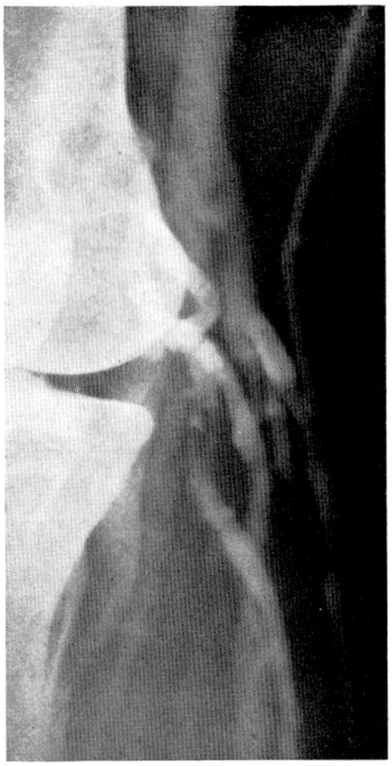

Fig. 1.16. Confused conditions at the junction of the popliteal veins with the popliteal.

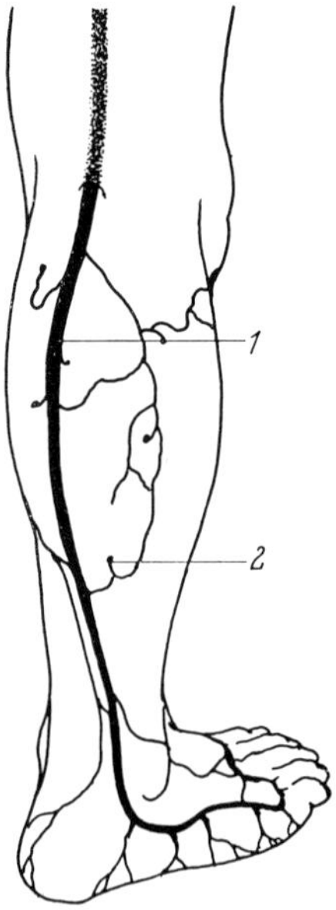

Fig. 1.17. Scheme of the small saphenous vein. (From May, R., and R. Nissl: Technik der Phlebographie und das Normalbild der Venen. In: Lehrbuch der Röntgendiagnostik, vol. I, 6th ed. H. R. Schinz, W. E. Baensch, W. Frommhold, R. Glauner, E. Uehlinger, J. Wellauer (eds.). Thieme, Stuttgart 1965. p. 349.)
1 Small saphenous vein
2 Constant perforating vein

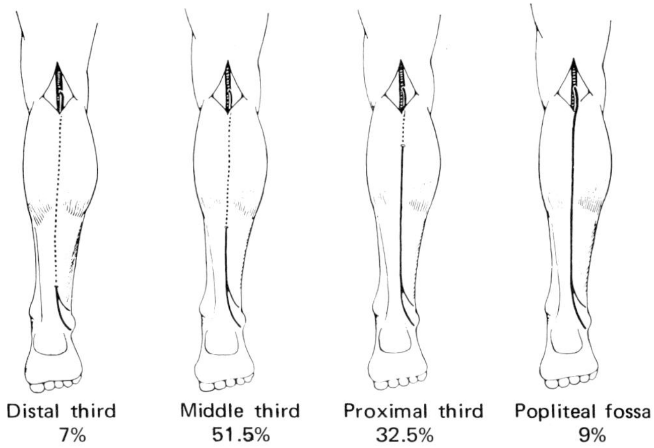

Fig. 1.18. Penetration of the leg fascia by the small saphenous vein. (After Moosmann and Hartwell.)

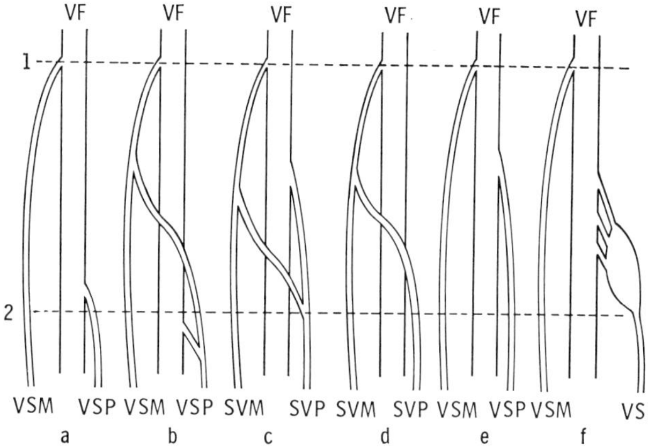

Fig. 1.19. Variations in the junction of the small saphenous vein. (After Mercier, Fouques, Portal and Vanneuville.)
VF Femoral vein
VSM Great saphenous
VSP Small saphenous
1 Level of saphenous hiatus
2 Level of popliteal fold

of cases) the junction was observed by us to be below the popliteal fossa. In 5.92 per cent it was level with the popliteal space or up to 3 cm above it. In the remainder, 13.89 per cent, it lay more than 5 cm above it; the highest junction found was 14 cm above the popliteal space.

Mercier et al. (1967) report variations in the entry of the small saphenous vein in a scheme obtained from a small number of examinations (Fig. 1.19), where the junction of the small with the great saphenous seen in Figure 1.19*b*, *c* and *d* corresponds with small saphenous-femoropopliteal type II and the variant in Figure 1.19*e* and *f* corresponds with the small saphenous-femoropopliteal type III and IV of May and Nissl (1959, 1966, 1968).

Typically the small saphenous joins with the popliteal vein not in a straight line from dorsally below but by way of shallow loop from laterally dorsal (Figs. 1.20 to 1.22).

Vodopivec (personal communication) assumes from autopsy material that the degree of the S-shaped junctional loop of the small saphenous vein depends on the position of the tibial nerve. If the tibial nerve runs superficially, the small saphenous vein enters the popliteal vein in a rather straight line from dorsally below. If the tibial nerve lies deeper, however, near the popliteal vein, the small saphenous vein forms the S-shaped loop of entry around the nerve. The closer the relation between the tibial nerve and popliteal vein, the more pronounced is the S-shaped loop.

Cibor and Cencora (1968) likewise observed relations between the junction of the small saphenous vein and the tibial nerve. They noted the division of the sciatic nerve to be 3 to 8 cm above the entry of the small saphenous vein. They found the entry of the small saphenous vein lateral to the tibial nerve in 63.5 per cent of cases, and medial to it in 36.5 per cent. It was difficult to specify exactly the connection of small saphenous vein and tibial nerve because it depended on the height of the patient. The S-shaped junctional loop is particularly distinct when there are varicosities of the small saphenous vein and may be a distinguishing mark for a very superficial, high-joining gastrocnemial vein. It is often difficult to determine by phlebography whether such a vein is the small saphenous or a gastrocnemial vein. In one-sixth of all cases the small saphenous vein does not flow into the popliteal but enters a femoropopliteal vein directly on the dorsal aspect of the thigh. It is now known that the variants of the small saphenous vein and its continuation into the femoropopliteal are persisting ontogenetic and phylogenetic atavisms, which have been described in detail by Kandel (1967).

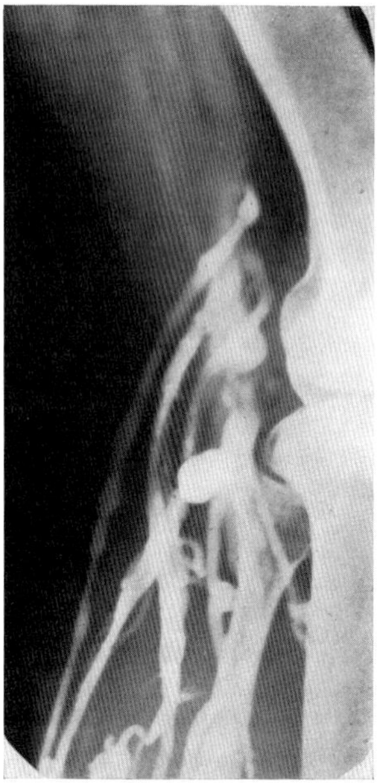

Fig. 1.20. Typical S-shaped junctional loop of the small saphenous seen from the laterodorsal aspect; separate junction of the gastrocnemial veins with the small saphenous vein.

The femoropopliteal vein joins the small saphenous and gastrocnemial veins on the dorsal aspect of the thigh in 36.08 per cent of cases. The junction of the small saphenous and the gastrocnemial veins and that of the femoropopliteal is subject to a number of variations, knowledge of which may be important in surgery for varicosities. In our material we found separate entry of the small saphenous and the gastrocnemial veins into the popliteal in 31.96 per cent (Fig. 1.23*a*). In 31.96 per cent of cases the small saphenous and gastrocnemius veins enter the popliteal jointly (Fig. 1.23*b*), and in 36.08 per cent a femoropopliteal vein is present. Perusal of the material revealed six types of femoropopliteal vein (Fig. 1.24).

In type I (3.66 per cent), the small saphenous vein receives a small branch from the dorsal aspect of the thigh just before entering the popliteal vein (Fig. 1.24*a*). In type II (2.29 per cent), the small saphenous does not enter the popliteal vein but winds around the inner aspect of the thigh, flowing into the great saphenous as a posterior medial ramus at different levels; van Limborgh (1962, 1963) calls it the medial accessory vein (Fig. 1.24*b*). In type III (17.35 per cent), the small saphenous has no connection with the popliteal, flowing directly into the femoropopliteal, which runs into the gluteal musculature (Fig. 1.24*c*). In type IV (7.3 per cent), the small saphenous continues directly as the

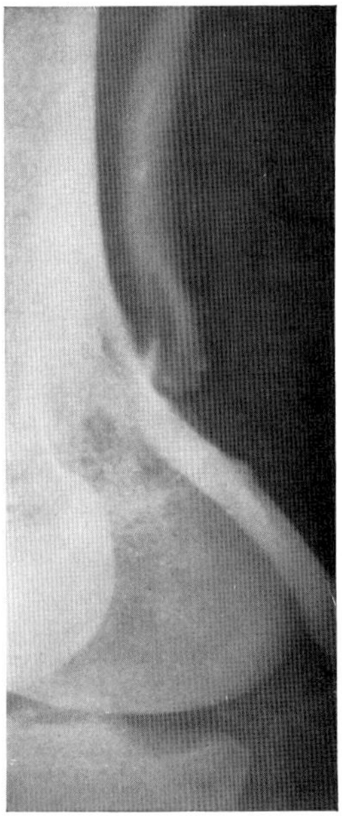

Fig. 1.21. Typical S-shaped junctional loop of an insufficient small saphenous from laterodorsally.

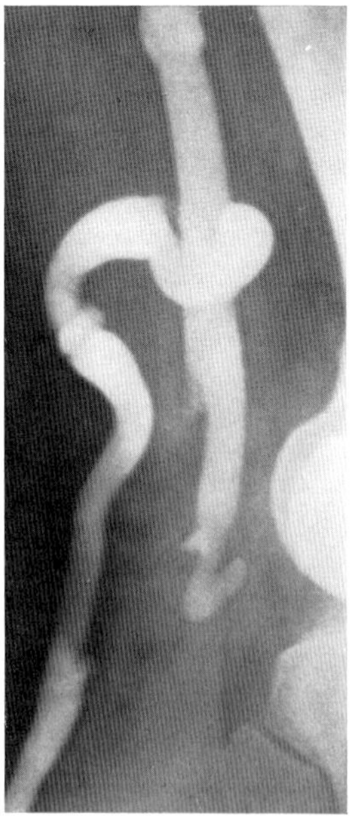

Fig. 1.22. Markedly varicose small saphenous joining rather high with a pronounced S-shaped loop.

femoropopliteal vein. This joins the femoral by one of the posterior communicating veins at different levels. At the bifurcation of the posterior communicating vein, a small branch enters the femoropopliteal from above (Fig. 1.24*d*). In type V (4.57 per cent), a larger vein—arising from the small saphenous—enters the gluteal muscles on the dorsal aspect of the thigh, a short distance in front of the junction of the small saphenous with the popliteal, to flow into the sciatic vein (Fig. 1.24*e*). In type VI (0.91 per cent), the small saphenous and femoropopliteal veins are both well formed and flow separately into the popliteal (Fig. 1.24*f*).

According to van Limborgh (1962, 1963), types II, V and VI may have as many as seven posterior communicating veins with the femoral. In all the types where the small saphenous joins the popliteal, it may join separately or together with gastrocnemial veins.

The anomaly of a bifid small saphenous vein is extremely rare; it was observed only twice in our 800 phlebograms (Fig. 1.25).

Considering the cases of bifid small saphenous vein in the literature more closely, it becomes clear that there usually is a single lesser saphenous and a rather proximal gastrocnemial vein. The *gastrocnemial veins*, which also join the popliteal, will be treated together with the *soleus veins* since they form a functional unit supplying the musculature of the calf. Basically, the veins of

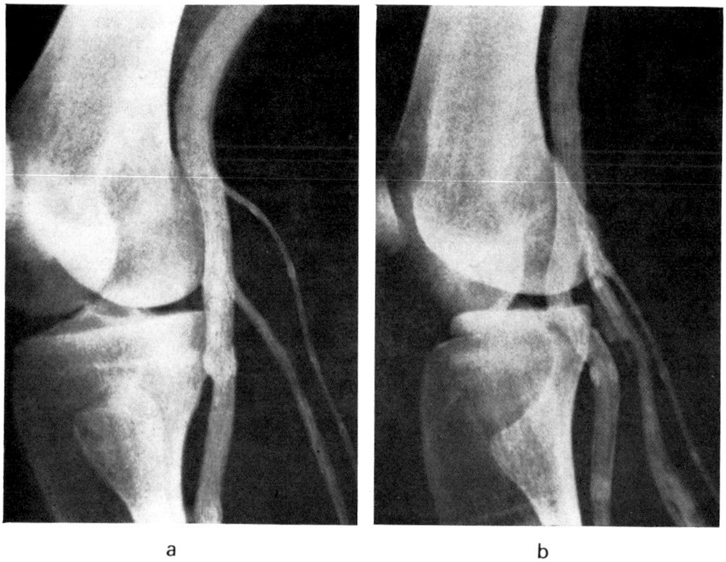

Fig. 1.23. Junction of the small saphenous and gastrocnemial veins with the popliteal: separately (31.96 per cent) (*a*); and together (31.96 per cent) (*b*).

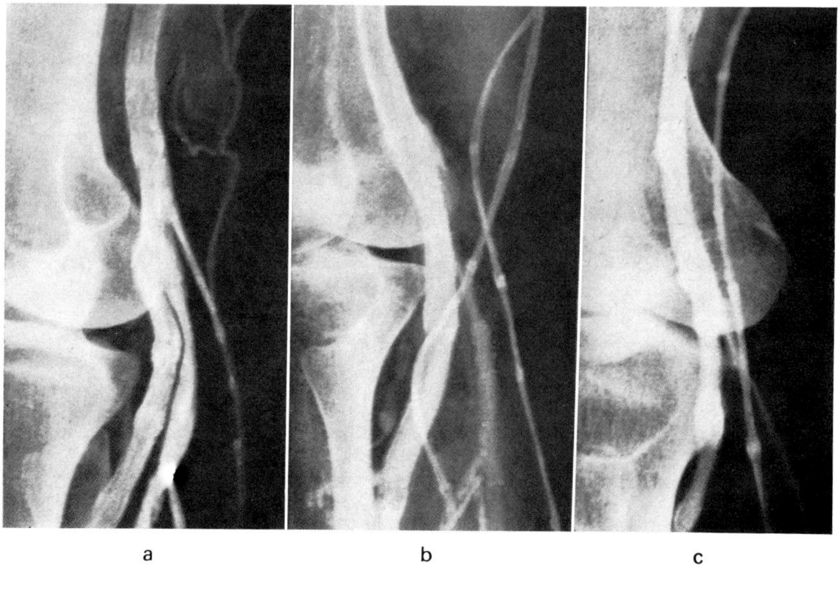

Fig. 1.24. Variations of the junction of the small saphenous in the presence of a femoropopliteal vein, types I to VI (*a* to *f*).

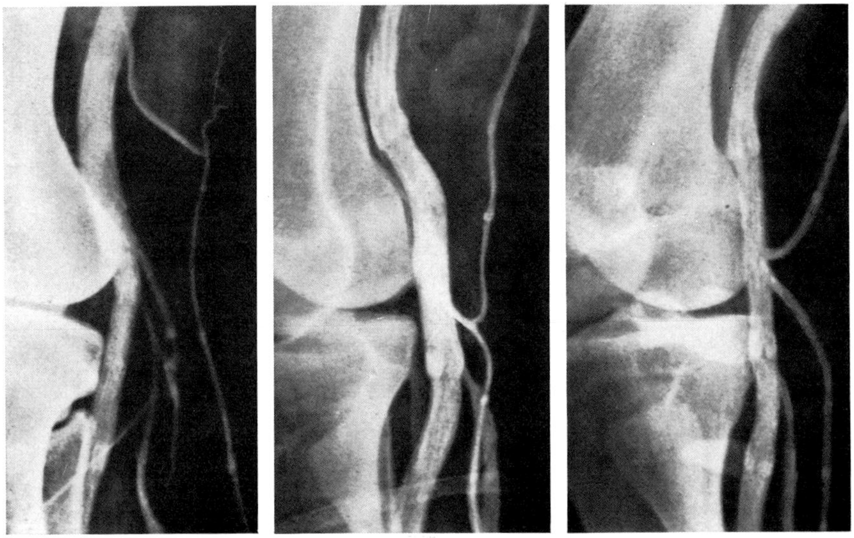

d e f

Fig. 1.24.

gastrocnemius and soleus are perforating veins (Linton, 1938, 1959).

Their special anatomic structure—they are amply provided with valves—as well as their important function as the "venous heart" of the leg is reason to consider them as a separate group of leg veins. It is the Swedish school that called attention to the significant role of the calf veins for venous

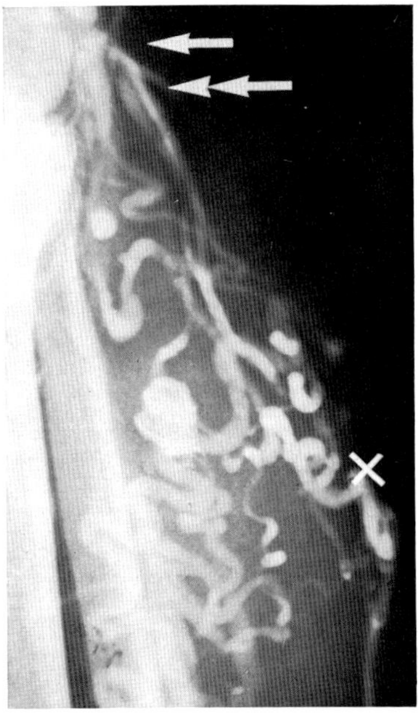

Fig. 1.25. Double small saphenous vein. The superficial small saphenous (←), only poorly visualized, flows directly into the popliteal; the slightly more distal second small saphenous («—) flows into the popliteal together with the gastrocnemius veins; insufficient gastrocnemius point (x), with small saphenous insufficient distal to the gastrocnemius point.

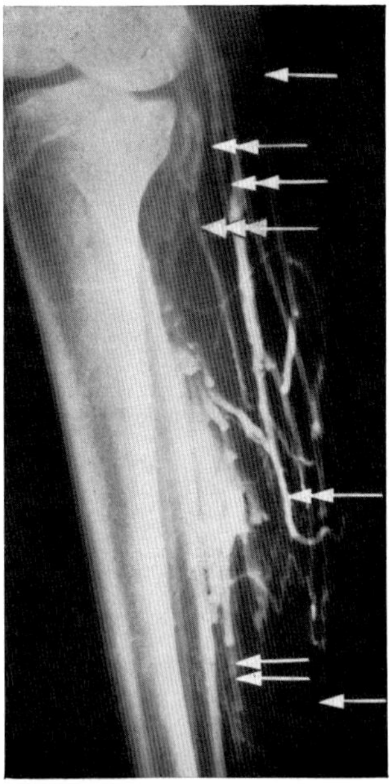

Fig. 1.26. Lateral view of the leg in a normal ascending phlebogram. Filling of sufficient muscle veins from superficial veins via communicating veins, the small saphenous veins (←), the medial gastrocnemial veins («—), the lateral gastrocnemial veins (⋘) and the deep leg veins (⇇).

drainage from the leg. Phlebography is meant to demonstrate—in addition to the deep veins—whether the muscular pump of the calf muscles is effective. Bauer (1960a, b, c) calls this the "venous heart" of the leg. Testing the muscle pump ("venous pump") is essential in dynamic or functional phlebography of the deep leg veins. Gullmo (1964) made the most important investigations of the function and morphology of the calf veins.

Assessment of the sufficiency or insufficiency of calf veins that are apparently normal requires phleboscopic observation of the direction of flow of the contrast medium (Figs. 1.26 and 1.27). According to Gullmo, normal veins are found in the gastrocnemius and soleus muscles only in patients under 25 years old. Later, signs of increasing degeneration are the rule. We believe that this age limit is too low, having seen patients aged 30 years who had completely sufficient gastrocnemial veins. Gullmo drew attention to the fact that the wide veins formerly described as "venous sinuses" are varices, i.e., pathologic changes. The veins in the gastrocnemius, commonly two in each head, join proximally to form one trunk (Fig. 1.28). They lie at different levels in the muscle, emerge ventrally from the gastrocnemius heads and enter the popliteal vein without an S-shaped loop from dorsal at an acute angle laterally and medially. Similarly, they may form a common trunk distally, which is typical for these pumping veins, according to Gullmo. Unlike the small saphenous vein, which con-

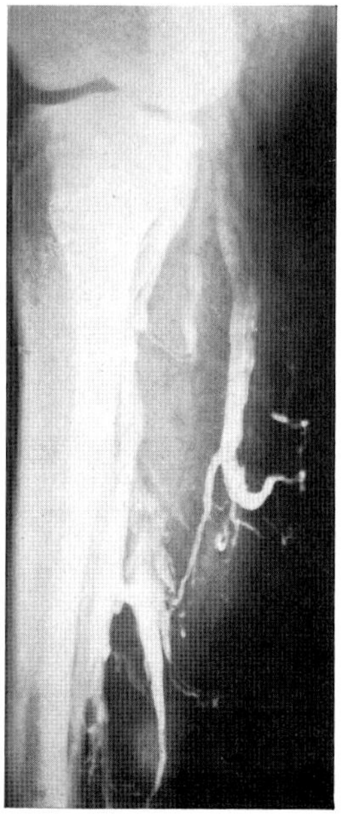

Fig 1.27. Partially insufficient gastrocnemius and soleus veins.

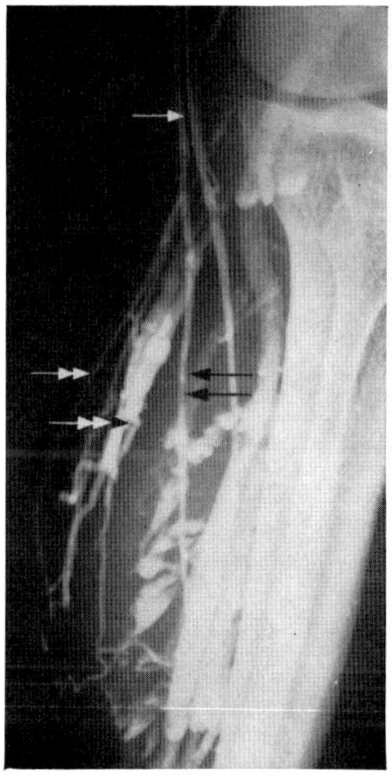

Fig. 1.28. Gastrocnemial veins in a phlebogram. Great saphenous vein, double (→), small saphenous vein (→→) and medial (→→→) and lateral (⇇) gastrocnemial veins.

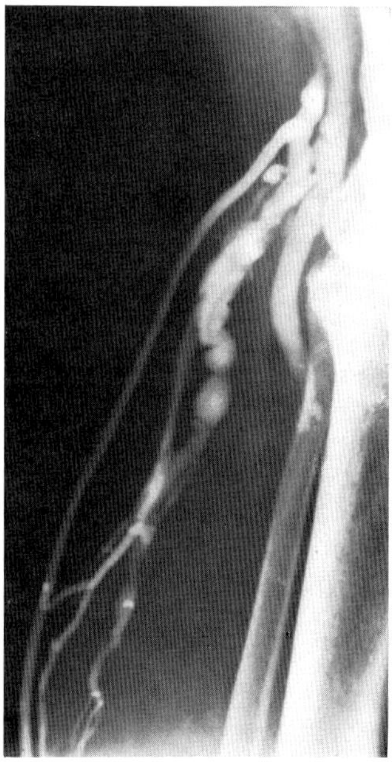

Fig. 1.29. Separate junction of the small saphenous and gastrocnemial veins (32 per cent of all cases). Typical S-shaped junctional loop of the small saphenous, and insufficient gastrocnemial veins; the bilaterally double gastrocnemial veins join to form one trunk proximally and distally.

tains only a few valves, the veins in the gastrocnemius and soleus muscles are amply supplied with regularly placed valves that give them the appearance of arcades. On lateral view of leg and knee joint, the gastrocnemial veins run very superficially into the musculature of gastrocnemius, approximately parallel with the small saphenous vein (Fig. 1.29). As mentioned before, the distal portion of the small saphenous is frequently insufficient below its entry into the fascia. This partial insufficiency may be contributed to by the communicating vein connecting the small saphenous with a vein to the gastrocnemius, which may be insufficient. We have designated this site the "gastrocnemius point" and stressed the distinction between a *sufficient* and an *insufficient* gastrocnemius point (Fig. 1.30). The venous blood from the soleus is drained at several levels; one or two veins that course longitudinally in the center of the muscle usually receive the major portion. The soleus veins enter the deep leg veins a good handbreadth or more distal to the gastrocnemius veins (Fig. 1.31). The upper portion of the soleus is drained in part by small accessory veins that flow into the gastrocnemius veins. As already described, these muscle veins begin to degenerate around the twenty-fifth year of life and come to resemble sinuses (Fig. 1.32).

Lateral Superficial Veins of the Lower Limb

The system of the great and small saphenous veins is supplemented by another, little known, system, that of the lateral superficial veins of the leg. Their development and anatomy have been described by Albanese et al. (1969).
Their course is that of an X, crossing at the

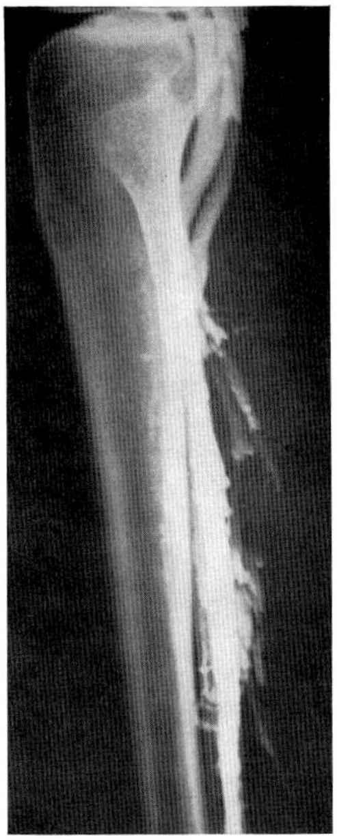

Fig. 1.31. Lateral view of the leg in a normal ascending phlebogram of the deep leg veins. The muscle veins are only weakly represented since their valves are sufficient and the contrast medium cannot flow distally.

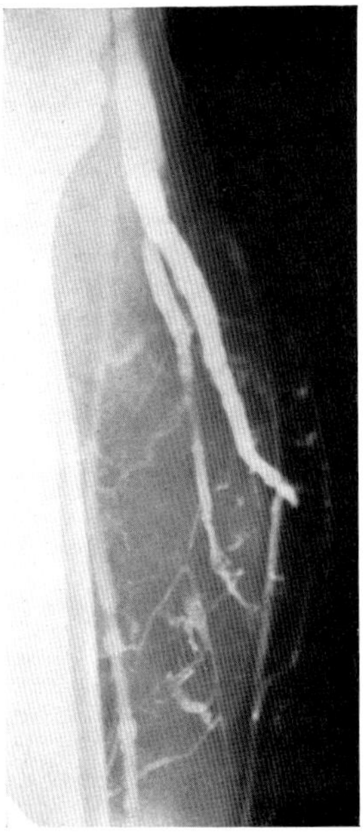

Fig. 1.30. Small saphenous vein insufficient distal to the gastrocnemius point.

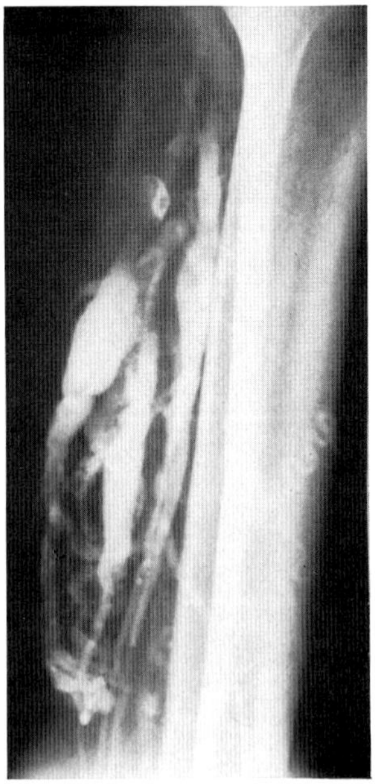

Fig. 1.32. Marked varices of the soleus veins.

lateral side of the knee. This X may be incomplete, in which case it corresponds to an upright or reversed Y, a parenthesis sign or an S.
These veins drain via mostly constant perforating veins into the deep layers (Fig. 1.33).

—The posterior branch from the thigh enters the sciatic or profunda femoris vein.
—The anterior branch from the thigh enters the inferior lateral circumflex vein of the femur.
—The crossing point drains via the perforating veins into the superior and inferior lateral veins of the knee, terminating in the popliteal vein.
—The posterior branch from the leg joins the posterior peroneal veins via the perforating veins.
—The anterior branch from the leg drains via several perforating veins into the anterior tibial vein and, in the region of the malleolus, into the anterior peroneal veins.

Communicating Veins and Perforating Veins

The deep and superficial venous systems of the lower extremity are separated by the fascia and joined solely by communicating and perforating veins piercing the fascia. The valves in these veins are so directed that with normal function the blood can flow only from the superficial to the deep venous system. There are both direct communicating veins, which join the deep veins, and indirect veins (called perforating veins by Linton [1938]), which join the muscle veins. In practice, there is no difference in their appearance on phlebography, and the terms perforating and communicating are used synonymously.
The best descriptions were given by Raivio (1948) and Linton (1953a,b); more recently van Limborgh (1962, 1963) studied the communicating veins in great detail. Itemization of the communicating veins and the nomenclature of van Limborgh follow below (Figs. 1.34 to 1.36). These veins may become insufficient. Hence, if any of them are to be neutralized by operation for varices, we consider it essential to demonstrate the communicating veins by phlebography, emphasizing the most important communicating veins that tend to become insufficient.
Van Limborgh divides the communicating veins of the leg, knee and thigh into a medial, lateral and posterior group.

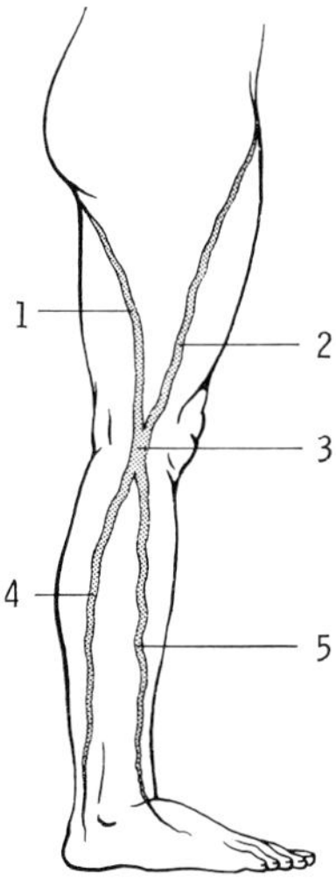

Fig. 1.33. Drawing of the lateral superficial veins of the lower extremity.
1 Posterior branch to the thigh
2 Anterior branch to the thigh
3 Crossing point
4 Posterior branch to the leg
5 Anterior branch to the leg

Communicating Veins of the Leg

Medial Communicating Veins of the Leg

Anterior medial communicating veins of the leg (*cma*). One to six veins, usually four, run from the anterior ramus of the great saphenous vein to the posterior tibial veins.

Intermediate medial communicating veins of the leg (*cmi*). This group comprises between five and ten veins, usually eight, which run from the main trunk of the great saphenous to the posterior tibial veins.
One of the most proximal of these is frequently insufficient. A varix in the main trunk of the great saphenous indicating insufficiency is usually seen on the medial aspect of the knee joint, one handbreadth below it. It was described in detail by Boyd (1948).

Posterior medial communicating veins of the leg (*cmp*). These veins number from three to six, usually five. They originate from the posterior ramus of the great saphenous and flow into the posterior tibial veins. The distal of three of these are the most important from the clinical point of view because when they are insufficient leg ulcers may result. They are known as *Cockett's veins* (Fig. 1.37).

Lateral Communicating Veins of the Leg

Anterior lateral communicating veins of the leg (*cla*). Numbering between two and five, usually four, these veins originate from an anterior accessory branch of the anterior ramus of the great saphenous and flow into the anterior tibial veins. They rarely become insufficient.

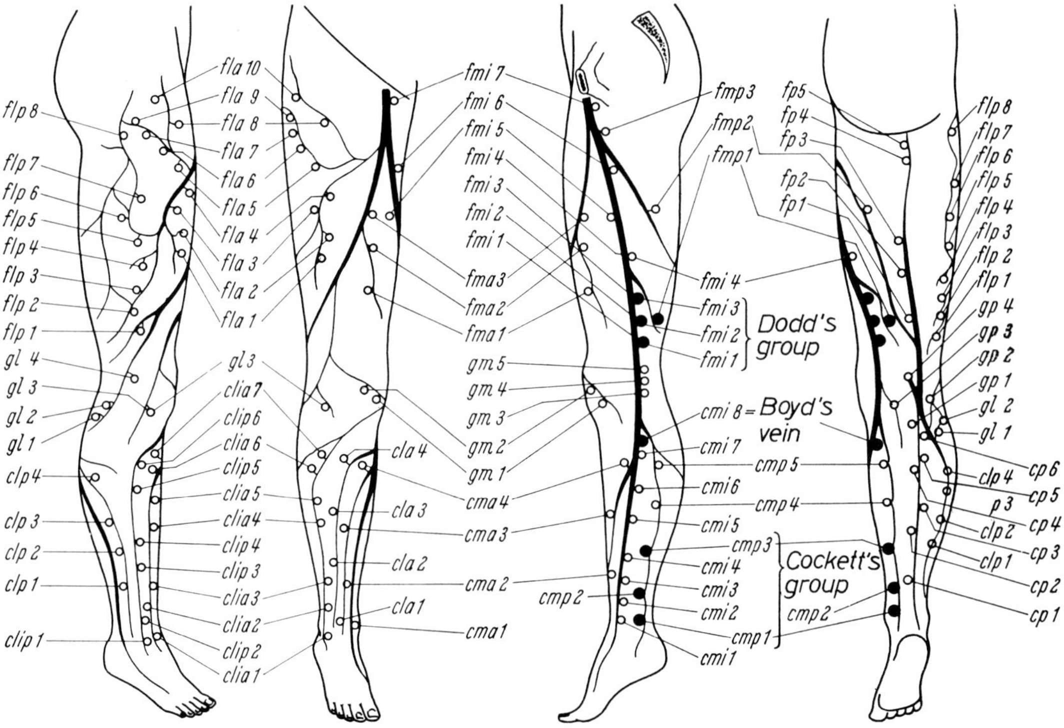

a b c d

Fig. 1.34. Diagram and nomenclature of the communicating veins of the lower extremity. External surface (*a*), anterior surface (*b*), internal surface (*c*), and posterior surface (*d*). (After van Limborgh.)

cma	=	Vv. communicantes cruris mediales anteriores
cmi	=	Vv. communicantes cruris mediales intermediae
cmp	=	Vv. communicantes cruris mediales posteriores
cla	=	Vv. communicantes cruris laterales anteriores
clia	=	Vv. communicantes cruris laterales intermediae anteriores
clip	=	Vv. communicantes cruris laterales intermediae posteriores
clp	=	Vv. communicantes cruris laterales posteriores
cp	=	Vv. communicantes cruris posteriores
gm	=	Vv. communicantes genu mediales
gl	=	Vv. communicantes genu laterales
gp	=	Vv. communicantes genu posteriores
fma	=	Vv. communicantes femorales mediales anteriores
fmi	=	Vv. communicantes femorales mediales intermediae
fmp	=	Vv. communicantes femorales mediales posteriores
fla	=	Vv. communicantes femorales laterales anteriores
flp	=	Vv. communicantes femorales laterales posteriores
fp	=	Vv. communicantes femorales posteriores

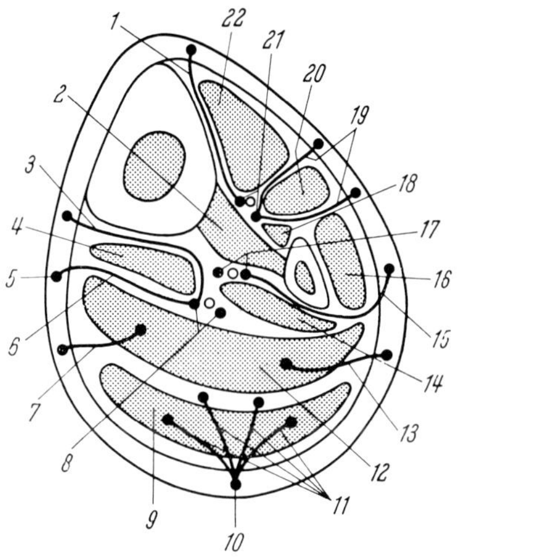

Fig. 1.35. Cross section of the middle third of the leg showing the position of the communicating veins. (After van Limborgh.)

1 cla = V. communicans cruris lateralis anterior
2 M. tibialis posterior
3 cma = V. communicans cruris medialis anterior
4 M. flexor digitorum longus
5 V. saphena magna
6 cmi = V. communicans cruris medialis intermedia
7 cmp = V. communicans cruris medialis posterior
8 Vv. tibiales posteriores
9 M. gastrocnemius
10 V. saphena parva
11 cp = Vv. communicantes cruris posteriores
12 M. soleus
13 clp = V. communicans cruris lateralis posterior
14 M. flexor hallucis longus
15 clip = V. communicans cruris lateralis intermedia posterior
16 M. peroneus longus and M. peronaeus brevis
17 Vv. peroneae
18 M. extensor hallucis longus
19 clia = Vv. communicantes cruris laterales intermediae anteriores
20 M. extensor digitorum longus
21 V. tibiales anteriores
22 M. tibialis anterior

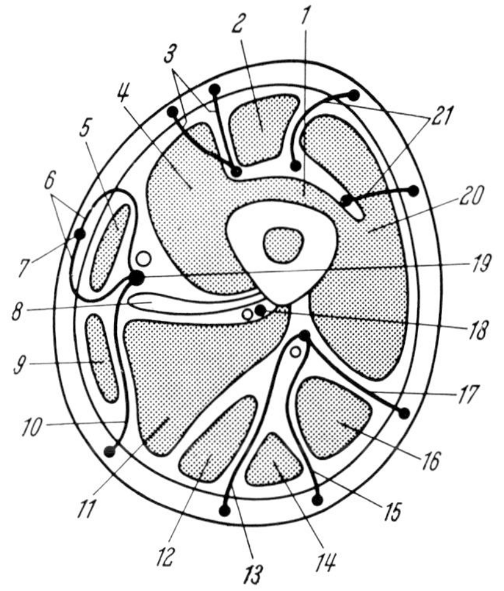

Fig. 1.36. Cross section through the middle third of the thigh, showing the position of the communicating veins. (After van Limborgh.)

1 M. vastus intermedius
2 M. rectus femoris
3 fma = Vv. communicantes femorales mediales anteriores
4 M. vastus medius
5 M. sartorius
6 fmi = Vv. communicantes femorales mediales intermediae
7 V. saphena magna
8 M. adductor longus
9 M. gracilis
10 fmp = V. communicans femoralis medialis posterior
11 M. adductor magnus
12 M. semimembranosus
13 fp = V. communicans femoralis posterior
14 M. semitendinosus
15 fp = V. communicans femoralis posterior
16 M. biceps femoris
17 flp = V. communicans femoralis lateralis posterior
18 V. profunda femoris
19 V. femoralis
20 M. vastus lateralis
21 fla = Vv. communicantes femorales anteriores

Intermediate lateral communicating veins of the leg. These are divided into (1) the *anterior intermediate lateral communicating veins of the leg* (*clia*), five to ten veins, usually seven, that course from a branch of the anterior ramus of the great saphenous between the anterior tibial muscle and the extensor digitorum longus to the anterior tibial veins; and (2) the *posterior intermediate lateral communicating veins of the leg* (*clip*), four to ten veins, usually six, running from the most posterior branch of the anterior ramus of the great saphenous in front of the soleus muscle to the peroneal veins.

Their intermediate branches are often insufficient in the presence of marked varicose changes on the lateral aspect of the leg (Fig. 1.38).

Posterior lateral communicating veins of the leg (*clp*). Their number varies between two and five; usually there are four. They derive from an external branch of the small saphenous and flow into the veins of gastrocnemius and soleus.

Posterior Communicating Veins of the Leg (cp)

Their number varies from two to eight, six being most common. They originate from the main trunk of the small saphenous and drain into the veins of the gastrocnemius muscle.
The posterior lateral and the posterior communicating veins of the leg play a greater part if the muscle veins of gastrocnemius and soleus are degenerated (Fig. 1.39).

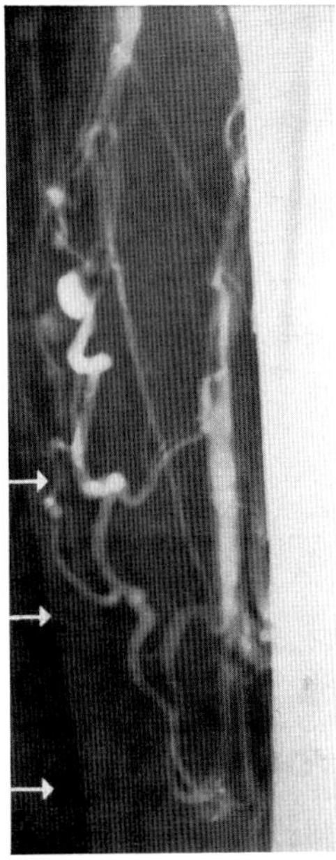

Fig. 1.37. Insufficient posterior medial communicating veins of the leg (Cockett's group).

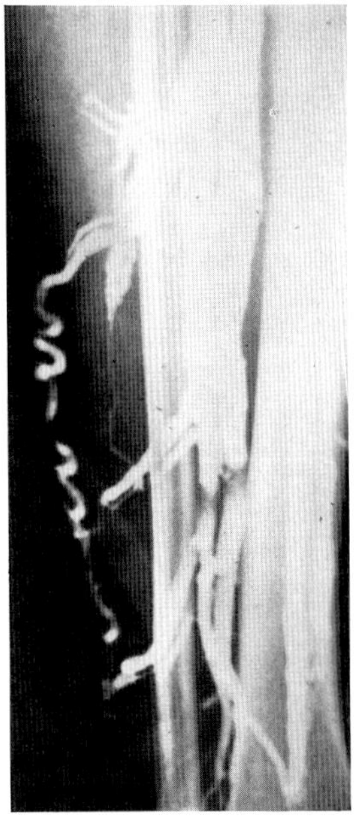

Fig. 1.38. Partially insufficient posterior intermediate lateral communicating veins of the leg.

Communicating Veins of the Knee

Medial Communicating Veins of the Knee (gm)

Their number ranges between two and six, and is usually five; they run from the great saphenous to the popliteal vein.

Lateral Communicating Veins of the Knee (gl)

These are two to six veins, usually four. They run from the external aspect of the knee to the popliteal.

Posterior Communicating Veins of the Knee (gp)

Two to seven veins, usually four, flow from the lesser saphenous or its smaller branches into the popliteal. Clinically, the communicating veins of the knee are of minor significance.

Communicating Veins of the Thigh

Medial Femoral Communicating Veins

Van Limborgh (1962, 1963) divided these into three groups.

Anterior medial communicating veins of the thigh (fma). Their number ranges between one and four, usually three, and they originate from the accessory saphenous vein and its branches and flow into the muscle veins of the extensors of the thigh.

Intermediate medial communicating veins of the thigh (fmi). Their number varies between four and eight, and is usually seven. They run from the main trunk of the great saphenous into the femoral vein.
Clinically the most important of these is the group at the level of the adductor canal, which is the first to become insufficient with varicose changes. Usually these are two or three veins, known as *Dodd's group*; they cause relapses after elimination of varices (Fig. 1.40).

Posterior medial communicating veins of the thigh. Their number ranges from one to five, usually three; they derive from a dorsal branch of the great saphenous and flow into the femoral vein. These veins also belong to *Dodd's group*.

Lateral Communicating Veins of the Thigh

Anterior lateral communicating veins of the thigh (fla). Their number varies between six and twelve; usually there are ten.

Posterior lateral communicating veins of the thigh (flp). Their number ranges between three and nine; usually eight are found. Both venous groups are rarely of clinical importance. They originate in a subcutaneous venous plexus in the musculature of the thigh.

Posterior Communicating Veins of the Thigh (fp)

These are four to seven veins, usually five. They derive from the femoropopliteal and drain into the femoral or a large perforating vein on the dorsal aspect of the thigh.
The communicating veins do not directly continue the superficial venous system. Gullmo (1964) observed small, siphon-like venous loops, intercalated between superficial and communicating veins. He called them "drainage loops." Their task is to collect venous blood from the subcutaneous veins and propel it rhythmically into communicating veins. This is well seen by phleboscopy. Furthermore, the looplike arrangement of the "drainage loops" permits movement of the muscle fascia against subcutaneous tissues without overstretching the communicating veins.

Veins of the Pelvis

From the viewpoint of the vascular surgeon, the *parietal veins* are of greatest interest among pelvic veins (Figs. 1.41 to 1.43). The veins that supply the viscera are so closely connected with pathologic changes in these organs that their treatment is usually the province of the abdominal, gynecologic or urologic surgeon. Further discussion of them is therefore dispensed with.
The *common femoral vein* continues as the *external iliac vein* along the inguinal ligament. It lies medial to and slightly below the artery of the same name at the inner aspect of the psoas major muscle. Just above the inguinal ligament, the external iliac vein receives the twofold deep circumflex vein of the ilium, a constant anastomosis of the obturator and inferior epigastric veins. The paired roots embrace the external iliac artery. Anastomoses with the superior epigastric and paraumbilical veins are important substitutes should the external iliac become occluded. At the junction with the common iliac vein, the external iliac vein is crossed by the

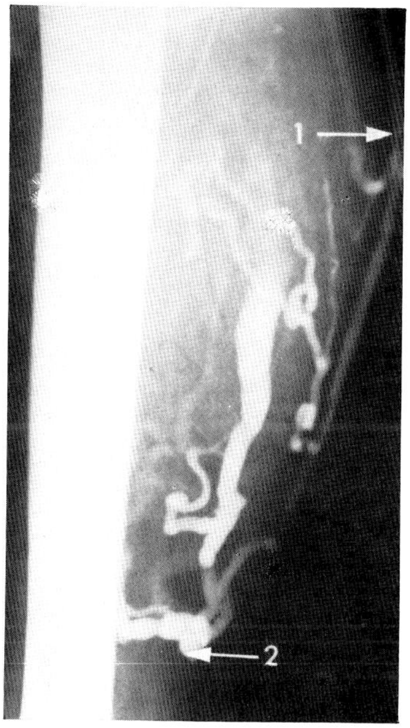

Fig. 1.39. Insufficient posterior communicating veins of the leg.
1 Insufficient gastrocnemius point
2 Soleus blow-out

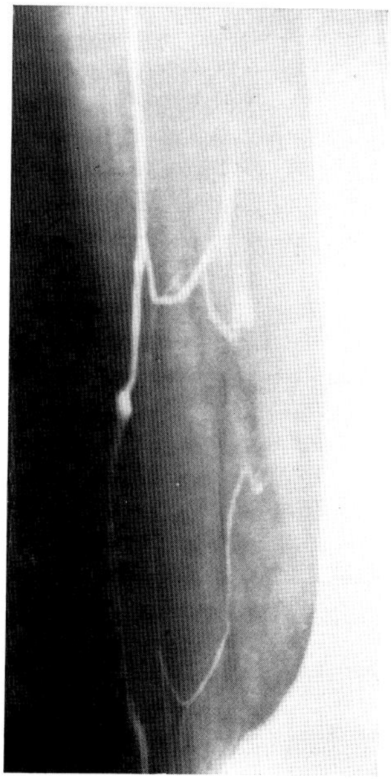

Fig. 1.40. Intermediate medial femoral communicating veins (Dodd's group).

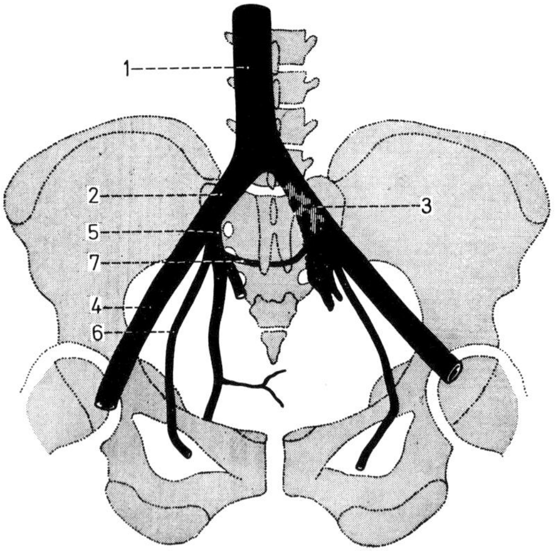

Fig. 1.41. Phlebography of the pelvis.
1 Inferior vena cava
2 Common iliac vein
3 Normally invisible zone (*zone normalement invisible*)
4 External iliac vein
5 Internal iliac vein
6 Obturator vein
7 Vein of the presacral plexus

internal iliac artery and by the ureter in front of it. The *internal iliac vein* encloses in its short trunk a plexus of visceral veins: the internal pudendal (and in women the uterine and vaginal venous plexuses), the vesical and the rectal venous plexuses.
Further thick *parietal veins* are the iliolumbar, the superior and inferior gluteal veins, the obturator vein and the superior and inferior lateral sacral veins.
At the level of the sacroiliac junction, the external and internal iliac join to form the *common iliac vein*, right and left. Since the inferior vena cava lies to the right of the vertebral column, the left common iliac vein is longer than the right. It usually receives the median sacral vein. The right common iliac vein lies dorsal to the homonymous artery; the left common iliac vein, caudal to the common iliac artery. Furthermore, they receive the ascending lumbar veins, which continue cephalad into the azygos and hemiazygos veins. The small branches are not demonstrable by routine roentgenography. They assumed importance only as collaterals when drainage is impaired, as after ligation of the *inferior vena cava*, when the collaterals can easily be studied (Figs. 1.44 to 1.46).
The distribution of the valves in the pelvic veins can be seen in Figure 1.47.

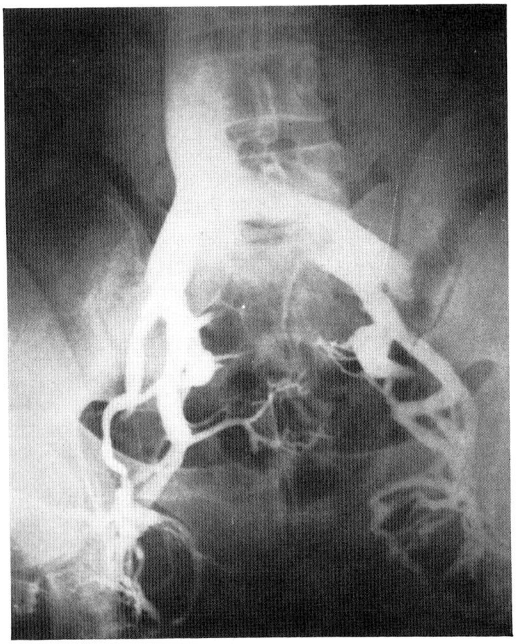

Fig. 1.42. Intraosseous demonstration of the pelvic veins from both ischial tuberosities.

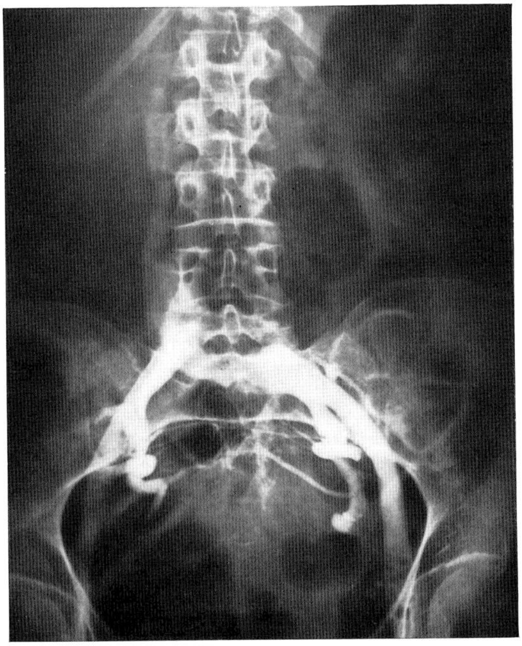

Fig. 1.43. Demonstration of the pelvic veins after direct puncture of the veins.

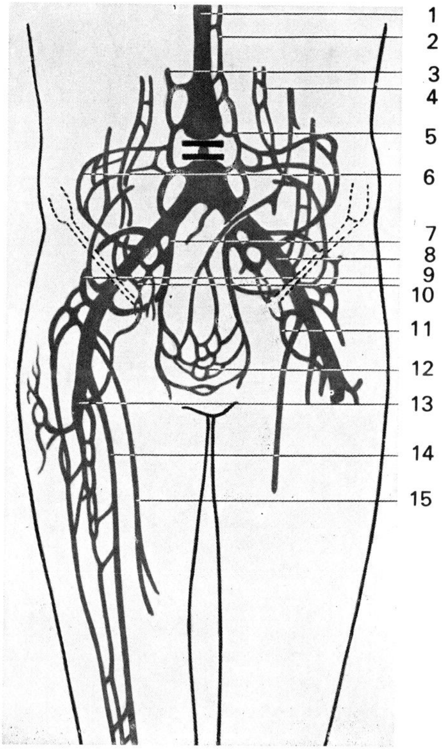

Fig. 1.44. Drawing of the pelvic veins and their collaterals. (After Owens.) Formation of collaterals after ligation of the vena cava.

1 V. cava inferior
2 V. hemiazygos
3 V. azygos
4 V. epigastrica profunda
5 V. iliolumbalis and V. lumbalis ascendens
6 V. circumflexa ilium profunda
7 V. iliaca interna
8 V. iliaca externa
9 V. glutea
10 V. obturatoria
11 V. circumflex femoris medialis
12 Plexus venosus rectalis
13 V. femoralis superficialis
14 V. profunda femoris
15 V. saphena magna

Two anatomic details are surgically important:

—The pelvic vessels—veins and arteries—are closely apposed by common, artfully intertwined vascular sheaths. Their structure was demonstrated by May (cited by Sieglbauer, 1966).

—Arteries cross the veins at two sites, and this presents the risk of compression. The left external iliac vein is superimposed by the left iliac artery in its cranial portion. On the right, the vein lies dorsal to the artery.

—The left common iliac vein is pressed against the fifth vertebra by the right common .iliac artery. The two vessels lie close together in this area.

May and Thurner (1956) studied in detail, on autopsy material from 430 cases, the architecture of pelvic veins in this region. They noted changes at the junction of the left common iliac vein with the cava which they called "pelvic vein spur" (Fig. 1.48).

Three basic types of this pelvic vein spur are distinguished:

—The simplest deviation (group I), in terms of the degree of formation, is shown in Figure 1.49 as an inconspicuous slender membrane, arising from the medial or lateral wall like a sail into the lumen and thus narrowing it. In 27

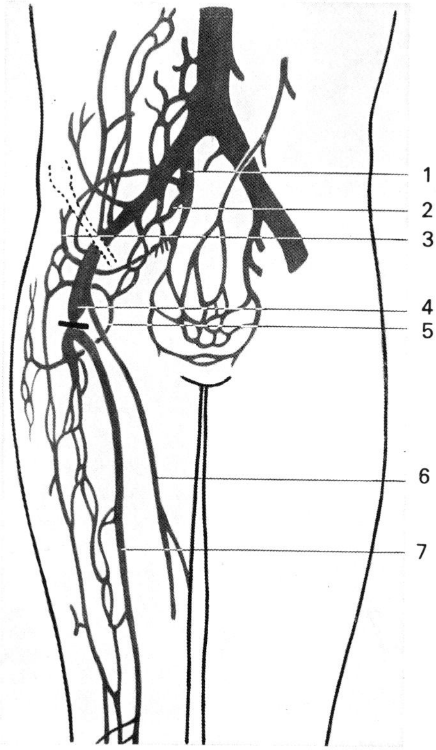

Fig. 1.45. Formation of collaterals after ligation of the common femoral vein. (After Owens.)

1 V. iliaca interna
2 V. obturatoria
3 V. glutea
4 V. femoralis communis
5 V. circumflexa femoris medialis
6 V. saphena magna
7 V. femoralis superficialis

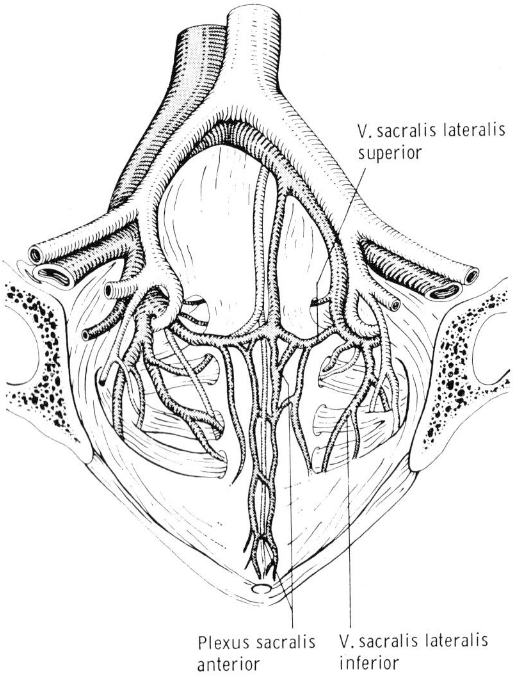

Fig. 1.46. Presacral veins. (After Cordier and Rousseau.)

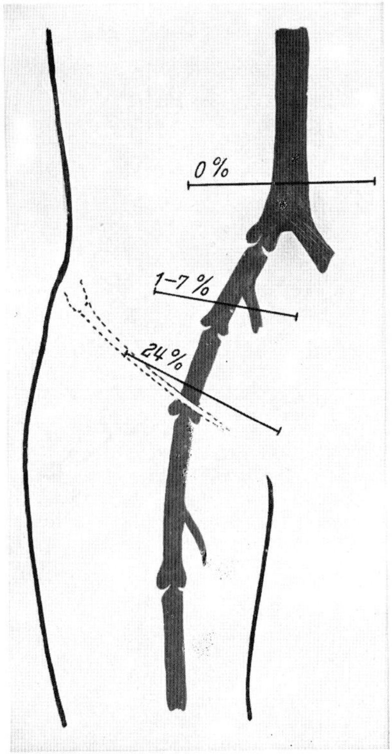

Fig. 1.47. Valves of the pelvic veins. (After Basmajian.)

of 430 cases, this type of spur formation was seen opposite the division of the cava, that is, topographically on the left side or at the upper pole of the entry of the left common iliac vein. The spur is not related to a venous valve, which, if present, has an entirely different shape; this can be seen in a healthy vein. The sail formation arising from the point of division, that is, from the medial wall toward the lumen of the left common iliac vein, was observed in 32 cases. The extent of the spur formation is subject to marked variation, but the spur always occupies a strictly dorsoanterior position. Membranes lying across or frontally in the lumen were not seen. Very faint, crested, tender thickening of both the medial and lateral inner walls of the vein may be seen; or the formation may be condensed to strong sails that occlude half the lumen or more. At times, the spur is divided and appears as a lattice, from which fact it is clear that the anomalies are not systematic but simply variants of one and the same cause. May and Thurner (1956, 1957) speak of a medial or lateral spur.

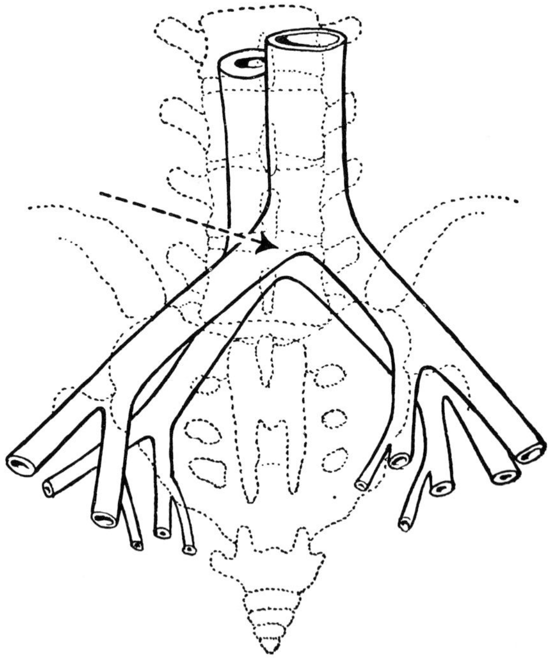

Fig. 1.48. Inferior vena cava. Dorsal aspect, site of pelvic vein spur (→).

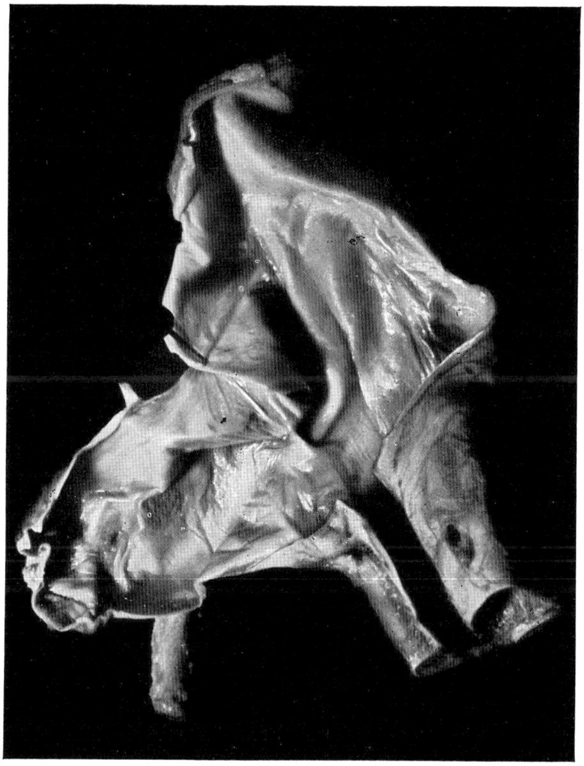

a

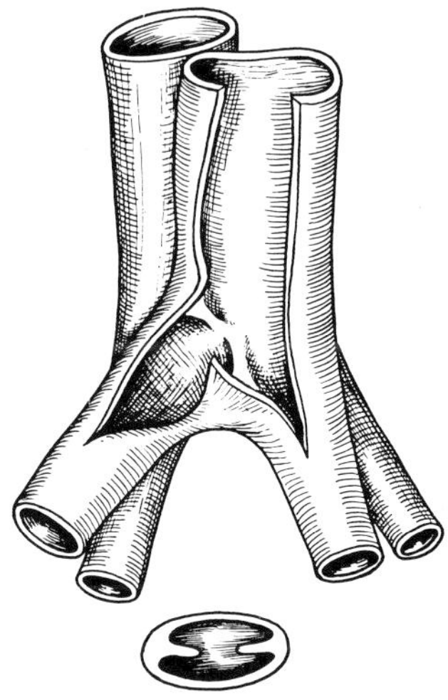

b

Fig. 1.49. Lateral pelvic vein spur. Anatomic preparation (*a*); simplified sketch (*b*).

—Another type (group II) of venous anomaly in the left common iliac vein does not differ in principle from that described above, but does offer a different picture to the observer. The anomaly could be described as a weir with bridge piers, which protrudes into the bloodstream and divides it, in the center of the lumen. It also occupies a strictly dorsoanterior position (central venous spur) (Fig. 1.50).
This type of spur also differs in size, may be duplicated and may divide the lumen of the common iliac vein into differently sized fields, presenting a picture of a system of vascular tubes. The anterior and posterior walls of the vein correspondingly show the insertions of the spur as trough-shaped retractions. This anomaly was observed 17 times.

—A third anomaly (group III; four cases seen)—in effect certainly the most important one—presents to the observer almost complete occlusion of the left common iliac vein at the junction with the inferior vena cava. The anterior and posterior walls of the vascular tube are usually approximated to a few millimeters, the remaining lumen being divided by numerous slender bridges with intercalary, almost dentate, clefts, so that there is a peculiar, quilted split in the lumen. Frequently, thin buttresses were demonstrated peripheral to the venous junction. May and Thurner (1956) call this partial obliteration (Fig. 1.51).

In addition to the three basic forms described, intermediate types are observed that may be explained by biologic variety. The discussion of the formation of venous spurs by May and Thurner (1965) deviates in some respects from that of McMurrich (1906), and especially from that of Krumbhaar and Ehrich (1943), because of the attempt to establish, by lucid, morphologically directed means, recognizable deviations for clinical purposes. We attribute special significance to discernible spur formation, particularly with regard to the steadily enhanced chances of treatment of varicosities and thromboses. Detailed histologic examinations of this vascular spur have apparently never been performed; only Krumbhaar and Ehrich (1943) mentioned them briefly. The spur is supposed to consist for the most part of elastic tissue with some collagen fibers and smooth muscle cells. Inflammatory cell infiltration has never been seen. In our opinion, histologic findings provide the

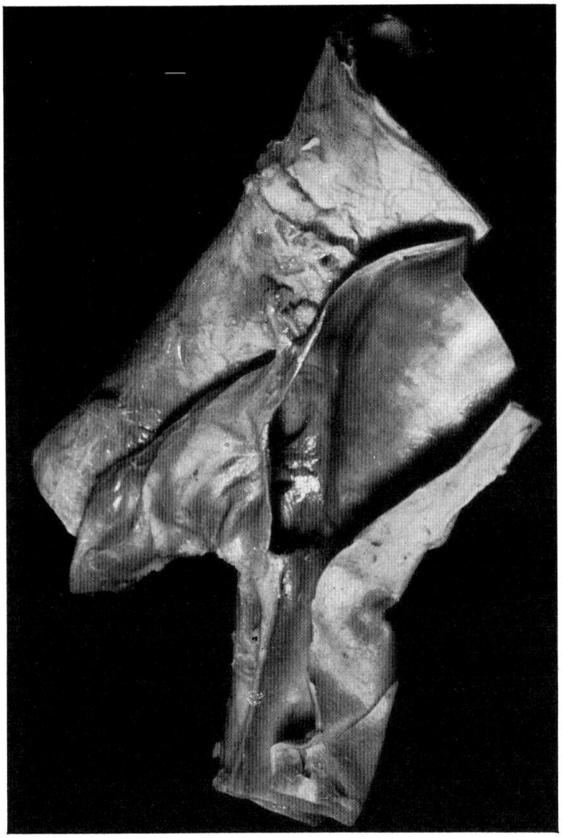

a

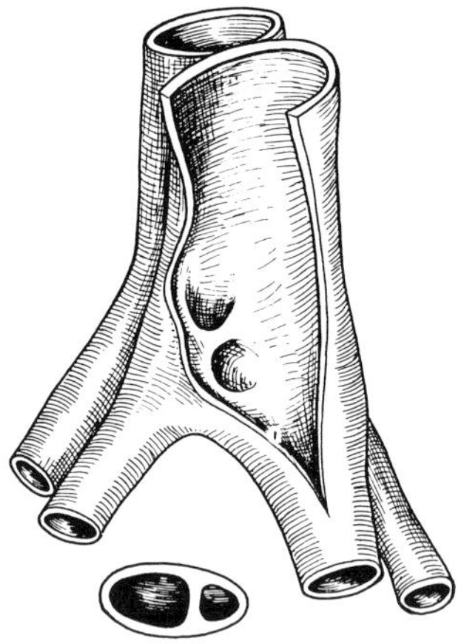

b

Fig. 1.50. Central pelvic vein spur. Anatomic preparation (*a*); simplified sketch (*b*).

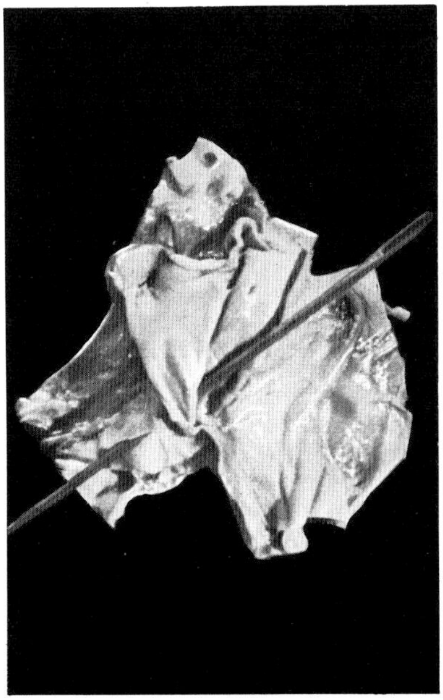

a

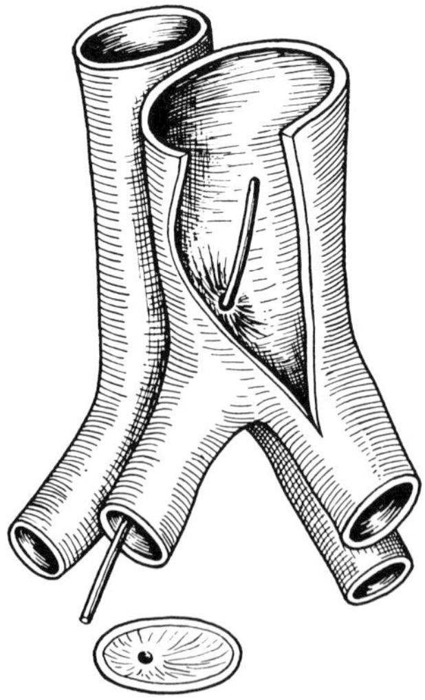

b

Fig. 1.51. Partial obliteration by a venous spur. The lumen is almost completely obliterated ("quilted"), and that remaining is divided by slender bridges. Anatomic preparation (*a*); simplified sketch (*b*).

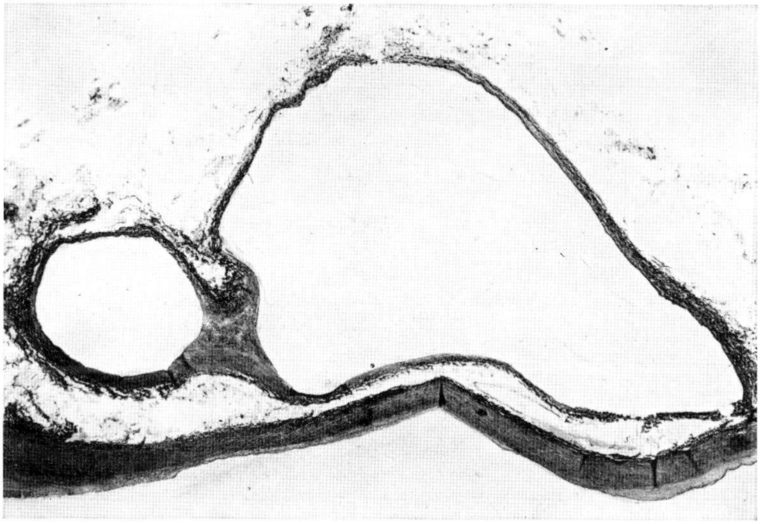

Fig. 1.52. Histologic section through the left common iliac vein at the level of a central spur.

key to the etiology of spurs; this is why we devoted special attention to it.

The results of histologic examination of several central spurs in the left common iliac vein (Figs. 1.52 to 1.54) can be summarized as follows:

Strands of tissue of varying width dividing the venous lumen show an endothelial layer on the luminal aspect. Spur tightly knitted to the anterior, slightly thickened, and posterior normal venous walls, but clearly defined. No demonstrable layering of the venous wall. Where adherent, the venous wall was pierced by numerous capillaries surrounded by occasional lymphocytes. Spur basically composed of fibrocytes with ample collagen. In the tissue, numerous capillaries loosely surrounded by plasma cells and lymphocytes. Resorcin-fuchsin staining revealed that the elastic fibers of the venous wall were not involved in the spur formation but represented a border between vein and spur tissue.

The consequences arising from the histologic findings are especially important. If the deviations were explainable on an ontogenetic basis, one would expect them to consist of smooth muscle fibers surrounded by elastic fibers. But the opposite is true. By and large, the spur consists of loose connective tissue, which indeed shows endothelial differentiation toward the lumen, but only occasional elastic fibers. Apparently the spur

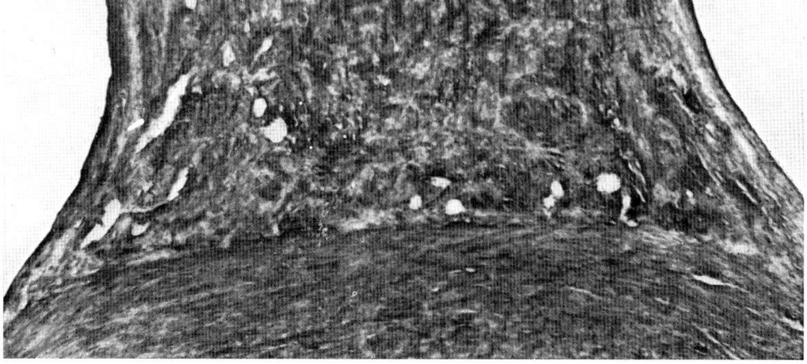

Fig. 1.53. Partial magnification of Figure 1.52. Base of the central spur with portions of the venous wall.

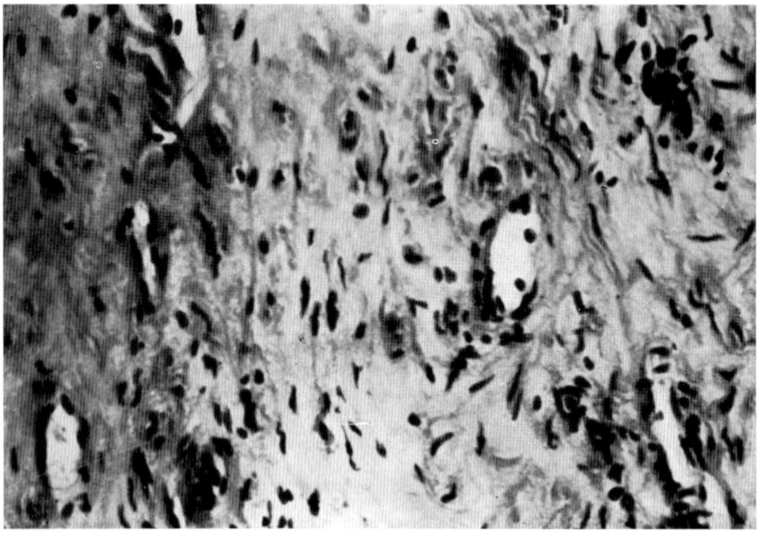

Fig. 1.54. Microscopic picture of the spur on higher magnification. It shows mainly fibrocytes with much collagen tissue.

consists of only one cell proliferation, arising from the intima of the vein, which is supplied by ingrowing capillaries (branches of vasa vasorum). Hemosiderin, which would indicate an organizing thrombosis, is not found. This proves that the spurs in the common iliac vein are a deviation that took place in extrauterine life. The lower segment of the inferior vena cava with its division into the iliac veins rests immediately on the hard anterior surface of the last lumbar vertebra. It is conceivable that the right common iliac artery, which crosses the left common iliac vein in front, almost touches both the anterior and posterior walls of the common iliac vein during its pulsation and that this produces chronic irritation of the venous intima. This might set up proliferation of endothelium. Both walls may therefore grow together and divide the lumen (spur formation) or produce sail formation at the margin. This somewhat resembles changes seen in callosities. Support for this hypothesis is the indication that venous spur formation is found predominantly in women (additional pressure by the pregnant uterus and marked lordosis).

If therefore our investigations originated from a desire to prove inadequate Virchow's explanation (1891) for the predominance of left-sided pelvic thromboses as due to interference with the stream by the crossing artery, we must qualify this by saying that in the last analysis the close topographic relation of the two vessels *is* the cause —though in a different sense—because it is responsible for the formation of a vascular spur.

Beside this explanation for the development of a vascular spur, which is probably correct, other explanations lose force. Kaufmann (1922) reproduced a picture of almost complete obliteration of the left common iliac vein from the Basel collection and explained this finding as result of a recanalized thrombus. Kaufmann spoke of a sinuous conversion of the left common iliac and internal iliac vein. Basically such an attempt at explanation should not be rejected, but morphologic findings argue against this supposition since the histologic picture fails to show blood pigment in addition to the other tissue structures. We assume that the development of the venous anomaly cannot be explained in this way, nor can it be ascribed to connections with venous disease (Schilling, 1936). Likewise, the findings refute the hypothesis that developmental or acquired disorders of the valves cause the described changes.

Several conclusions may be drawn from the diagnosis of spur formation in the left common iliac vein.

May and Thurner (1956) believe that they explain spur formation correctly: that it acts as a weir in the bloodstream, like bridge piers in a river where similar conditions of stream and eddies result (Aschoff, 1925). Stenosis of the venous lumen follows spur formation, no matter which type. As a consequence of this constant stoppage of normal venous drainage from left limb and pelvic area, while arterial flow into both limbs and both sides of the pelvis are preserved, slight overpressure in the veins of the left lower extremity is to be expected. This does not mean that the cause of varicosities or thrombus formation in these regions is thus established, but only that the additional venous hypertension is the cause of the left-sided varicose and thrombotic manifestations when a general disposition or demonstrable venous disease is present. If we accept this, the dictum of Virchow (1851), that each lasting dilation of a vessel is due to the blood pressure acting on an altered vessel wall, still applies today.

Spur formation in the left common iliac vein does not in any way make it possible to predict the nature of the venous dilatation or where in the pelvis or limb it will appear.

Any change dividing or narrowing the lumen of a vein naturally raises the problem of thrombosis and embolism. Three factors are responsible for the development of thrombosis (Kaufmann, 1922; Aschoff, 1925):

—changes in the bloodstream;
—changes in the wall; and
—changes in the composition of the blood.

Since spur formation in the left common iliac vein causes both a change in the bloodstream and a change in the wall, it is understandable that it represents a latent risk should there be a change in the composition of the blood (due to surgery, malignant growths, and so forth). Spur formation could also play a part in the limitation of a thrombus. There are certain preferred locations in the legs for the development of thromboses.

Virchow (1848) and later Aschoff (1925) mentioned favorite sites, and Neumann (1938) detailed them in his segmental hypothesis. A thrombus that continues to grow in a vein may at certain points stop growing or show discontinuity. Aschoff (1925) (see also Brass, 1941) wrote: "Right-sided thrombosis extends to Poupart's ligament, whereas on the left it extends to a point where the left iliac vein is compressed by the right iliac artery." This observation teaches that because of anatomic conditions there are limits to the spread of thrombosis that are exceeded only exceptionally, and that furthermore the correctness of this assumption is clearly proved by the anatomic situation in the left lower extremity. Evidently, only in rare cases, can a spur be considered to be the site of origin of thrombosis, although we have seen cases of this nature. But it constitutes the limit to progressive thrombosis in the area of the femoral vein, possibly being caused by it. Neumann's (1938) maxim, "Resistance due to perivascular architecture which has to be overcome by the circulation simultaneously forms the limits of thrombosis," should be supplemented on the basis of our findings that the endovascular architecture specifically may limit thrombosis.

Table 1.1 Incidence of Different Types of Pelvic Vein Spur

Cases examined	430
women	142
Spur group I	59
Spur group II	17
Spur group III	4
Embryos and newborn	88
Spur combined with thrombosis in the leg veins	31

Finally, we believe we have found spur formation to be the essential cause for the preponderance of left-sided pelvic thromboses.

From the data in Table 1.1, it follows that the percentage incidence of the groups with 95 or 99 per cent probability lies within certain limits (Table 1.2).

Table 1.2 Incidence of Spur Formation in Pelvic Veins

Probability	95%	99%
Frequency of spur formation	15.1–22.4	13.9–23.6
Incidence in group I	62.7–81.9	59.6–85.0
Incidence in group II	12.9–30.5	10.1–33.3
Incidence in group III relative to the figure 80	1.0–11.0	0 –12.6
Incidence of thrombosis in patients with spurs	28.5–49.6	25.2—52.9

In our material, spur formation was observed on the left side without exception.

For comparison, the figures of McMurrich (1906): Of 107 cases, 35 spur formations (32.7 per cent), of which 91.4 per cent were on the left. Figures of Krumbhaar and Ehrich (1943): Of 399 cases, 95 spur formations (23.8 per cent); in children and infants, 4.7 per cent; with the addition of doubtful cases, 17.3 per cent; in children above 10 years, 33.8 per cent.

Comparative examinations of 112 oxen did not reveal the spur formation seen in man, but in eight cases there was fenestration of the left common iliac vein and a frequently accompanying parallel vein, the size of a small finger. No such finding was observed in the right iliac vein.

At times the angle of bifurcation of the inferior vena cava is so low that the right common iliac artery conceals it. This venous compression is seen in the roentgenogram as a contrast medium defect, the "normally invisible zone" (*zone normalement invisible*) of Guilhem and Baux (1954).

Valves in Perforating and Communicating Veins

The valves in the communicating veins between the superficial and deep venous systems are arranged so that reflux of venous blood can take place only from surface to depth if they are sufficient (Fig. 1.59). Raised pressure in the deep venous system thus cannot be transmitted to the superficial system; the valves neutralize it. The valves are arranged both epifascially and subfascially (Raivio, 1948).

Valves of the Muscle Veins

The veins of gastrocnemius and soleus have dense arcades of valves that begin to show marked degeneration after the twenty-fifth year of life, according to Gullmo (1957), or after the thirtieth year, according to our own observations.

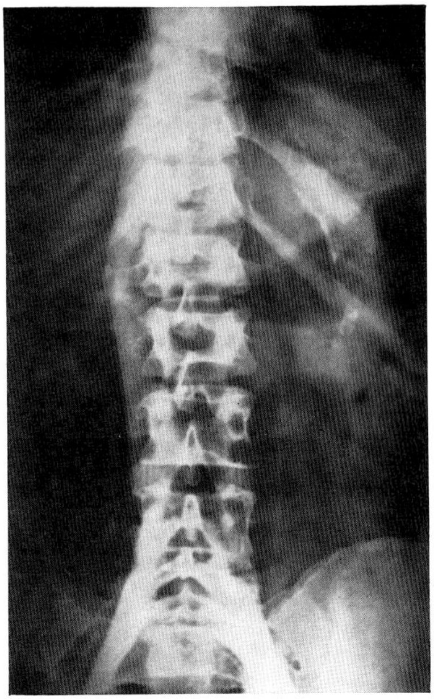

Fig. 1.61. Phlebogram of the inferior vena cava.

Inferior Vena Cava

The two common iliac veins join to form the *inferior vena cava* on the right and ventral to the intervertebral disk between L4 and L5 behind the beginning of the common iliac artery (Fig. 1.60). It lies in its course on the right anterior surface of the vertebral column and is clearly separated from the aorta. Below the diaphragm it runs ventral to the right renal and adrenal arteries and the right lumbar and right inferior phrenic arteries. At the diaphragm it penetrates the foramen venae cavae cranially, the aorta piercing the aortic hiatus. The distance here is almost 3 cm. In the liver, the inferior cava is embedded in the sulcus venae cavae. The length of the venous trunk distal to the diaphragm varies with that of the body and is around 20 cm; the diameter is around 3 cm.

The inferior vena cava is extended between two fixed points, the site of penetration of the diaphragm and the junction of the two common iliac veins. Since it lies in loose connective tissue without a common vascular sheath, completely independent of the aorta, it is not only freely movable but stretches with the movements of the diaphragm. It forms a slight arch, convex to the right. It rests on the vertebral column at L2 and L3 and turns ventrally to flow into the right atrium.

The vein never has valves.

The *smooth contour of the inferior vena cava on a roentgenogram* shows a slight depression at the posterior wall at the level of L2 due to *impression by the right renal artery*. In addition, there are filling defects caused by the junctions with the renal and hepatic veins at the level of L1 and L2 (Fig. 1.61).

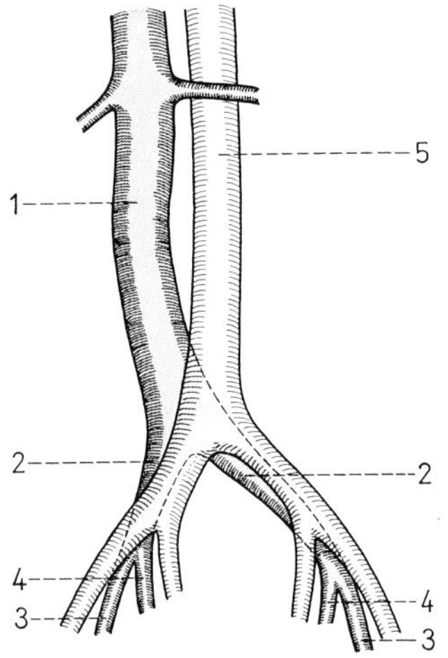

Fig. 1.60. Topography of the inferior vena cava.

1 V. cava inferior
2 V. iliaca communis
3 V. iliaca externa
4 V. iliaca interna
5 Aorta

Branches of the Inferior Vena Cava

Parietal branches

—Inferior phrenic veins; and
—Four lumbar veins connecting with the ascending lumbar vein.

Visceral branches. Description of these branches is beyond the scope of this book. There are three hepatic veins, the renal veins and the testicular veins, of which the right flows into the vena cava and the left into the renal vein.

Anomalies of the Inferior Vena Cava

Congenital Transverse Membranous Occlusion of the Vena Cava Just Below the Diaphragm

This very rare malformation was dealt with in detail by Kimura et al. (1962, 1963), who reported more than 30 cases in Japan alone. It appears possible that the anomaly is more common in Japan since only individual cases have been reported from other countries. An earlier description was given by Bennett (1950), and the anomaly was probably first described by Meyer (1903).

For details on diagnosis, clinical picture and therapy, see page 202ff.

Topographic Anomalies of the Inferior Vena Cava

These anomalies are due to developmental arrest. The key to the understanding of these malformations is knowledge of the embryologic development of the inferior vena cava. It has been described by Grünwald (1938) and by Elke and Ludin (1965) (Fig. 1.62).

In the third to eighth embryonal weeks the *symmetric primary venous system* is transformed by unequal differentiation and involution to the *asymmetric secondary venous system.* Essential to this transformation is the predominant position of the right supracardinal vein, the intersubcardinal segment and the hepatic segment of the inferior cava primordium.

The development of the large body veins is intimately involved with the development of the heart. The asymmetry in the development of the heart begins toward the end of the third embryonic week at the cardiac tube. Formation of the systemic and lung veins follows in the next 4 weeks. At the same time, the basic phase of cardiac development occurs, with torsions, loop formations and septations caused by the embryonic bloodstream.

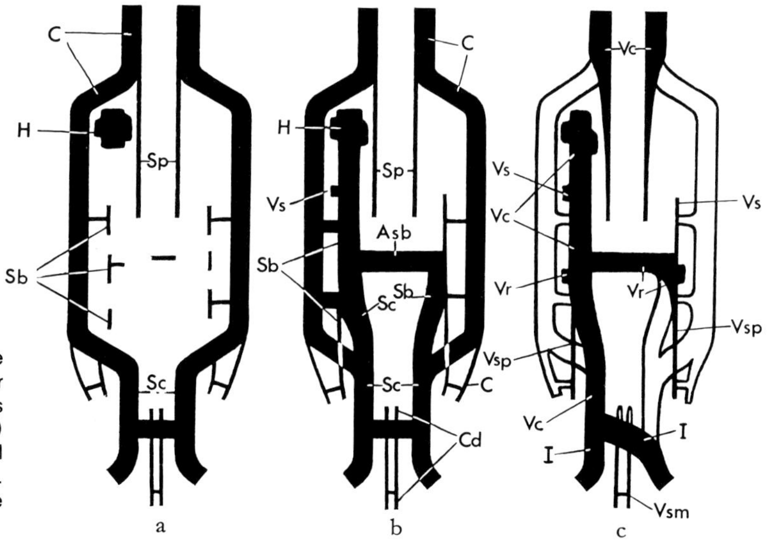

Fig. 1.62. Diagram of the development of the inferior vena cava and its tributaries in man. (After Grünwald.) Primary stage (*a*); transitional stage (*b*); definitive stage (*c*). The obliterated portions are thinly outlined.

Asb = Intersubcardinal anastomosis
C = Cardinal vein
Cd = Caudal vein
H = Common hepatic vein
I = Common iliac vein
Sb = Subcardinal veins
Sc = Sacrocardinal veins
Sc-Sb = Connection of sacrocardinal with subcardinal veins

Sp = Supracardinal veins
Vc = Caudal cava vein
Vr = Renal vein
Vs = Suprarenal vein
Vsm = Median sacral vein
Vsp = Testicular vein
Vt = Longitudinal thoracic veins (azygos and hemiazygos, not in final stage yet)

It is understandable, therefore, that malformations of the inferior vena cava are so often combined with cardiac malformations.

Three-Phase Development of the Inferior Vena Cava

The first important venous anlagen (caudal cardinal veins) appear in human embryos of 4 to 6 mm length as two long vascular trunks, running lateral and dorsal to the mesonephros; they can be followed to the caudal terminations of the mesonephros. At this stage, they represent the only venous trunks that run cranially from the abdominal and pelvic areas. The cardinal veins are further complemented in embryos 7 to 13 mm in length by the appearance, in the region caudal to the origin of the umbilical arteries, of the sacrocardinal veins, which flow into the cardinal veins near their termination. Their source is the leg anlagen. These venous systems are bilaterally symmetric but are at first separate. In embryos of 10 mm length, the caudal veins develop medial to the sacrocardinal veins along the caudal aorta, but are also connected with the sacrocardinal veins. One of these anastomoses later forms the important link between the two sacrocardinal veins. This stage of development is known also as the *primary* venous system.

With the formation of the subcardinal veins, which appear at first to be segmented but later join to form one trunk on each side, a new developmental phase begins. The subcardinal veins connect with the sacrocardinal veins and, by several branches, also with the still existing caudal cardinal veins. They receive blood from several organs and, by way of the sacrocardinal veins, that from the pelvis and lower extremities. Since the blood has better chance of drainage in the subcardinal veins than in the caudal cardinal veins, the latter become unimportant and atrophy. Originally the subcardinal veins end blindly cranially, but the right connects with the vena hepatica revehens communis (v. cava caudalis primitiva) to form the *secondary* venous system.

The blood from the left subcardinal vein flows into the right subcardinal by an anastomosis that soon develops further. Asymmetry in favor of the right side is a noteworthy feature of the secondary venous system.

The asymmetric development is not restricted to the cranial portions of the subcardinal veins (intersubcardinal anastomosis) but also includes the sacrocardinal veins; of these, the left, lying between the intersubcardinal anastomosis on the one side and the deeper anastomosis between sacrocardinal and caudal veins on the other side, completely atrophies. Destruction of the left sacrocardinal vein cranial to its connection with the caudal veins signifies transition to the final state (embryos of 20 mm length). According to Clara (1940), the inferior vena cava is composed of three sections. The cranial is formed by the vena hepatica revehens, the next section by the markedly dilated right subcardinal vein and the last one by the right sacrocardinal vein. Contrariwise, on the left, only the distal portion of the left common iliac vein develops, whereas the proximal portion of this vein has already arisen in the primary venous system from the anastomosis between the sacrocardinal and caudal veins.

Clinical Signs

Hemodynamic disorders are produced only by incorrect junction, chamber anomalies or transposition of the great vessels. Other anomalies of the inferior vena cava remain silent.

Agenesis of the Inferior Vena Cava

In *agenesis of the inferior vena cava* the azygos vein (v. thoracica longitudinalis dextra) increases considerably in size. According to Elke and Ludin (1965), the orthograde junction of the azygos vein is revealed by anteroposterior tomography of the region of the right main bronchus. If, however, the inferior and superior venae cavae are closed, this bypass blood flow does not take place. Powerful deep and superficial collateral veins are formed via visceral veins, especially the portal system, and veins in the abdominal and thoracic wall in the direction of the subclavian vein.

Isolated Anomalies

Isolated anomalies of the inferior vena cava are found in about 0.3 per cent of all cases, and anomalies combined with congenital malformations of the heart in about 0.6 per cent.

Many accounts of individual cases are found in the literature, but we refer mainly to excellent summaries that contain precise references (Fuchs, 1964; Elke and Ludin, 1965; and Sarma, 1966).

Left-Sided Infrarenal Inferior Vena Cava

The *left* supracardinal vein has remained instead of the *right*. The vessel runs laterally on the left of the aorta to the junction with the left renal vein. There, as the medial portion of the left renal vein (which originated from the subcardinal vein), it crosses the vertebral column from left to right and courses paravertebrally on the right (see Fig. 10.8*b*, p. 208).

Bilateral Infrarenal Inferior Vena Cava

The supracardinal veins have remained bilaterally. Two broad veins run along either side of the aorta and join at the level of the kidneys (see Fig. 10.8*a*, p. 208).

Preureteric Inferior Vena Cava

The right ureter lies behind the cava; this causes the risk of ureteric stasis. The proximal portion of the right ureter runs laterally on the right of the inferior vena cava, crosses it dorsally in the middle and flows distally on the medial side of the cava to the bladder. *Cause:* The postcardinal vein has been preserved and the supracardinal has regressed.

Absence of the Inferior Vena Cava (Continuation of the Inferior Vena Cava in the Azygos Vein)

The prerenal segment of the inferior vena cava is connected with the junction of the azygos and the superior vena cava. Hence the hepatic veins enter the right atrium by the normal orifice of the inferior vena cava.

Apart from these four basic anomalies numerous individual variations have been reported in the literature that can be decoded with knowledge of embryonic development.

Junctional anomalies with the heart are not discussed here; they belong to the realm of cardiac surgery.

References

Ahlberg, N. E., O. Bartley, N. Chidekel, K. O. Edlundh: Roentgenological diagnosis of pelvic varicosities in women. Acta obstet. gynec. scand. Suppl. 7 (1964) 120

Albanese, A. R., A. M. Albanese, E. F. Albanese: Lateral subdermic varicose vein system of the legs. Its surgical treatment by the chiseling tube method. Vasc. Surg. 3 (1969) 81

Aschoff, D.: Vorträge über Pathologie. Fischer, Jena 1925

Askar, O.: The short saphenous vein. J. cardiovasc. Surg. 4. (1963) 126

Askar, O.: On the surgical anatomy of the communicating veins of the leg. J. cardiovasc. Surg. 4 (1963) 138

Askar, O., M. Abou-El-Ainen: The surgical anatomy of the deep fascia of the human leg. J. cardiovasc. Surg. 4 (1963) 114

Basmajian, I. V.: The distribution of valves in the femoral external, iliac and common iliac veins and their relationship to varicose veins. Surg. Gynec. Obstet. 95 (1952) 537

Bauer, G.: Observations on the technique of phlebography. Acta radiol. 26 (1945) 577

Bauer, G.: Venous insufficiency in the leg. Nord. Med. 63 (1960a) 251

Bauer, G.: Dynamic intraosseous phlebography. Nord. Med. 63 (1960b) 253

Bauer, G.: Flebografia dinamica intraossea. Angiologia 12 (1960c) 85

Bennett, I. L.: A unique case of obstruction of inferior vena cava. Bull. Johns Hopk. Hosp. 87 (1950) 290

Bergstrand, I., C. A. Ekman, R. Köhler: Inferior venacaval obstruction in hepatic cirrhosis. Acta radiol. 2 (1964) 2

Bevan, P. E., S. H. Green, F. A. R. Stammers: Low termination of the internal saphenous vein. Brit. med. J. 1956/1, 610

Boyd, A. M.: Discussion on primary treatment of varicose veins. Proc. roy Soc. Med. 41 (1948) 633

Brass, K.: Aufbau und Entwicklung der Beinvenenthrombose. Frankf. Z. Path. 56 (1941) 74

Brecher, G. A.: Venous Return. Grune & Stratton, New York 1956

Burch, G. E.: A Primer of Venous Pressure. Kimpton, London 1950

Caron, J., G. Bonte: La phlébographie azygos. J. Radiol. Electrol. 43 (1962) 259

Cibor, Z., A. Cencora: La veine saphène externe, données anatomiques. Phlébologie 21 (1968) 297

Clara, M.: Entwicklungsgeschichte des Menschen. Quelle & Meyer, Leipzig 1940

Cockett, F. B.: The pathology and treatment of venous ulcers of the leg. Brit. J. Surg. 179 (1955) 260

Cockett, F. B., H. Dodd: The Pathology and Surgery of the Veins of the Lower Limb. Livingstone, Edinburgh 1956

Cordier, G., J. Rousseau: Les anastomoses entre les veines sacrées et le veines hémorrhoidales. Presse méd. 64 (1956) 845

Derra, E., F. Loogen, P. Satter: Anomalien der unteren Hohlvene. Dtsch. med. Wschr. 90 (1965) 689

Dodd, H.: The varicose tributaries of the superficial femoral vein passing into Hunter's canal. Postgrad. med. J. 35 (1959) 18

Dodd, H., A. P. Calo, M. Mistry, A. Rusford: Ligation of ankle communicating veins in the treatment of the venous ulcer syndrome of the leg. Lancet 1957/II, 1249

Dos Santos, I. C.: Sur quelques vérités premières oubliées ou méconnues de l'anatom-physiologie normale et pathologique du système veineux. Amat. lusit. 7 (1947) 5–32

Elke, M., H. Ludin: Drainage der unteren Körperhälfte bei Agenesie und erworbenem Verschluß der Vena cava caudalis. Fortschr. Röntgenstr. 103 (1965) 665

Fuchs, W. A.: Vena cava inferior. In: Handbuch der medizinischen Radiologie, Vol. X, L. Diethelm, O. Olsson, F. Strnad, H. Vieten, A. Zuppinger (eds.), Springer, Berlin 1964.

Grünwald, P.: Die Entwicklung der Vena cava caudalis beim Menschen. Z. mikr.-anat. Forsch. 43 (1938) 275

Grupp, G., I. Grupp, H. Spitz: Collateral vascular pathways during experimental obstruction of aorta and inferior vena cava. Amer. J. Roentgenol. 94 (1965) 159

Guilhem. P., R. Baux: La Phlébographie Pelvienne. Masson, Paris 1954

Gullmo, A.: The strain obstruction syndrome of the femoral vein. Acta radiol. 47 (1957) 119

Gullmo, A.: Periphere Venen. In: Handbuch der medizinischen Radiologie, Vol. X 3, L. Diethelm, O. Olsson, F. Strnad, H. Vieten, A. Zuppinger (eds.), Springer, Berlin 1964

Haeger, K.: The surgical anatomy of the sapheno-femoral and the sapheno-popliteal junctions. J. cardiovasc. Surg. 6 (1962) 420

Haserbroeck, K: Über die Bedeutung der Arterienpulsation für die Strömung in den Venen und die Pathogenese der Varizen. Pflügers Arch. ges. Physiol. (1916) 163

Helander, C. G., A. Lindbom: Roentgen examination of the inferior vena cava in retroperitoneal expanding processes. Acta radiol. 45 (1966) 289
Hilty, H.: Die makroskopische Gefäßvariabilität im Mündungsgebiet der Vena saphena magna des Menschen. Schwabe, Basel 1955
Kandel, R.: Chirurgisch-anatomische Eigentümlichkeiten bei der Behandlung der varikösen Vena saphena parva. Zbl. Phleb. 6 (1967) 313
Kanematsu, T., S. Okubo: A case of complete obstruction of vena cava inferior in the hepatic part. Trans. Soc. Path. Jap. 18 (1928) 395
Kappert, A.: Der heutige Stand der Venenforschung. Ciba Symp. 15 (1967) 113
Kaufmann: Lehrbuch der speziellen pathologischen Anatomie. De Gruyter, Berlin 1922
Keen, J. A.: The collateral venous circulation in a case of thrombosis of the inferior vena cava and its embryological interpretation. Brit. J. Surg. 29 (1941) 105
Kimura, C., H. Shirotani, M. Hirooka, M. Terada, K. Iwahashi, S. Maetani: Membranous obliteration of the inferior vena cava in der hepatic portion. J. cardiovasc. Surg. 4 (1963) 87
Kimura, C. Shirotani, T. Kuma, M. Hiroka, K. Hagashi, K. Tsunekawa, S. Matsuda: Transcardiac membranotomy for obliteration of the inferior vena cava in the hepatic portion. J. cardiovasc. Surg. 3 (1962) 393
Kobak, M., M. Lev: Anatomy of the deep venous system of the popliteal fossa and lower leg. Arch. Surg. 68 (1954) 350
Krumbbaar, E. B., E. E. Ehrich: A frequent obstructive anomaly of the mouth of the left common iliac vein. Amer. Heart J. 26 (1943) 737
v. Lanz, T., W. Wachsmuth: Praktische Anatomie, Vol. I/4. Springer, Berlin 1938
Ledderhose, G.: Die Bedeutung der Venenklappen und ihre Beziehungen zu den Varizen. Zbl. Chir. (1904) 1325
van Limborgh, J.: L'anatomie du système veineux de l'extrémité inférieure en relation avec la pathologie variqueuse. Folia angiol. 8 (1961) 3
van Limborgh, J.: La nomenclature des veines communicantes des l'extrémité inférieure. Rapport du Comité de Nomenclature de la Société Béneluxienne de Phlébologie. Selbstverlag Anat. Inst., Amsterdam 1963
van Limborgh, J., D. A. Banga, J. H. Meijerikenj, H. H. Luigies: De venae communicantes van het been. Ned. T. Geneesk. 106 (1962) 3
Linton, R. R.: The communicating veins of the lower leg and the operative technic for their ligation. Ann. Surg. 107 (1938) 582
Linton, R. R.: The post-thrombotic ulceration of the lower extremity: its etiology and surgical treatment. Ann. Surg. 138 (1953a) 415
Linton, R. R.: The surgical treatment of the postthrombotic syndrome with ulceration of the lower extremity. De Smedt, Brüssel 1953b
Luke, I. C.: The deep vein valves. Surgery 29 (1951) 381
McMurrich, J. P.: The valves of the iliac vein. Brit. med. J. 1906/II, 1699
Maranta, E. F. Camponova, M. S. Del Buono: Die Beckenangiographie. Fortschr. Röntgenstr. 101 (1964) 229
May, R.: Die Rolle der Vv. perforantes bei der Varizenoperation. 5 (1964) 455
May, R., R. Nissl: Die Phlebographie der unteren Extremität. Thieme, Stuttgart 1959
May, R., R. Nissl: Varizen der Vena gastrocnemia. Fortschr. Röntgenstr. 103 (1965a) 229
May, R., R. Nissl: Technik der Phlebographie und das Normalbild der Venen. In: Lehrbuch der Röntgendiagnostik, Vol. I, 6th Ed.; H. R. Schinz, W. F. Baensch, W. Frommbold, R. Glauner, F. Uehlinger, J. Wellauer (eds.). Thieme, Stuttgart 1965b.
May, R., R. Nissl: Phlebographische Studien zur Anatomie der Beinvenen. Fortschr. Röntgenstr. 104 (1966) 171
May, R., R. Nissl: Phlebographische Studien uber die Venen der Kniekehle und der Wade. Fortschr. Rontgenstr. 109 (1968) 614
May, R., J. Thurner: Ein Gefaßsporn in der V. iliaca comm. sin. als wahrscheinliche Ursache der überwiegend linksseitigen Beckenvenenthrombose. Z. Kreisl.-Forsch. 45 (1956) 912
May, R., J. Thurner: The cause of the predominantly sinistral occurrence of thrombosis of the pelvic veins. Angiology 5 (1957) 419
Mercier, R., Ph. Fouques, N. Portal, G. Vanneuville: Anatomie chirurgicale de la veine saphène externe. J. Chir. 93 (1967) 59
Meyer, A.: On a case of complete fibrous obstruction (congenital) of both superior and inferior venae cava in a young man of 18 years: first recorded case. Med. Rec. 63 (1903) 806
Moosmann, A., W. Hartwell Jr.: The surgical significance of the subfascial course of the lesser saphenous vein. Surg. Gynec. Obstet. 118 (1964) 761
Nagayo, M.: Über die Obliteration der Haupstätte der Lebervenen und der unteren Hohlvenen im heparen Abschnitt derselben. Mitt. med. Fak. Tokyo 9 (1911) 1
Netzer, C. O.: Die Strömungsverhältnisse im tiefen Venensystem beim postthrombotischen Syndrom. Zbl. Chir. 35 (1958a) 1968
Netzer, C. O.: Die normale und krankhaft veränderte Venenströmung in den unteren Gliedmaßen. Habil.-Schrift, München 1958
Neumann, F.: Ursprungszentren und Entwicklungsformen der Beinthrombose. Virchows Arch. path. Anat. 301 (1938) 708
Osler, W.: Case of obliteration of vena cava inferior with great stenosis of orifices of hepatic veins. J. Physiol. 13 (1878) 291
Ota, S.: Obstruction of the hepatic portion of the inferior vena cava. Trans. Soc. Path. Jap. 20 (1930) 57
Owens, F. M.: Vena cava ligation in thromboembolic disease. Lancet LXXI, 1951, 435
Pleasants, J. H.: Obstruction of inferior vena cava with a report of 18 cases. Johns Hopk. Hosp. Rep. 16 (1911) 363
Porstmann, W., S. Platzek: Obliteration der Vena cava superior et inferior bei einem 19j. Patienten. Fortschr. Röntgenstr. 101 (1964) 90
Powell, T., R. B. Lynn: The valves of the external iliac femoral and upper third of the popliteal veins. Surg. Gyner. Obstet. 92 (1951) 453
Raivio, E.: Untersuchungen über die Venen der unteren Extremitäten mit besonderer Berücksichtigung der gegenseitigen Verbindungen zwischen den oberflächigen und tiefen Venen. Ann. Med. exp. Fenn. 26 (1948) 1
De la Riega, E., E. Kuhn: Alleinige persistierende linke obere Hohlvene. Z. Kreisl.-Forsch. 54 (1965) 734
Saphir, O., M. Lev: The venous valve in the aged. Am. Heart J. 44 (1952) 843
Sarjeant, T. R.: Surgical Anatomy on the Treatment of Venous Stasis. Surg. Clin. N. Amer. 44 (1964) 1383
Sarma, K. P.: Anomalous inferior vena cava – Anatomical and clinical. Brit. J. Surg. 53 (1966) 600
Schilling, R.: Über Phlebosklerose. Virchows Arch. path. Anat. 262 (1936) 658
Sen, P. K., G. Kinare, M. D. Kelkar, G. B. Parkular, J. Mehta: Congenital membranous obliteration of the inferior vena cava. Cardiovasc. Surg. 8 (1967) 344
Sieglbauer, F.: Lehrbuch der normalen Anatomie des Menschen. Urban & Schwarzenberg. Wien (1944)
Sieglbauer, F.: Anleitung zum Präparieren ganzer Leichen. Selbstverlag, Anat. Inst., Innsbruck 1966 (S. 137)
Sparks, A. L., H. Fox: Occlusion of the entire inferior vena cava. Arch. Path. 26 (1938) 519
Stanton Sherman, R.: Varicose Veins: Anatomy, Reevaluation of Trendelenburg Tests and an Operative Procedure. Surg. Clin. N. Amer. 44 (1964) 1369
Sternberg, C.: Über Obliteration der vena cava inferior und Thrombose der venae hepaticae. Verh. dtsch. path. Ges. 10 (1906) 131
Stevens, M. E., W. Knox, K. Stewart, J. Walter: Ligation of the inferior vena cava. I. Amer. med. Ass. (1965) 578
Swart, B.: Azygoserweiterung bei fehlender Vena cava inferior und Situs inversus mit Laevokardie. Fortschr. Röntgenstr. 97 (1962) 523
Verneuil, A.: Du siège réel et primitif des varices du membre inférieur. Gaz. hebd. Sci. méd. Bordeaux 2 (1855) 811
Virchow, R.: Über die Erweiterung kleinerer Gefäße. Virchows Arch. path. Anat. 3 (1851) 427
Wanke, R.: Chirurgie der großen Körpervenen. Thieme, Stuttgart 1956
Williams, A. G.: The formation of the popliteal vein. Surg. Gynec. Obstet. 97 (1953) 769
Winckler, G.: Les veines du pied. Arch. Anat. (Strasbourg) 37 (1923) 175

2 Experimental Venous Surgery

J. Kunlin and A. Kunlin

Introduction

In this chapter we will discuss progress in venous surgery, especially with regard to repair of veins and shunts by angioplasty or prostheses. A complete survey of all experiments on the leg veins will not be given; well-known problems, such as venous injury and thrombosis, have largely been omitted, but those experiments that are of importance for experimental surgery are cited.

As recently as 15 years ago, transplantation of one vein onto another was regarded as an intervention that was destined to fail. In the last few years, interest in certain kinds of bypass has gradually increased; the attempt to make an important venous trunk functional again has received increased attention.

Historical Aspects

By the end of the 19th century several surgeons had employed angiorrhaphy and achieved some success with arteries in animal experiments (Briau and Jaboulay, 1896, Petit, Glück, 1898). Carrel (1902) was the master of advanced techniques of anastomosis and perfected them. Jensen (1903) succeeded in suturing a canine vein by means of a ring. Hoepfner (1903) transplanted with success an autologous and a homologous artery on the carotid of dogs, using Payr's ring technique.

Carrel and Guthrie (1906) created experimental venous surgery. In their paper, which dealt chiefly with transposing venous segments into arteries, they also mentioned transplantation of part of the inferior vena cava to the same vein of another dog. In the same article Carrel and Guthrie described the vascular patch and end-to-side anastomosis (Fig. 2.1).

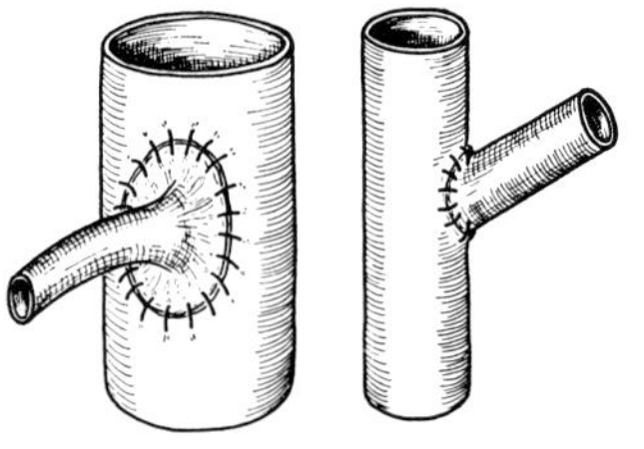

Fig. 2.1. Lateral anastomoses after Carrel and Guthrie.

Although they were engaged in restitution of the arterial stream and organ transplantation rather than with pure venous surgery, their work remains remarkable as the precursor because it anticipated most of the future areas of application.

Despite this experimental progress, little plastic surgery was carried out on man in the first half of the 20th century, apart from substitution of a few arterial aneurysms by venous transplants. In this period, only two examples of venous repair are to be found: grafting of a sheep's vein to a popliteal of man (Doyen, 1909); and transplantation of a saphenous vein to the contralateral femoral (Coenen, 1913). In both cases, no proof of patency was furnished by the authors. Important works and books on vascular surgery from that time do not mention plastic surgery of the venous system at all (Delbet, 1906; Morestin, 1906; Lejars, 1906; Lexer, 1913; Villard and Perrin, 1913; Moure, 1914).

Nevertheless, laboratory trials were undertaken. Borst and Enderlen (1909) attempted in vain to replace the jugular vein of a dog by a homotransplant of the carotid. Jeger and Israel (1913) set themselves the problem of restoring the inferior vena cava at the level of the renal veins; the result was only partially successful. Apparently not a single publication appeared for 37 years until the communication of Southwick (1950) on portacaval shunt by an arterial homograft. Portacaval transplants were performed on man by means of an autoplastic vein by Blakemore and Lord in 1945, but no experimental data seem to have been published for this, or for the splenorenal grafts Rousselot (1952) carried out on man.

Anatomy and Physiology of the Veins

A few basic facts that must be considered in venous surgery should be emphasized.

Vascular Structure

The *venous wall* is thin, consisting of elastic connective tissue, and contains a number of smooth muscle fibers, depending on the location of the vessel. The veins around the neck, the visceral veins and the caval veins are poor in muscular elements and barely contractile. Their lumina, kept patent by fixation to neighboring tissues, permits only passive variations due to endovenous pressure and pressure by surrounding tissues. This is particularly true of veins in the neck and thorax. On dissecting the jugular vein or superior vena cava, one can easily see how they become inflated and collapse with the rhythm of respiration. This situation, although unfavorable for venous surgery, would appear to promote stenosis of anastomoses. Experience has shown that this is not so, however.

On the other hand, the veins of the extremities, especially the superficial veins, are muscular and contractile. Their diameter can be reduced to a third of its original dimension. The muscular structure is a disadvantage in surgical manipulations. Vasoconstriction at the level of a suture may be a source of failure and, in fact, the results of surgery of the femoral vein are possibly less favorable than those of operations on the jugular because of enhanced vasoconstriction.

The *endothelium* plays an essential part in venous patency. Endothelial changes due to certain factors were studied by Robertson et al. (1954, 1957), Ferrero and Mairano (1955), Fontaine et al. (1956), Gottlob and Zinner (1962, 1973), Fallon (1972), Acland (1973).

At the beginning of this century Guthrie noted that a venous graft is preserved better in Ringer-Locke solution than in isotonic saline. Venous stasis and even freeing of the vessel causes minor structural changes of the endothelial cells that must be ascribed to injury. Catching hold of the vein with forceps or clamp, or temporary ligature, causes disappearance of the endothelium after 24 hours. Disconnection of the vessel between two ligatures produces complete destruction of the endothelium in 2 to 6 days. A clot forms after 3 days, but liquefies later. Infusion of water has no damaging effect. However, injection with hypertonic solutions (10 per cent sodium chloride solution, hypertonic glucose solution or various sclerosing media) destroys the endothelium in 2 hours (Fontaine et al., 1962).

Regeneration generally follows quickly—0.5 to 1 mm per day (Sinapius, 1966). The endothelial cells enlarge to twice or three times their diameter, and blood elements that are fixed to the traumatized zone begin to cover the defect from the second day. Amitotic cell divisions are frequently observed (Zinner and Gottlob, 1961). Mitoses of endothelial cells were only exceptionally seen (Altschul, 1954; Poole et al., 1958). Connective tissue cells may be involved in this regeneration, but not monocytes (Sinapius, 1966). The endothelial lesions may trigger thrombosis, but their significance should not be overestimated. The whole intima is removed for several centimeters during endophlebectomy, as will be shown later. Nevertheless obliteration does not generally follow since thrombolytic mechanisms are stimulated.

The part *venous valves* play in angiorrhaphy or grafting is unknown. Comparative studies of valve-bearing and valveless transplants in the area of normally valved veins would be of interest.

With arterial plastic surgery, a large *caliber* undoubtedly improves chances of success, but this is not the case with veins. All experimenters found to their surprise that repair of the inferior vena cava was much more difficult than that of the jugular or superior vena cava. No doubt other factors play a part, such as intra-abdominal pressure and poor drainage in the inferior vena cava. Results always depend on technique and suture material.

Nonetheless, the differences in success between various veins appear gradually to decrease with better and more refined techniques. The importance of appropriate form of substitutes should also be kept in mind (Mikhailov, 1969).

Venous Hemodynamics

Circulatory Factors

The venous system collects the capillary blood and conducts it to the heart. At the same time, it acts as a depot for a considerable quantity of blood, especially in the spleen, liver, skin and lungs. The body can mobilize this blood under physiologic and pathologic conditions. The capacity of the venous system is three or four times that of the arterial system. Approximately 60 per cent of the total blood accumulates here.

The venous circulation (Fig. 2.2) is sustained by arterial pulsation. The blood pressure declines distally to 20 mm Hg. At the termination of the capillary network, the pressure in the capillaries is only 8 mm Hg. The pressure gradient between the origin of the veins and the right atrium is therefore small. Venous flow is supported by several factors. The peripheral venules receiving blood contain valves and are muscular. Contractions of their walls support the transport of blood, according to some authors. But their actual importance must be doubted. Pulsations of neigh-

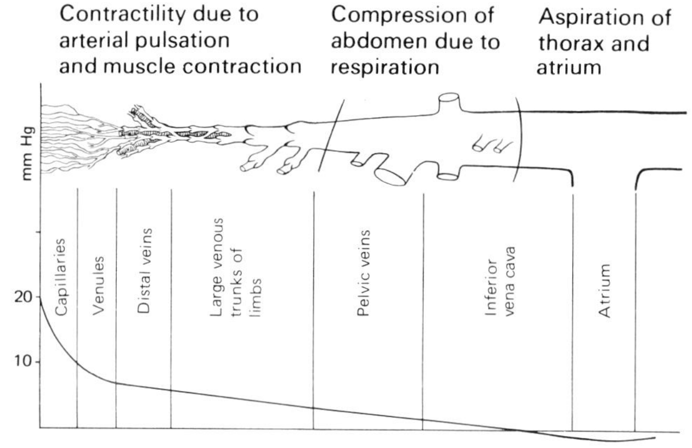

Fig. 2.2. Scheme of venous circulation.

boring arteries appear to play some part. The musculature has special importance for the venous circulation. The changes in volume caused by muscle contractions compress the neighboring veins and propel the blood centrally, corresponding with the position of the valves. The intra-abdominal pressure is raised by diaphragmatic movements with each respiration. This causes compression of visceral veins which, in conjunction with the simultaneous drop in intrathoracic pressure, favors drainage of the blood toward the heart. Venous pressure is increased by muscular activity. This favorable factor is made use of in postoperative treatment (exercises, the Valsalva maneuver).

Gravity plays a part that is not to be overlooked since hydrostatic pressure supports the venous pressure. It facilitates backflow in the veins of head and neck, in the brachiocephalic trunk and in the superior vena cava. Circulation in these regions is "isogravitational," whereas it is "antigravitational" in the lower extremities, abdomen, and inferior vena cava, at least in man. The effect of gravity is neutralized when the subject is recumbent. It plays a considerably smaller part in animals than in man (Table 2.1). The caliber of the veins is much greater than that of the arteries. Since the volume of blood that reaches the heart is identical with that ejected by the aorta, the flow velocity in the veins is ipso facto much less than in the arteries (Table 2.2). The flow velocity increases in the direction of the heart.

Table 2.1
Venous Pressure of the Anesthetized Dog on the Operating Table

Femoral vein	10 to 15 mm H_2O
External jugular vein	0 to 5 mm H_2O
Inferior abdominal vena cava	4 to 8 mm H_2O
Thoracic inferior vena cava	0 to −2 mm H_2O
Superior vena cava	+2 to −2 mm H_2O

Table 2.2 Blood Flow Velocity

Femoral vein	6.2 cms^{-1}
Renal vein	4.3 cms^{-1}
Mesenteric vein	8.5 cms^{-1}
External jugular vein	14.7 cms^{-1}
Large arteries	20–30 cms^{-1}

The experimental work of Wright et al. (1973, 1974) about the relation between venous stasis and arterial flow in the canine leg must be mentioned. The ligation of the femoral vein induces a 50 per cent drop in arterial flow. This demonstrates the importance of repairing not only the artery but also the vein in cases of severe vascular injuries (Barcia et al., 1972; Wright et al. 1973, 1974).

In all, low pressure and low flow velocity are the characteristic factors of venous circulation that present the chief problem in venous surgery. On the other hand, it is seen that an arteriovenous fistula inserted near a venous prosthesis augments the chances of patency because pressure and local outflow increase.

Local Factors

Any irregularity of caliber or any impediment in the bloodstream produces local turbulence which favors the deposition of fibrin, not only at the site of the obstruction but also some distance away. Thus fibrin deposits develop on the spur of an arterial bifurcation or that of a collateral, especially if the vessel loses its elasticity. As soon as it becomes prominent, an atheromatous plaque causes a fibrin deposit on it and in the area of the whirl. These hemodynamic disturbances and their sequelae have been mentioned or studied in anastomoses (Szilagyi, 1960) and in arteries (Palma, 1952, 1959, 1962; McDonald, 1960; Dos Santos, 1964; Schlicht, 1963, 1966; Malan, 1966, 1967, 1969). But they are also found in veins, where they appear to be of less importance because of the lower pressure and flow.

On the rabbit's vein opposite an aortocaval fistula Fallon et al. (1972) described a small zone free of endothelium destroyed by the violent arterial inflow. Abnormal cells are present in the neighborhood: they have several nuclei which is proof of regeneration of the endothelium. Thickening of the intima develops also, particularly if the vein used for the arteriovenous connection is implanted at an angle less than 90° (Bond et al. 1975). This can lead to progressive narrowing and obliteration. Could it not be a useful condition in humans with a-v fistula made for venous reconstruction thereby doing away with the second operation to suppress the a-v communication which is generally indispensable?

When a portacaval anastomosis or an H-shaped ilioiliac venous anastomosis is applied, a small crescentic fibrin spur usually forms on the distal commissure of the anastomosis (Fig. 2.3). This sickle-shaped bulge, sometimes associated with small strands, was repeatedly observed by us in experiments on dogs; it was also seen by Olivier (1951) in man at the junction of the left common iliac vein. According to May (1959), these spurs form during life. They have been considered by other authors to be congenital malformations: they were found in 80 cases among 430 autopsies of adults, but in none of 88 embryos or newborns (May and Nissl, 1959). Histologic examination confirms May's view. These new formations can be regarded mainly, if not always, as secondary organization of fibrin depots or bridges caused by local whirls in the circulation. The fact that the right common iliac artery frequently compresses the terminal segment of the left common iliac vein favors their development.

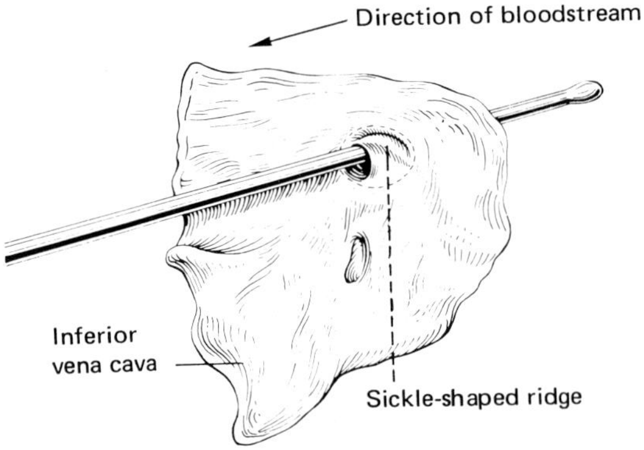

Fig. 2.3. Sickle-shaped ridge at the junction of a portacaval graft. Preparation from the dog: this bulge developed at the caval aspect $6\frac{1}{2}$ months after portacaval anastomosis.

The consequence is that whirl formation must be avoided during surgical intervention. The type of anastomosis is therefore not unimportant. End-to-end anastomosis is undoubtedly superior to end-to-side junction, which may cause turbulence. However, other advantages of the latter give it an important place in plastic surgery at present.

Furthermore, great differences in caliber should be avoided, although the reason is somewhat obscure. Some authors achieved better results when the prosthetic material had a slightly larger caliber. On the other hand, Van der Stricht and Lejeune (1964) recommend a somewhat smaller graft, which, in their opinion, retains patency longer since the flow velocity is greater. The experiments of Silvestri (1968), using the jugular to replace the cavae, seem to speak in favor of this. A mechanical suture was employed, which favors results in any case.

Clotting Factors

The state of the circulation is certainly important for successful vascular surgery, but it is difficult to determine its precise effect because it is so difficult to separate thrombosing and thrombolytic factors.

In the healthy person, thrombosing and thrombolytic tendencies balance harmoniously. Fibrin deposits form from circulating fibrin in all vessels, but they are quickly dissolved by enzymes secreted by the vessel wall. Zehnder (1947) and Fontaine et al. (1956) noted in animals that a thrombus that forms in an isolated vessel between two liguatures is lysed generally. Dissolution of a thrombus obliterating the whole lumen has frequently been observed also in man. This phenomenon is hardly ever demonstrable in arteries. Nevertheless we observed with surprise an empty vessel lumen of some centimeters in length between two organized thrombi in a patient with arteriosclerosis. The lumen was filled with a pink fluid and a gelatinous mass,

which was very soft and adhered only loosely to the intima. The intima was a little dull.
This phenomenon of pathophysiologic interest will be discussed later, in the section on recanalization of thrombosed veins.

Bioelectric Phenomena of Clotting

Among the factors that safeguard the circulatory balance, special attention has recently been paid to electric phenomena. Abramson (1928, 1942) showed that all blood cells have a negative surface charge and move toward the positive pole on electrophoresis. Sawyer and Pate (1953) stressed the importance of electric phenomena in the formation of a thrombus. Normally, an electrode lying in the lumen of a vessel has a negative charge, whereas a second one, in contact with the adventitia, is positive. Conditions are reversed when thrombosis sets in: the inner electrode becomes positive, and the outer negative.
If electrodes are placed on vessel walls, one connected with the positive, and the other with the negative pole of a battery, thrombosis forms only at the positive side. Heparin in the usual dosage neutralizes the positive charge and prevents clotting, but dicumarol does not (Schwartz, 1959), nor does dextran, which works only by increasing the blood flow (Sawyer, et al. 1973).
These studies are very important for the selection of material for vascular prostheses or heart valves. Sawyer et al. (1965b) tested tubes of metal and plastic. The silver tubes thrombosed after as little as 1 to 3 hours; Tuffier had noticed this previously (1915). Platinum is obliterated in 48 hours. Also, stainless steel and copper cause rapid thrombosis. Their inner surface, which is in contact with the blood, is in fact positively charged. On the contrary, magnesium and aluminum tubes are charged negatively (less than 0.5 V) and remain patent up to $1\frac{1}{2}$ years despite their progressive alteration.
Gott et al. (1961) tested rigid prostheses of plastic material covered with colloidal graphite and carefully polished. They were introduced into the inferior and superior thoracic vena cava by a small incision and fixed by ligature. They were removed after 2 hours and the degree of thrombosis was assessed. Ten different kinds of plastic material were thus tested. Tubes of polyethylene, Teflon, and methyl methacrylate–silicon caused thrombosis almost without exception after 2 hours. But the methyl methacrylate–graphite tubes yielded an ideal patency in 70 per cent of the subjects. In the remaining 30 per cent there was moderate or very little thrombosis.
Similar results are obtained if the tube is connected with the negative pole of a battery of 3 V (5 mA during 1 hour). Connection with the positive pole is always followed by thrombosis.
Whiffen et al. (1964) used graphite tubes prepared with benzalkonium, which permits heparin to be bound with graphite.
Wright and Johnston (1966) tested this material in hemodynamic disorders by using polycarbonate-graphite tubes of a caliber considerably smaller than that of the caval veins in which they were tested. They remained patent for more than 3 months.
These tubes are rigid and were tested particularly with regard to their usability for cardiac surgery. They are completely useless for vascular surgery, in which the tubes have to be pliable. Meanwhile Lessinger et al. (1966) were successful in fixing heparin to certain materials from which flexible vascular prostheses can be made without incorporating graphite, which is poorly absorbed by these materials. In a later trial, Gott et al. (1968) were able to apply heparin, fixing it to 15 polymers and also caoutchouc, polyvinyl, polyethylene, teflon and soft silicon. When these materials were used without impregnation, thrombosis occurred after 2 hours. With the addition of heparin, they remained patent throughout the trial, which lasted for 2 weeks.
Fraser et al. (1968), in long-term observations (1 year) on the superior vena cava of dogs, achieved better results with benzalkonium and heparin-impregnated Dacron prostheses than with those impregnated with graphite-benzalkonium-heparin (7 of 10 patent, but with slight, noninterfering stenoses). The comparative series using autoplastic veins (half of them with an enlarged transplant, a "double panel graft") yielded a result of 9 of 10 patent. It is interesting to note that fixation with heparin evidently lasts a long time—but we do not yet know how long. On the other hand, it is evident that anticoagulants can act only locally and are restricted to the surface of the plastic tube that is in contact with the blood. According to the studies of the authors mentioned, the antithrombotic effect may be caused by factor XI, the Hageman factor, being fixed to the heparinized plastic surface. This hypothesis is compatible with the views of Salzman et al. (1967), who performed tests with a heparinized cellulose membrane. Grode et al. 1969).
Najjar et al. (1970) tested TDMAC-heparin—fixing Dacron prostheses in the laboratory; the results were encouraging. In order to avoid hemorrhage, this material was first introduced into a second Dacron prosthesis. Both were sewn to the vessel together. So far as we know the

period of observation has not exceeded 2 months. Nelsen et al. (1970) tested newer nonheparinized tubes, which consist of an electronegative plastic material. This synthetic material is anticoagulant but is not suitable as yet for the preparation of supple vessel prostheses because of mechanical faults.

These investigations, which are still under way, may possibly promote the development of new vascular prostheses, which should be constructed so that they do not permit blood loss. This is not an easy problem to solve without impeding organization of the prosthetic wall by ingrowing connective tissue.

Technique of Experimental Venous Surgery

Operative technique is decisive. The quality of the anastomosis or the graft depends on meticulous care.

Venous Anastomoses

Suture

Carrel's (1902) specifications for constructing an anastomosis still hold: strict asepsis, careful removal of adventitia, gentle manipulation, finest needles and thread (monofilament plastic is the best at present), simple continuous suture without much tension, to avoid narrowing of the lumen, frequent rinsing with isotonic glucose or Ringer-Locke solution (Fig. 2.4).

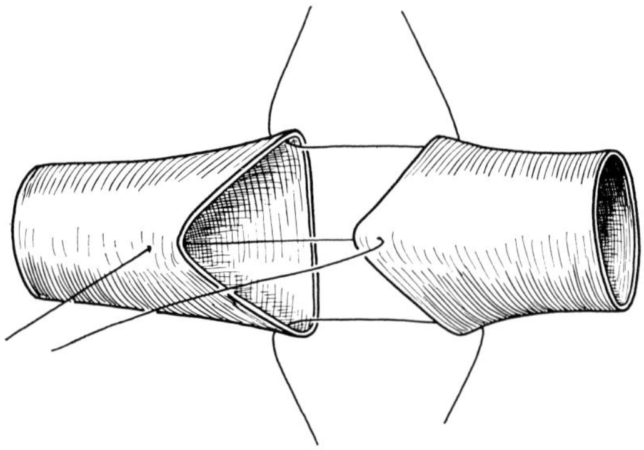

Fig. 2.4. Tripartite suture of Carrel. It facilitates suturing and permits greater precision.

For vessels of small caliber, oblique interrupted sutures help prevent stenosis by scarring (Dobrowolskaia, 1912; Kunlin, 1953a; Sauvage and Wesolowski, 1955). Mistakes can also be avoided by using a loupe or operating microscope.

Microsurgery

Jacobson and Suarez (1960) were the first to use an ocular microscope with a six- to forty-fold magnification. It is advisable to use special clamps with firm support in order to immobilize the field of vision and the margins of the sutures. Very fine instruments, as used by ophthalmologists, or specially constructed ones are required. A pneumatic needle holder with pedal control was devised by Salmon and Assimacopoulos (1965), for exclusion of unavoidable movements of the hand with the usual needle holders.

The requirement of the finest suture material stimulated production of special needles and sutures.

In 1950 I applied two arteriovenous fistulas with stainless steel wire of 0.1 mm diameter, whose oblique end, obtained by scissoring, served as the needle. In both cases the anastomosis burst. The artery tore because the extremely smooth steel wire does not stick and severs the vessel during pulsation. However, steel wire has proved useful with veins (Eadie and DeTakats, 1966).

Recently, very fine needles of stainless steel (Acland, 1971) or quartz (Bunke, 1967) were designed for suturing vessels with a diameter of 0.8 to 1 mm. The smallest diameter is 0.075 mm. The suture is a monofil with a diameter of 0.025 to 0.012 mm. Because of the difficulty of inserting it, attempts were made to produce needles with a diameter of 0.7 mm from the end of the suture (nylon with a diameter of 0.017 mm), onto which metal was applied by a physicochemical process (Bunke, 1967).

In order to save time (which is important in some cases), Bunke (1967) soldered the nylon filament with a heated forceps instead of knotting it.

Vogelfanger and Beattie (1967) reduced the size of their stapler and achieved a high rate of success with arteries and veins with a diameter of 1 to 2 mm.

Nevertheless, the results are slightly worse than those obtained by hand and a surgical microscope, for Jacobson and Katsumura (1965) were successful with all their venous autografts with a diameter between 1 and 1.8 mm. In order to diminish the time of suturing, they spread the stitches far apart in certain cases and glued the gaps together (see vessel adhesives, p. 44). But in these cases, the suture line has to stretch during application of the glue so that the vessel takes on normal shape after removal of the clamps.

Stenosis is a risk without this precautionary measure.

Technical Details

Anastomosis with a Vitallium tube, which actually is a slight modification of an ancient method (Abbe, 1894; Payr, 1904), was tried by Blakemore and Lord (1945), using new material, but it does not yield satisfactory long-term results. Nonoxidizable tubes were used by Kunlin (1952), Carter (1962) and Arnulf (1965). They are split so that they can later be removed, which is recommended. But reoperation is always risky and should be avoided.

Suspension of the suture was proposed. At first the sutures were suspended from the most resistant tissues close to the anastomosis, in order to counter cicatrization and resulting stenosis (Jensen, 1903; Kunlin, 1953). Later they were anchored to a Vitallium ring. Enerson (1957) used a nylon ring; Lewis (1958), a Teflon one (Figs. 2.5 and 2.6). Baumann (1973) surrounded the suture with plastic netting.

The disadvantage of rings is that they may tilt and compress the vein. This raises the risk of thrombosis. Hence we designed rings that cannot tilt. Connected rings (for transplantation) were not satisfactory, because the whole was too rigid. Best results were obtained with simple rings with a stabilizing flange that lies on the vessel and is fastened to the venous wall (Fig. 2.7).

It is important to select a ring that is scarcely larger than or the same size as the vein. The ring must be notched so that the sutures cannot slip.

McLean et al. (1959) inserted 0.5 cm rings made of Lucite into an Ivalon prosthesis. Mitsuoka and Howard (1968) used the same idea (Fig. 2.8), as did also Ohara and Kijima (1973), and Leshnower (1974).

The rings of Donetzki (1958) are provided with hooklets by which the vessel ends are suspended (Fig. 2.9).

Selker and Carney (1967) applied rings similar to Donetzki's to small arteries (caliber 1.5 to 2 mm) by means of a loupe.

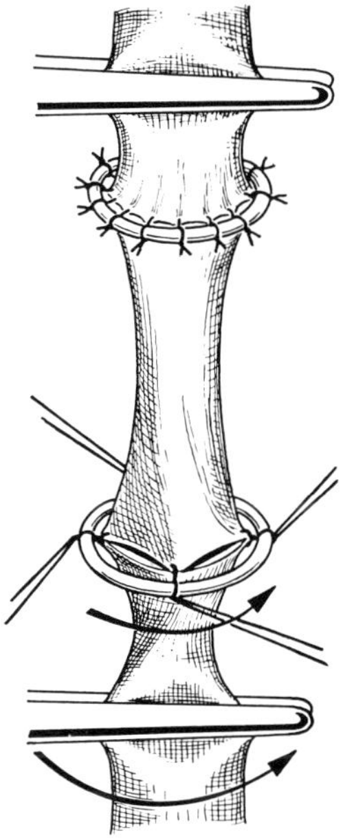

Fig. 2.6. Technique of ring suspension used by Kunlin. The surface of the rings is provided with flanges so that the rings do not slide. The grooves are not shown. (From Kunlin, J.: J. Chir. (Paris) 85 (1963) 305.)

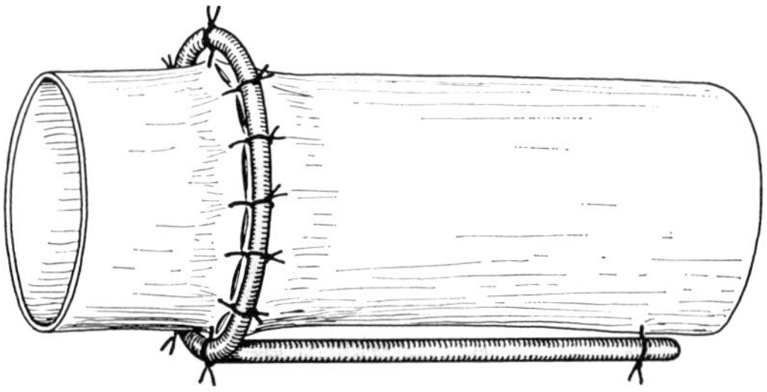

Fig. 2.7. Pedicled ring for stabilization. The pedicle is fastened to the vessel wall.

Mechanical sutures were devised in order to shorten the time of suturing; they avoid the anastomotic narrowing at the same time.

Nakayama (1962) uses two flattened rings of stainless steel. They are provided with small tips on which the upturned edges of the vessel are pierced. The rings are adapted by special forceps, the tips fitting into the intervening holes; the

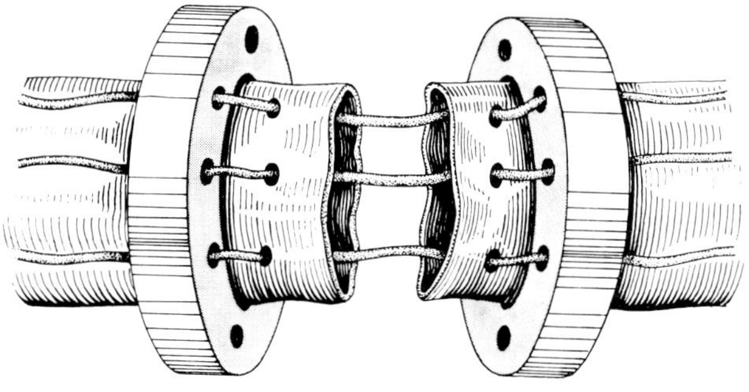

Fig. 2.5. Suspension of the suture by Jensen's method.

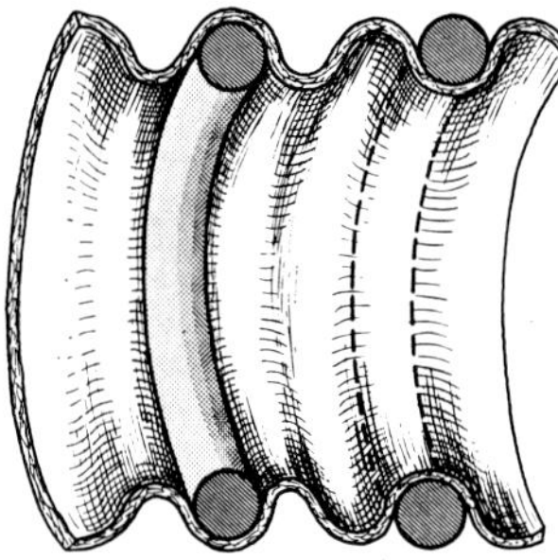

Fig. 2.8. Prosthesis with inner or outer plastic rings.

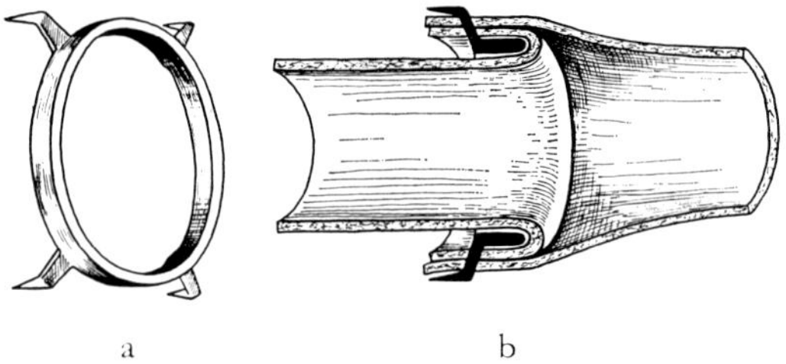

Fig. 2.9. Donetzki ring (*a*) and section through an anastomosis with a Donetzki ring (*b*). (From Kunlin, J.: J. Chir. (Paris) 85 (1963) 305.)

ends are turned back, so that the rings are fixed to one another (Fig. 2.10).

The rings of Marchal et al. (1967) follow Nakayama's design and are suitable for large-caliber veins, as for example the vena cava. These authors join the rings with a glue of gelatin, resorcinol and formaldehyde.

Clamping permits rapid anastomosis and, because the clips are semirigid, causes slight stretching. Gudov (1950) and Androsov (1956) were the first to use tantalum clips for angiorrhaphy. This method had already been employed by Petz 40 years ago for suturing large organs such as the stomach and intestines. Other clip suturing instruments were developed in Hungary, Canada, Japan and the United States. The appliance of Takaro (1960) permits anastomosis of prostheses. These clips appear to be the best mechanical aid known today; they do not tilt as rings can do, which then compress the vessel and produce stenosis and thrombosis of the anastomosis. Inokuchi et al. (1974) also used the mechanical suturing apparatus for lateral anastomoses.

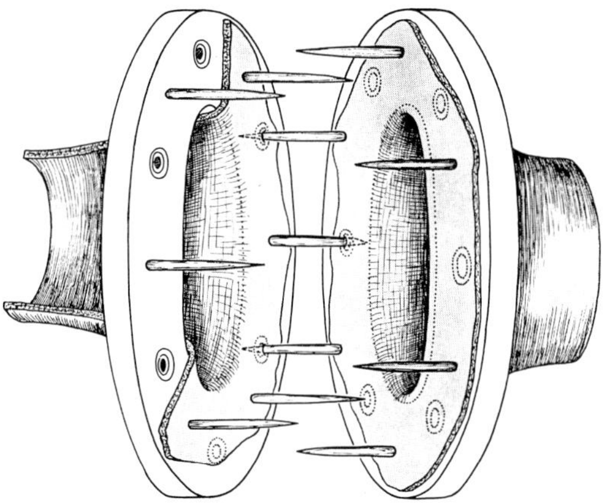

Fig. 2.10. Nakayama's rings.

Vessel Adhesives

The method of gluing vessels was first used by Healy (1952), but it needs to be perfected. At present, a stay has to be introduced into the vessel lumen and must be removed by an incision after a few minutes. It is very important to prevent the adhesive from entering the interior because of the risk of thrombosis.

Several reports have been published on joining of vessels by gluing; using methyl-acrylate and ethyl-, butyl- or propylcyanoacrylate (Carton, 1960; Buda, personal communication, 1965; Healy, 1967; Bauchhenns, 1968). Intraparietal calcifications developed in a few cases when butyl acrylate was used (Souther, 1971). Adhesives available today still produce marked reactive inflammation that culminates in distinct sclerosis. This procedure has to be improved for clinical use.

The search continues for the ideal adhesive, which should have the following properties, according to Healy:

— The adhesive should also permit arterial anastomoses that can withstand a pressure of 30 cm Hg.
— The inflammatory reaction should not be greater than that of silk sutures.
— The substance should have optimal viscosity to permit use of small quantities that will not enter the vessel lumen.
— The time needed for gluing should be neither too long nor too short; the optimum would be 30 seconds, with elimination of the substance within a few months.

Electrocoagulation

Heat produced by an alternating current creates strictly localized coagulation of the cut margins, which are seized by a special electrode forceps (Sigel and Acevado, 1962). The electric impulse is automatically released for a very restricted, previously determined period and applied with optimal strength to the tissue to be coagulated.

Joining of the cut edges is relatively assured and the method is certainly faster than manual suturing. The authors do not give details but histologic sections referred to in their publication make it appear that the method is suitable for veins.
Under certain conditions a *laser beam* can coagulate tissues and sever them. Strully et al. (1967) used it for lateral arteriovenous anastomoses, without clamping and in combination with adhesives. Will this method be suitable for venovenous anastomosis? Apparently no report is available so far.

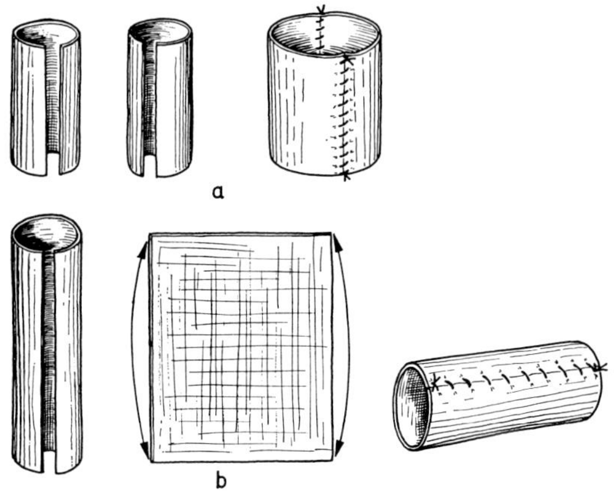

Fig. 2.11. Means of enlarging a venous graft. (*a*) The diameter can be doubled, tripled, or enlarged as a "composite graft" as desired (suggested by Jeger, Lexer and Henle and developed by Deterling and Bhonslay). (*b*) The diameter is enlarged as desired but the length remains limited to three times the initial diameter (after Muren et al.). (From Kunlin, J.: J. Chir. (Paris) 85 (1963) 305.)

Substitutes for Veins

Organic Grafts

Fresh venous autografts. The simplest procedure is *reposition.* The venous segment, which must be completely disconnected from its surroundings, is resected between two clamps, repositioned and, after turning in some cases, sutured.
Frequently, the jugular or femoral vein is replaced by the contralateral vein, in whose place it is grafted during the same procedure.
If a large-caliber vein like the cava is to be replaced and a graft of the same size is required, it must be pieced together, as suggested by Jeger (1913), Lexer and Henle (1913) and developed by Deterling and Bhonslay (1955) (Fig. 2.11), or the maneuver of Muren et al. (1956), called "cross-turned autograft" after Ouchi and Warren (1961), must be used. The latter procedure has the advantage that only one suture line is required but the disadvantage that the length of the graft is limited (Fig. 2.11*b*).
Y-shaped grafts have been devised to replace a bifurcation, as that at the junction of the two renal veins, in the dog by Earle et al. (1960) (Fig. 2.12).
Similarly, two grafts joined like the barrels of a gun, with a common mouth (Kunlin, 1963) (Fig. 2.13) have been used, but the fact that fibrin is easily deposited on the distal spur is a serious drawback.

Grafts of preserved veins. McReynolds (1967) showed in dogs that autoplastic venous segments, conserved under the skin, remain patent and maintain their normal structure. They were successfully substituted for the femoral artery in animals after several weeks. DeWeese (1967) used this method of preservation for arterial surgery in man, but it does not appear to have been used for venoplasty.

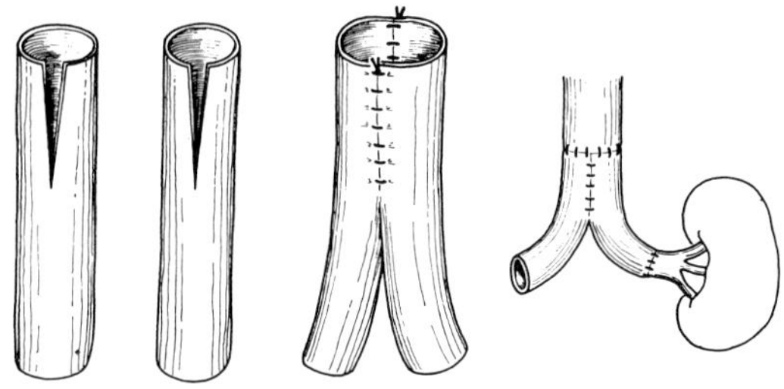

Fig. 2.12. Y-shaped graft. It permits replacement of renal veins. (From Kunlin, J.: J. Chir. (Paris) 85 (1963) 305.)

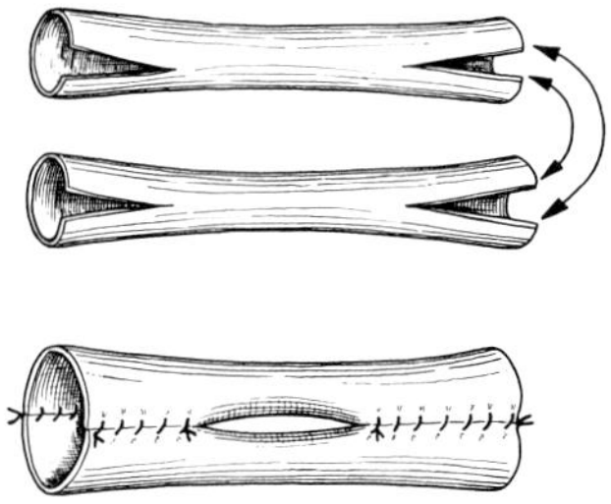

Fig. 2.13. Duplicated graft with common junction. (From Kunlin, J.: J. Chir. (Paris) 85 (1963) 305.)

Fresh arterial autografts. Moore and Riberi (1958) replaced the superior vena cava by the abdominal aorta of the same animal. This in turn was replaced by a homograft during the same operation. The results were excellent.

Fresh or preserved venous homografts. Frequently two surgical teams perform the same operation on two animals simultaneously. Lyophilization, by desiccation with silicic acid, used by Payrau and Pouliquen (1960) for preserving corneas, has been successfully undertaken by us (in two cases), and by Smith et al. (1975).

Although venous homografts have only a very weak antigenic effect after 4 months (Schwartz et al., 1967), it is safer to employ an autograft (see p. 45).

Arterial homografts. After preservation by deep-freezing, arterial homografts are frequently being used. Southwick (1950) was the first to report experience with them.

Arterial heterografts. Bovine aorta preserved in alcohol was used by Moore et al. (1960); the aorta of a stillborn calf was used by Epfelbaum and Dimaria (1965). Collagen tubes prepared with bovine (Rosenberg et al. 1966, 1970, Dale et al. 1969) or pig arteries were transplanted by Fujiwara et al. (1974).

Organic autoplastic tubes. Pedicled tubes for the right atrium have been joined to the superior vena cava (Moore and Yong, 1964). Others, made from portions of the inferior vena cava, have been employed for replacement of the renal vein (Gillot et al., 1967). It should be noted that these are not grafts but transpositions like the experimental azygos vein shunts made by Gerbode et al. (1949) for superior vena caval occlusion.

Tubes made of pericardium (Jones et al., 1958; Riberi and Moore, 1958) or peritoneum (Collins et al., 1960) have been grafted onto the superior and inferior vena cava but have always failed, except with a-v fistula (Baumann, 1972).

Padula et al. (1969) grafted organic autologous tubes that had previously developed around an implanted Silastic cylinder to the superior vena cava with 80 per cent success, and to the inferior vena cava with good results in 50 per cent of the cases. However, Smith et al. (1975) had only 14 per cent success on the inferior vena cava with that material.

We had formerly grafted such synthetic vessels to the femoral artery of dogs (Kunlin, 1953). In conjunction with Testart, we attempted to graft the human great saphenous vein, after pre-implantation as substitute, to the veins of the animal (p. 47). Even homoplastic trachea has been employed on the venae cavae by Todd et al. (1963) with astonishing results.

Surprisingly, the small intestine, completely separated from its mesenteric insertion, yielded excellent results as a graft (Rothoff and Haering, 1964; Matsumoto et al., 1966) when it was everted like the finger of a glove and after its mucosa, and in some cases also the seromuscularis, had been peeled off. Fraser et al. (1968) were successful with such a graft to the superior vena cava in only two of 12 trials. Lawler et al. (1971), also using homologous small intestine, had better results in the superior vena cava; their failures were restricted to the inferior vena cava, sometimes after the graft had been patent for a short time. Rodolico et al. (1967), Vieville (1969) and we (with Testart, 1967), had the same experience on the vena cava inferior. On the same vein Hart et al. (1969) had better results with the pediculate, normally irrigated ileum, but with only three months follow-up.

Vascular Prostheses

The difficulties in storing organic grafts for man, combined with the good results with synthetic prostheses in arterioplasty, stimulated similar experiments with veins. More or less rigid *synthetic tubes* were used initially. Lucite (Daniel, 1952), polyethylene (Witz, 1954), Amylan and silicon (Ohara, 1957) were tested. Later, woven or knitted prostheses of nylon (Deterling, 1955) and Orlon (Sauvage, 1955), and then of Dacron (Collins et al., 1960) and Teflon (Bower, 1960; East, 1960; Sewell, 1960) were tried. Teflon or Dacron is flexible enough that it can be crimped, so that the prosthesis can be deflected without snapping (Fig. 2.14). More recently, woven elastic silicon prostheses (Ashton, 1969), silastic-

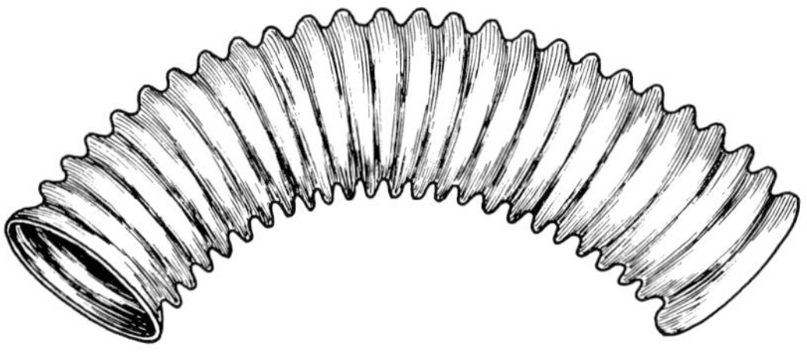

Fig. 2.14. Flexible vascular prosthesis.

Teflon (Anlyan, 1964) and silicon-Dacron prostheses (McCaughan, 1969) have been used.

Ivalon, an elastic, spongy, plastic material produced in boiling water, unfortunately had to be abandoned since it caused marked reactions and was subject to changes.

Metal tubes of magnesium (used by Payr in 1900), aluminum or stainless steel were anastomosed with the vena cava by Sawyer et al. (1965b) during studies on bioelectric properties of the vessel wall and the blood (p. 41). These, as well as the *graphite tubes* of Whiffen and Gott (1965), woven Teflon or Dacron prostheses saturated

with graphite-benzalkonium-heparin (Fraser et al., 1968), TDMAC – Dacron prostheses (Grode 1969, Najjar and Gott, 1970) and newer non-heparinized tubes consisting of electronegative plastic material (Nelsen et al., 1970), are not yet suitable for vascular surgery (p. 42). Preimplanted homoplastic prostheses were also tested (Inokuchi and Ono, 1966). McCann (1967) obtained good results with Dacron or nylon prostheses covered with aluminum powder.
A new prosthesis made with polytetrafluorethylene (Gore-tex) has been tested on the venae cavae superior and inferior, and on the external iliac vein with rather satisfactory results (Soyer et al., 1972; Fujiwara et al., 1974; Smith et al., 1975). We have to wait for long-term rates. Methylmethacrylate copolymerized onto crimped woven Teflon by irradiation was very satisfactory on large veins (Hasegawa et al., 1973). In addition we must mention the thread (Gravens et al., 1973) and the prosthesis rendered bactericidal by impregnation with silver nitrate, both with and without zinc and allantoin (Clark et al., 1974); at present, this has only been tried on arteries. Leshnower et al. (1974) tried a less porous Dacron prosthesis supported by an external polypropylene thread (folded around in the form of a spiral) for superior caval bypass to the right auricle with good results. In the control group done with classic Dacron, all thrombosed.

Patch

The patch is a graft that is not in the shape of a tube. A piece of organic or synthetic tissue is sutured to the edges of the longitudinal incision or the lateral injury of the vessel in order to widen the caliber or seal the wound. Carrel and Guthrie (1906) were the first to use a patch with an autoplastic vein (Fig. 2.15). Homoplastic dura mater was successfully employed by Petropoulos (1963). However, the most surprising results were achieved in the experiments of Csillag et al. (1960), who sewed into the vena cava patches of small intestine, stomach, kidneys, lungs (autologous or homologous), a caoutchouc lamella and even a philodendron leaf and the skin of a plum! Matsumoto et al. (1967) and Dogru et al. (1971) also grafted patches of small intestine. Kunlin and Testart successfully employed in dogs patches of a piece of the autoplastic sheath that had formed around a Silastic cylinder implanted subcutaneously several weeks previously.

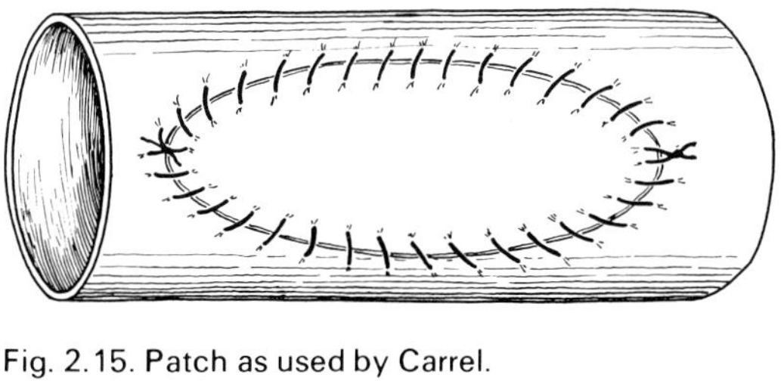

Fig. 2.15. Patch as used by Carrel.

Methods or Aids for Improvement of Grafting Results

Drugs

Antibiotics are frequently given during the first postoperative days. They seem to be especially useful when foreign materials have been used.
Anticoagulants. Most experiments have been performed without anticoagulants. However, some authors used them in comparative series (Zinicola, 1962; Baird et al., 1964; Foster et al., 1965; McLachlin et al., 1965, 1970; Eadie, 1966; Mikhailov, 1969; O'Hara, 1973).
The figures speak for themselves: without anticoagulants—14 successful among 60 cases; with anticoagulants—53 successful among 77 cases. Anticoagulants appear to be necessary for only 1 week, because by all reports, occlusions occurred in a few days in most cases. Nevertheless Hobson et al. (1973) had no better results with heparin or Dextran 40 in canine femoral vein replacement than without. With Dextran 40 on the vena cava inferior inserted prostheses, Todd et al. (1963) obtained no better results; Barnes et al. (1968) found it useful.
With Dextran 75 the permeability rates were improved in femoral vein grafting (Eadie and De Takats, 1966) and in transplanting pericardium tubes on the superior vena cava of dogs (Brais et al., 1973).
With dipyridamole the evolution of Teflon prostheses on the superior vena cava was very satisfactory according to Hasegawa et al. (1973).
Phenylbutazone slowed the secondary stenosis or obliteration of Dacron prostheses on the inferior vena cava (Calvert et al., 1976).
Fibrinolytics were applied in experimental grafting of the femoral or inferior cava vein by Demetz et al. (1961), Baird et al. (1964) and Eadie and De Takats (1966); only the last-named described better results when they were used. The evidence so far appears inadequate to base a conclusion on. Nevertheless it is remarkable that none of the authors reported cases of hemorrhage, which was observed on experimental arterial Dacron grafts until two months after operation (J.-L. Fontaine et al., 1974).
The fibrinolytic properties of snake venom are

being studied (Rahimtoola et al., 1970; Pitney et al., 1971; Ehrly et al., 1973). Postlethwaite et al. (1977) with subcutaneous administration of Arvin (and a Dacron prosthesis on the rabbit inferior vena cava) achieved 7 permeabilities on 11 cases, instead of 100 per cent thrombosis without. The time of postoperative observation seems to be too short (28 days). Nevertheless the use of fibrinolytics appears to be a helpful method. It is remarkable that none of the authors reported cases of hemorrhage. Ligation-induced *hyperpressure* improved the results of suturing the azygos vein on the right auricle in Gerbode's work (1949). This device was also used by Gillot (1973) for long femorocaval grafts.

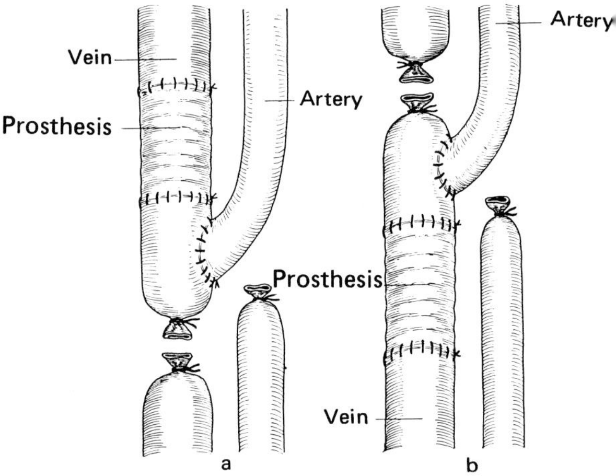

Fig. 2.17. Venous prosthesis with arteriovenous fistula. (*a*) Pressure in the prosthesis 15 cm H_2O; four failures in four cases; (*b*) pressure in prosthesis 50 cm H_2O; three successes in four cases. (After Bryant, Lazenby and Howard.)

Temporary Arteriovenous Fistula

This aid was suggested by Kunlin (1953b) in construction of a venous saphenoiliac bypass on a patient (Fig. 2.16), but unfortunately the fistula could not be established at the time because the femoral artery was thrombosed.

In 1958 we used the method in 2 cases, replacing the canine inferior vena cava and establishing a fistula between the right femoral artery and vein, but it was not successful (Kunlin, 1963). The basic idea was to raise venous pressure in order to prevent stenosis at the suture. In addition, we expected it to provide better nutrition and oxygen supply to the venous graft. The favorable results we achieved with the ring suture drew our attention away from these experiments. Bryant et al. (1958) were successful with implantation of a prosthesis into the femoral vein at the margin of the fistula only when the distal arterial segment had been interrupted. The prosthesis was also placed distally but in immediate proximity (Fig. 2.17). The width of the junction was intentionally restricted to 4 to 6 mm, in order to reduce the effect on the heart. If anastomoses are too narrow, spontaneous occlusion of the fistula is to be expected. It has sometimes happened and is, in this case, a happy occurrence if not too early.

Venous *pressure* is highest distal to the arteriovenous fistula (Fig. 2.18). It drops suddenly to almost zero at the level of the anastomosis, rises slowly to approximately 5 mm Hg after 10 to 15 cm in the direction of the heart, and finally declines to practically zero near the heart. These measurements show that the rise in pressure is moderate (Stansel, 1964; Holt, 1965; Dart, 1966; Dost, 1966; Mitsuoka, 1966; Yamagushi, 1968; Hobson, 1973). Therefore, it is *not* the *rise in pressure*, which is only small, that is operative and important but the striking *increase of the blood flow*.

In the special case of Bryant et al. (1958), who replaced the femoral vein by a prosthesis, the pressure was particularly high, between 50 and 60 cm H_2O, because the fistula lay proximal and, in addition, the femoral artery was ligated distally (Fig. 2.17*b*).

Outflow is raised considerably, three to eight times, depending on the site of the arteriovenous communication (Dean, 1964; Yamagushi, 1968;

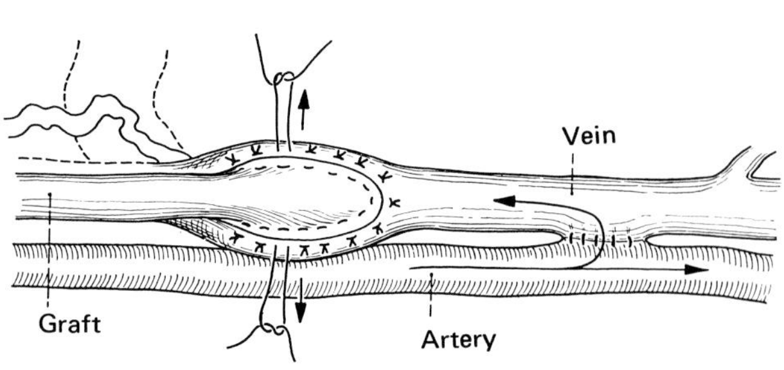

Fig. 2.16. Venous graft with arteriovenous fistula. (From Kunlin, J.: Congr. Soc. Int. Chir. Lisbonne 15 (1953) 875.)

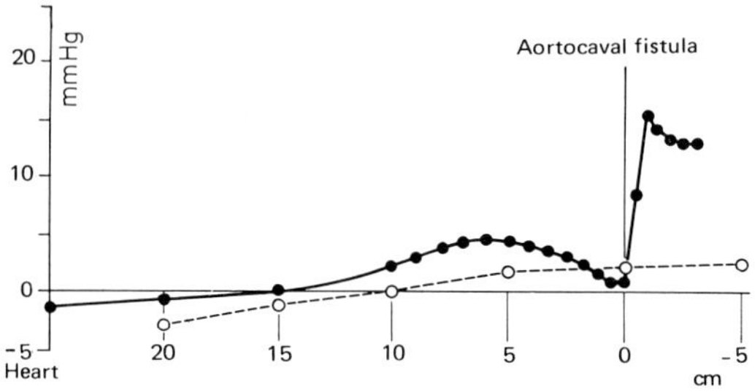

Fig. 2.18. Mean values of venous pressure in the dog. Normal (broken line) and with arteriovenous fistula (solid line). (After Dost.)

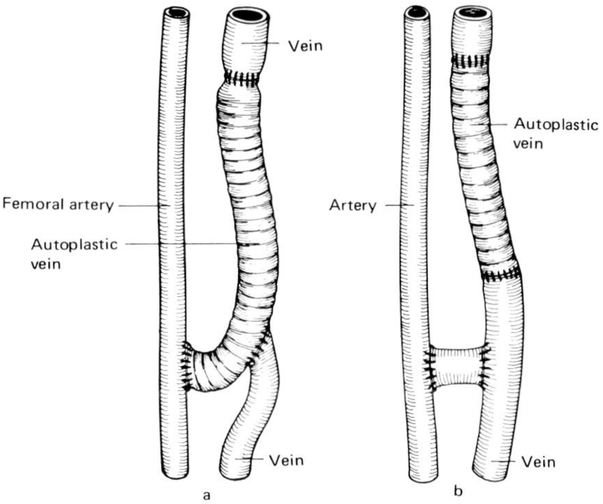

Fig. 2.19. Grafting with a K-shaped arteriovenous fistula (*a*); arteriovenous communication by means of a second autoplastic vein (*b*). (After Johnson and Eiseman.)

Aschberg, 1971; Lewin, 1971; Hobson, 1973) (Table 2.3).

Table 2.3 Venous Pressure and Outflow in the Infrarenal Cava Vein with and without AV Fistula (From Yamagushi, A., S. Eguchi, T. Iwasaki, K. Asano: J. cardiovasc. Surg. 9 (1968) 99)

Fistula	Outflow ($ml/kg\ min^{-1}$)	Pressure behind fistula ($mm\ H_2O$)
Without fistula	7.5	normally 4–8
With AV fistula		
distal aortocaval fistula	58.3	152
proximal aortocaval fistula	12.2	257
femoral fistula	23.4	65

Another sequel is *enlargement* of the vein. The caliber of the jugular vein that has been grafted onto the inferior vena cava in the bypass may be dilated more than two-fold (217 per cent mean, according to Steinmann et al., 1966). The enlargement continues beyond the anastomosis.

The *cardiac load* increases between 25 and 50 per cent (Holt, 1965; Part, 1966; Dost, 1966). As early as 3 weeks later, signs of overloading the heart become apparent on electrocardiography; they disappear with discontinuation of the arteriovenous fistula, however (Mitsuoka, 1966).

Mention should be made of the K-shaped fistula of Johnson and Eiseman (1969). Is it not possible that its unsatisfactory results can be ascribed to too early reoperation (Fig 2.19*a*)?

Johnson's other method (1969), which has also been used by Lewin et al. (1970), appears to be important: *use of a graft in construction of the fistula*. This makes surgical closure of the fistula much easier (Fig. 2.19*b*). Sisteron (personal communication) suggested applying a sufficiently strong delayed suture around this graft which can be tied from without several days later, without another operation. This ligature may also prove useful as guideline for reoperation.

There are various opinions about how long an arteriovenous fistula should function. Most authors claim that 2 weeks is sufficient. But in these cases, the grafts were short, the longest not exceeding 10 cm. With more extensive venous repair, the fistula ought not be discontinued before 2 months. In a patient with the postphlebothrombotic syndrome it was not removed until 4 months afterward (Kunlin, Pajot and Hadjiat, unpublished). Yamagushi et al. (1968) noted some calcification and ossification in the inserted prosthesis after substituting the inferior vena cava by means of an aortocaval fistula. They ascribed this to the extraordinarily great turbulence of the stream.

Sisteron (personal communication) had the idea of applying an arteriovenous fistula at the distal section of an important collateral artery. This procedure would not overload the heart as does the direct arteriovenous communication.

The problem remains whether the retrograde flow from the collateral artery is sufficient to safeguard the success of the transplantation. Experiments of Hadjiat are proceeding at present.

An arteriovenous fistula as a help for the superior vena cava replacement has also been used by Scheinin (1964).

Results of Experimental Venous Plastic Surgery

Hitherto, all experiments have been carried out in dogs. With refinement of technique, more and more experiments will be performed in smaller animals.
Almost all publications deal with *transplantation*, a procedure with more troublesome results than either *transposition* or anastomosis of a *pedicled angioplasty*, which is practically always successful.
In the majority of the experiments, the ends of the graft were connected with the receiving vessel by end-to-end suture. The bypass method was described in reports (Zinicola et al., 1962; Haimovici et al., 1963; Steinman et al., 1966), in which it is noted that the grafted vein retains its small caliber if the receptor vein is not ligated. End-to-side anastomosis on an extremity was employed distally in conjunction with a K-shaped arteriovenous fistula by Johnson and Eiseman (1969) and proximally with long venous transpositions by Gruenagel (1971), Gillot (1973) and Kunlin (p. 53).
The following evaluation of results refers only to experiments done with organic material and flexible, woven or knitted synthetic prostheses. Prostheses of nylon, Orlon and similar materials employed before 1960 were not suitable for venous replacement and have been abandoned.
It is remarkable that veins below the diaphragm are much more difficult to replace successfully than those above it. This is probably due to differences in hemodynamics and venous pressure in these two regions (p. 39). The great mobility of the portal and mesenteric veins of the dog renders the operation on these considerably more complex.
As regards the *technique of anastomosis,* manual suture is by far the most common (this is true also in man). Less frequently used were *rings* with tips or hooklets, "*suspended sutures*" and *mechanical sutures* (clips), although they yielded better results than simple suturing. This could be explained by the fact that tilting of rings that were *too broad* occurred so often. The stapling *suturing appliance* may on occasion be difficult to handle. In any case, application of this technique requires further study.
On insertion of tubes, the difference in success to be considered is that between long tubes (with or without an organic graft being introduced into its lumen) and small tubes used solely to facilitate anastomosis. The former are rigid and practically unusable. The latter are well tolerated but rarely applied.
The more refined the technique, the better the results. The microsurgical procedure is excellent since it reveals all the mistakes that might be overlooked by the naked eye.
The *temporary arteriovenous fistula* applied in addition to venous restoration appears to warrant more and more interest. Indeed, it increases the percentage of success more than do anticoagulants or fibrinolytics, which, as of now, improve it only slightly. Twelve different authors recorded 34 per cent successful results without arteriovenous fistula, but 81 per cent with arteriovenous fistula. The advantages of a fistula become still more obvious when comparisons are made of the results for replacement of the difficult inferior vena cava: only 26 per cent patency with prostheses without a fistula, but 80 per cent good results with arteriovenous union.
The behavior of various substituting materials was compared for all veins, regardless of site, and led to the following conclusions:

—fresh autoplastic material yields best results;
—homoplastic material is less favorable;
—heteroplastic material, rarely used, apparently is not to be recommended because of secondary stenosis and calcifications; and
—synthetic prostheses (poor results if employed on small veins and without addition of special measures) have produced remarkable results in anastomoses of large veins.

More experience is necessary for the definitive evaluation of the new Gore-tex prosthesis.
Trachea or bowel with peritoneum or pericardium constructed tubes are hardly commendable in spite of some interesting results. The use of artificial fibrous tubes developed around plastic seems to be premature.
The periods of observation varied greatly. For autoplastic material 2 to 3 months appears to suffice. Homoplastic and alloplastic material may cause stenosis or thrombosis even after several months. The experiments ought to be surveyed for 6 to 8 months before being classed as successful. Because of the frequency of recanalization following thrombosis, patency of venous grafts can be graded as successful only if several phlebograms have confirmed it to be lasting (Dale, 1961).
To sum up one can say that it is easier to successfully replace a large vein than to replace a small vein; a short segment, rather than a long one. The vena cava inferior is the least favorable of all. The results, however, are getting progressively better on all veins because of improved substitutes, finer techniques and additional methods (anticoagulation, av fistula).

Replacement of the Jugular and Femoral Veins*

Autografts

Manual suture: 63 per cent success for the jugular, 53 per cent for the femoral.
Microsurgery is 100 per cent successful, even on the small-caliber saphenous vein of the dog.
Insertion of tube: Owing to insufficient reported data, the results cannot be stated with certainty but only estimated at 70 per cent successful.
Ring anastomosis: 80 per cent patency.
Mechanical suture: 90 per cent patent.
Manual suture with arteriovenous fistula: 90 per cent patent.

Homografts

Venous homografts have rarely been tried on jugular or femoral veins, and only with manual suture. The results are worse by 20 per cent than those with autoplastic veins.

Prostheses

Almost all attempts with prostheses in the femoral vein foundered, even when arteriovenous fistula was used. There is one exception: three of four operations were successful when the fistula lay proximal and the vein was ligated across it (Bryant et al., 1958).

Replacement of the Superior Vena Cava

It should be emphasized that *ligation of the azygos* somewhat assists the course of grafting at the superior vena cava. Anastomosis to the atrium must be avoided to prevent secondary stenosis.

Autografts

Manual suture yielded about 40 per cent success with venous autografts. When the aorta was used to replace the superior vena cava, it remained patent in 100 per cent of cases.
Ring suture, *mechanical suture* and *arteriovenous fistula* between the carotid and jugular have only rarely been applied and cannot be accurately assessed. Results were improved, however.

Pedicled tubes from the atrium yielded good results; they are shorter than the other grafts, however.
The use of *autoplastic tubes* from pericardium or the aponeurosis of the rectus abdominis muscle resulted in failure.
Good results with *small intestine* were reported only once. Other authors report almost universal failure, as we found (experiments in conjunction with Testart).
The question whether fibrinolytic activity of the submucosa and seromuscularis exists was answered in the negative by evidence of experiments by Didon (Hôpital Foch, Paris-Suresnes).

Homografts

Venous homografts were successful in approximately 35 per cent with manual suture.
Preserved homoplastic aorta yielded no better results than the veins.
Todd (1963) reported seven successes with the *trachea* among 11 trials.
Ring anastomosis ("suspended suture"): Results are improved but only a small number of operations using this technique have been performed (two of ours were patent, with 50 per cent localized stenosis).

Heterografts

Manual suture: use of *alcohol-preserved bovine aorta* yielded nine patent vessels among 11 trials. In two cases, observed for 3 years, there was shrinkage and calcification (Moore, 1964).

Prostheses (only Dacron or Teflon)

Manual suture: Teflon was successful in approximately 60 per cent of cases, but Dacron in only 35 per cent. These figures were somewhat improved by use of *more rigid prostheses* or those *provided with rings*.
No report is available on *ring suture* or *mechanical suture*.
The success rate rose to around 85 per cent when *arteriovenous fistula* was used together with a prosthesis.
Because of insufficient experience, no final evaluation can be made on results with the recent graphite-benzalkonium-heparin-impregnated or TDMAC-heparin-Dacron prostheses, despite their promise.

*Statements made in 1968

Replacement of the Inferior Vena Cava

It should be mentioned first that replacement of the thoracic inferior vena cava yielded much better results than that of the abdominal inferior vena cava. In this respect, the former may be compared with the superior vena cava.

Autografts

Approximately 30 per cent of operations with fresh *venous material* and *manual suture* were successful.
Use of *autoplastic aorta* as graft yielded no more gratifying results than the vein, but this material was used by only one author.
Ring suture and *arteriovenous fistula* produced results twice as good (only one publication).
Successful application of *small intestine* (manual suture) was described in only one publication; others have reported poor results. Tubes of *peritoneum* or *pericardium* also were failures.

Homografts

Venous grafts, as well as fresh or preserved *aorta*, yielded few satisfactory results (between 20 and 25 per cent).
Results were better with *mechanical suture* or use of *rings* (only one publication). We were successful with the "*suspended suture*" (at the superior vena cava) twice in two attempts (see above), but Vieville succeeded only once in 12 trials.
Use of *arteriovenous fistula* and manual suture considerably enhances success (up to around 50 per cent).

Heterografts

Three publications are available describing use of vein, aorta and synthetic material prepared with bovine collagen (Breslau, 1965), but all yielded poor results.
Prostheses inserted following preimplantation were likewise unsuccessful (Inokushi, 1966).

Prostheses

Manual suture: Results of implantation of prostheses with manual suture are poor: the success rate with Teflon was a little better than that with Dacron, 10 per cent.
Prostheses with rings had roughly 30 per cent better chances.
Use of recent woven, *elastic, silicon prostheses* was successful in 50 per cent of cases (Ashton, 1969).
Mechanical suture: Results were better than with manual suture.
Use of *arteriovenous fistula along with manual suture* was followed by 80 per cent success. Better results are apparently obtained with the suprarenal abdominal vena cava than with the infrarenal vena cava (Najafi, 1967).
Prostheses prepared by homoplastic preimplantation were successful in only 45 per cent of cases (Inokushi, 1966).

Vena Cava–Atrial Bypass

Sewell (1960) reported good results with Teflon in animals.

Replacement of Renal Veins

Replacement of renal veins by autologous veins was successful 25 to 50 per cent of the time.

Replacement of the Portal and Superior Mesenteric veins

With *autologous* veins the success rate was 50 per cent; with *homologous* vessels or *prostheses*, 25 to 30 per cent (Daniel, 1952; Egdahl, 1956; Foster, 1965; Wimberley, 1968).
In six of our experiments with "suspended suture" we recorded only one success owing to 29°C hypothermia. The remaining five animals died of mesenteric infarction. One single vein was thrombosed. We ascribe these failures to inadequate hypothermia (31° to 36.5°C), apart from two technical errors (Kunlin and Lengua, unpublished).

Portacaval or Mesentericocaval Bypass Operation

Manual suture: *Autoplastic* material yielded good results in approximately 50 per cent of cases, as did "suspended suture".
With *mechanical suture* the results were better.
Homoplastic replacement vessels yielded good results in only 30 per cent of cases.

Portal Vein–Right Atrial Shunt

Patency remained satisfactory in 20 per cent of cases, with autoplastic veins. Gillot (1966) was successful in one case in which he used the *gallbladder in situ* as a graft.

Splenopulmonary Shunt

Gruenagel (1971) achieved good patency with "suspended suture" only when the graft was protected from interfering diaphragmatic contractions by a synthetic tube.

Patch

Success is easily obtained with small grafts, regardless of whether the material is autoplastic, homoplastic or alloplastic (see p. 47).

Long Venous Grafts

Most experiments have been carried out with short venous segments 2 to 5 cm long. Use of grafts of more than 10 cm long was described in one report (95 per cent successful) (Cerino et al., 1964).
We performed 14 venous graft procedures with material of 10 to 22.5 cm length between 1960 and 1963.

Long Autografts of the Jugular Vein

Manual ring suture. The results of reposition of nine jugular veins of dogs with an average length of 12.8 cm (between 10 and 18 cm) with "suspended suture" were (average time of observation, $3\frac{1}{2}$ months): total occlusion in one; severe stenosis (due to tilting of rings) in two; in one, limited obliteration in the distal third, but patency preserved in the proximal two thirds thanks to *formation of new collaterals* which flowed into the graft; and five patent grafts.
The results were less favorable than those we obtained by using shorter grafts of the jugular (average length 6 cm): in 25 cases, 22 patent vessels (88 per cent), after an average time of observation of roughly 9 months.
Mainly technical complications were responsible for the less favorable results with our long jugular grafts.

Extremely Long Grafts

We attempted 1964 to insert still longer venous grafts in relatively small dogs:

(1) Removal, followed by reposition of the jugular vein–brachiocephalic vein–superior vena cava. One animal died of shock at the end of the operation under these difficult conditions.
(2) Removal of both jugular veins, which were sutured end to end in order to obtain a long graft. Distally, the suture was applied near the origin of the jugular vein. Proximally, the anastomosis lay near the right atrium or at the end of the vena cava superior with suspended suture (Fig. 2.20).

With *anastomosis at the atrium* in three cases, with grafts 18 to 22.5 cm long, the results were: one death the following day, with the vessel patent and evidence of hemothorax; stenosis of the anastomosis at the atrium after a month in one animal; and in the remaining one, graft patent when checked phlebographically after 1 month, but already stenosis at the proximal anastomosis and neocollaterals at the graft. On removal after 8 months, the graft was still patent but showed marked stenosis in its proximal portion.
This insufficient series was complemented by further experiments during 1969 and 1970.
Anastomosis at the juxtacardial portion of the superior vena cava (Kunlin, Padovani, Testart and Alberti, unpublished) was done in 18 dogs. Graft length was 22.5 to 30 cm (average 26 cm), and graft diameter, 6 to 8 mm. Manual suture was used; the material was Tevdek or Monofil 6–0 or 7–0. No heparin was given. Antibiotics were administered for 4 days.
"Suspended suture" was used in only three dogs. The graft was pulled through paravertebrally in the depth of the field, parallel to esophagus, in order to avoid the dangerous zones of lower neck and upper thorax.
Distally, end-to-end anastomosis was made with the origin of the jugular vein, and lower, side-to-end anastomosis to the superior vena cava (in two cases end-to-end to the azygos vein); continuous suture without rings was used (except in three cases).
Of 18 dogs, two died after 1 week, one dog with infection and thrombosis, the other with pneumothorax following phlebography and patent graft. Of the 16 survivors, three had thromboses after 3 to 4 weeks (one with infection); — in one the graft was partly patent after 1 month, but obliterated after 11 months; and in 12 the results were excellent after 2 to 22 months (average 11 months). Phlebograms were taken repeatedly.
On removal of the graft, the lower anastomosis was infrequently slightly narrowed by a small, sickle-shaped fold at the distal side, formed as usual and produced by the stream of the two confluent veins. Neither the cava above the anastomosis nor the azygos was ligated during operation.
Small collaterals at the graft were visible at autopsy but not in the phlebogram.
These long grafts yielded the same good results as the short ones. No recanalization was observed.

Histologic findings (Audebraud, Hôpital Foch, Paris-Suresnes): Slightly thickened venous wall. There was commonly a more or less distinct dissociation of the elastic architecture. Some pictures revealed the presence of new collaterals.

In 1975/1976 we performed autoplastic jugular grafts (dogs, average weight: 16.5 kg, length of graft: 12.5 cm) between the canine superficial femoral vein and the iliac vein or the inferior vena cava (in two cases with double jugular vein; 20 cm length). The transplant was passed under the completely transected iliopubic ligament. The distal anastomosis was terminoterminal, the proximal was terminolateral. Simple continuous suture with plastic monofilament 7–0. No anticoagulation.

Results 13 cases: 1 death; 1 immediate thrombosis, technical fault probable; 11 excellent permeabilities after 2 to 7 months.

Gillot (1973) made the longest experimental grafts (40 to 45 cm) on big dogs (35 to 45 kg). He used both the jugular and the right femoral veins. Distal lateral anastomosis on the left femoral vein, proximal connection end-to-side of the suprarenal abdominal vena cava. In addition a distal arteriovenous fistula was established and an incomplete ligature was placed on the femoral vein above the distal anastomoses with the purpose of producing a certain amount of hyperpressure. Ten cases: 2 deaths (hemorrhage), 1 rupture, 7 permeabilities after 3 to 5 months.

Fate of Grafts after Transplantation

During the first experiments we were perplexed by the great number of failures of venous grafting. For lack of thinner thread, we used 3.0 or 4.0 silk. All our grafts of the inferior vena cava became obliterated, and there were stenoses in the grafts of the jugular vein. One success with

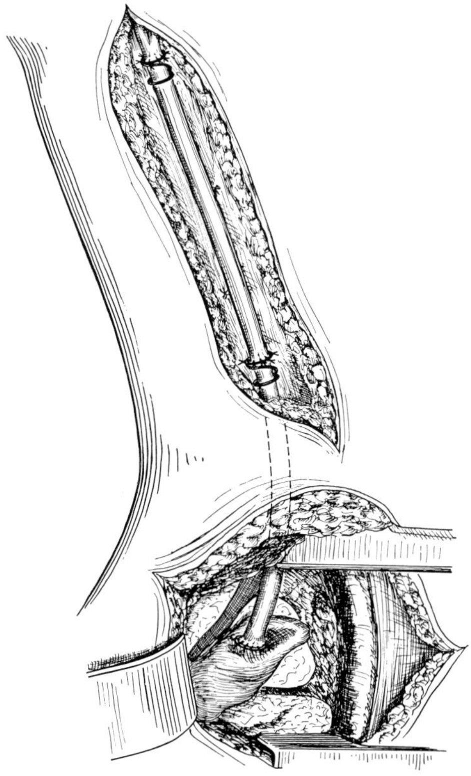

a

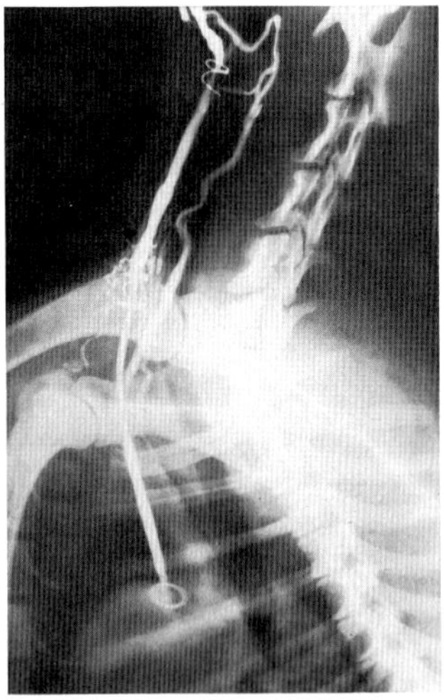

b

Fig. 2.20. Long graft (22.5 cm). Special spiral rings that cannot tilt (*a*) were tried. No longer used, they were later replaced by another model (see Fig. 2.7). Note the newly formed collaterals around the ring in the center of the phlebogram (*b*).

the femoral vein was perhaps due only to narrowing of the iliac vein, resulting in some degree of venous hypertension (Kunlin, 1963).

Study of the failures showed that massive thrombosis was rare, and only when grave technical errors were evident. The *main cause* was *progressive stenosis of the suture line*. After a suture is applied, fibrin is deposited in increasing amounts at the site of union of the vessels. The clots initially touch because of variations in pressure and rhythmic movements of the venous wall, and later are joined together by fibrin strands of varying thickness. At times, the clots remain stationary, or small elongated clots float in the bloodstream. A network of bridges and strands of highly variable thickness and formation is produced by partial fibrinolysis. As soon as this process has commenced, cicatrization of the suture sets in, causing stenosis and a constant threat to patency. These formations easily create fresh local thromboses. In animals that have died of disease or surgery, small fresh clots are found in these strands although the suturing was done several months before. Thus the anastomoses slowly become subject to a vicious circle. Stenosis forms step by step, terminating in obliteration (Fig. 2.21).

After some time, the graft suffers the fate of the anastomosis. The wall is thickened by fibrin deposits, and the lumen becomes increasingly narrower. Nevertheless, the vessel remains patent as long as the anastomosis remains patent and is obliterated only after total closure of the anastomosis. Occasionally the walls collapse and grow together. From time to time, the grafts are shortened to as little as 30 per cent of their original length.

If there is no interference, the anastomoses remain wide, without constricting strands. The wall of the graft remains soft, thin and transparent, its structure unchanged. The endothelium is partly preserved, partly regenerated. In the media and adventitia, slight fibrosis is witness of a transient inflammatory reaction. Muscle fibers have frequently disappeared. If valves are preserved, they show normal histologic structure.

The almost unavoidable fate of the graft—namely, obliteration due to progressive stenosis—caused many surgeons to search for means of preventing these complications, either by circular suspension or by creation of venous hypertension, especially by means of an arteriovenous fistula.

Refinement of the suturing technique and use of especially fine suturing material considerably improved results of grafting, so that progressive stenosis became much rarer. Knowledge of the mechanism of formation of the strands and bridges is nevertheless very instructive, since it provides understanding of the origin of the constrictions and occluding membranes frequently seen in human veins, even without trauma or surgical intervention.

The *organization of prostheses* of Dacron or Teflon in veins is comparable in every respect with prostheses that have successfully been applied in arteries. Fibrin deposits on the inner surface are thicker with Dacron than with Teflon. If the

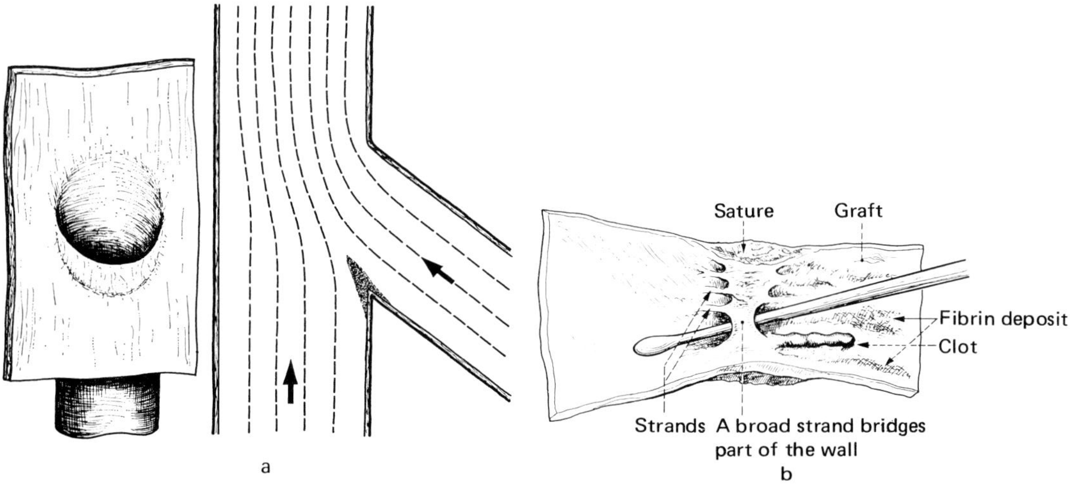

Fig. 2.21. Progressive stenosis of a venous anastomosis. (*a*) Diagram of a termino-lateral; (*b*) vessel opened, site of suture of a termino-terminal. (From Kunlin, J.: J. Chir. (Paris) 85 (1963) 305.)

prosthesis is to be removed a few weeks later, it will be found to have firmly grown to its surroundings, more so with Dacron than with Teflon. The neointima on Teflon is thinner. It consists of a layer of acellular, dense connective tissue covered with endothelium. The external surface consists of a fibrous adventitia with a few vessels. Reaction by macrophages around the plastic filaments is constant. The ideal prosthesis that does not cause a reaction has yet to be invented. Satisfactory organization of the wall of the prosthesis and a well formed neointima are by no means always found.

It is noteworthy that Mikhailov et al. (1969) described nerve fibers in the outer shell of prostheses after 1 month and even in the neointima after 3 months.

Rheosensitivity

The caliber of a transplanted vein, at least an autoplastic one, adapts itself to local conditions of flow. The process is the same as that seen daily in collateral arteries. If more blood flows through them, they enlarge. When the stream slows, the opposite occurs. Rheosensitivity is a peculiar phenomenon, surely independent of blood pressure and probably also of general nervous and hormonal influence. The main or sole factor that triggers the structural changes is the degree of the flow in the vessel. Dilatation or reduction is due to active cell synthesis or decay, the development of which appears to depend on as yet unknown local conditions.

Grafting of Venous Valves

DeWeese and Niguidula (1960) reported a series of 20 femoral autografts. The anastomoses were applied obliquely, and very fine suture material was used. Eleven of the grafts were patent, and the valves were competent in nine.

Grafting valve-containing venous segments was performed by seven teams (DeWeese and Niguidula, 1960; Kunlin et al., 1963, 1966; Cerino et al., 1964; Devin et al., 1964; Waddell et al., 1964, 1967; McLachlin et al., 1965; Aschberg et al., 1971 [with a-v fistula]. (Fig. 2.22).

Points of Importance

Heparinization for 2 days is followed by distinctly better results.

Grafting of autoplastic valved venous segments of 2 to 3 cm in length yielded good results in approximately 75 per cent of cases. Our own experience with *long jugular veins* (which occasionally contain two valves and average 9.7 cm in length), when grafted without special measures, showed less favorable results (success rate around 50 per cent).

It is very important to test valvular function at the end of the operation. We were surprised to note occasionally that valves in dogs were wholly or partially insufficient although no pathologic process was demonstrable. In tests of function of valves in the jugular vein during nine operations, the valves were competent in only four, were partially competent in four and totally incompetent in one.

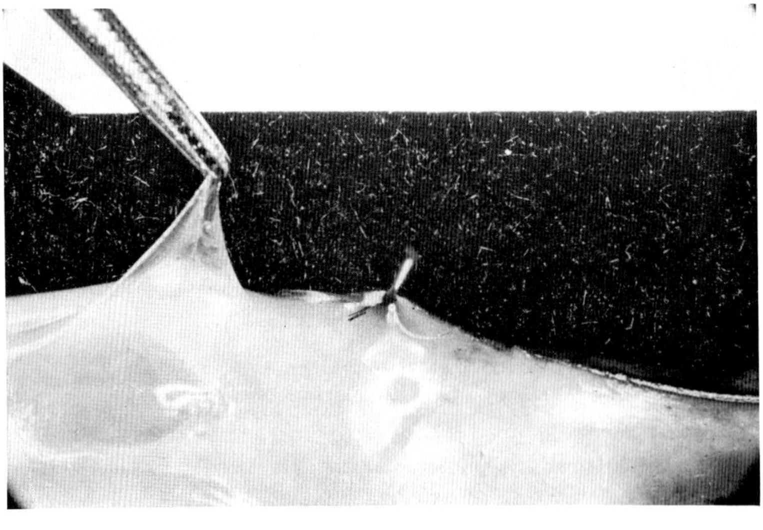

Fig. 2.22. Normal picture of a grafted autoplastic valve.

Recanalization of valvulate veins following thrombosis is associated with damage to the valves.

Homoplastic grafting of valves produced less favorable results. Of 34 homografts of valved femoral veins, ten remained patent during the short period of observation of 2 to 3 weeks, and competent valves were found only twice (Waddell et al., 1964).

Preservation of functional valves following thrombosis is probably difficult (as it is in nongrafted veins): after squeezing out the thrombosis produced by an electric current 2 days previously in the superficial femoral vein of a dog, valvular function was restored only exceptionally (McLachlin, et al., 1970). It has been stated that "preservation of valves in the presence of thrombosis is successful only through early fibrinolysis." It is possible to achieve this in man in some cases but not yet with certainty. No report on this specific problem in animals is known to us.

Recanalization of Thrombosed Veins

Recanalization of thrombosed veins in man has long since been described by pathologists. Modern methods of investigation have shown that this is practically a constant phenomenon. Linton and Hardy (1948) demonstrated recanalization of the thrombosed femoral vein of man in all 84 cases. Olivier (1949) observed recanalization in 36 of 40 ancient thromboses.

May (1967) took phlebograms of 100 veins, 1 year after thrombosis, in patients to whom no anticoagulants had been given. He found 10 per cent total occlusion, 70 per cent incomplete recanalization and 20 per cent full recanalization. Treatment with anticoagulants, especially long-term administration, enhances results.

Recanalization has also been observed in arteries but very rarely.

Unfortunately, recanalization of a thrombosed vein is practically never accompanied by restoration of valvular function. The valves remain adherent, retracted and incompetent (Beneke, 1890; Homans, 1916; Edwards and Edwards, 1935).

Several studies by systematic and repeated phlebography showed that numerous vein grafts thrombosed but became patent after some time. This occurred so frequently (Dale, 1961) that the question arises whether a considerable proportion of apparently successful grafts are simply recanalized. Can this really be called successful grafting? It is doubtful.

There are considerable differences in structure between a recanalized vein and a vein that has always been patent according to DeWeese and Niguidula (1960) and Waddell et al. (1967). Logically, therefore, the success of grafting is not as brilliant as statistics suggest, since the final figures naturally include the recanalized cases.

Experiments explaining the processes of recanalization. Venous ligature is almost always followed by shunting via collaterals. Every surgeon has experienced this when ligating varices. These collateral veins did not exist prior to ligation. Their considerable diameter soon destroys the favorable effect of the ligature. Streuter and Paine (1953) noted that the inferior vena cava of dogs was recanalized within 6 weeks, on average, depending on the strength of catgut used.

Miles and Young (1953) saw that to prevent this a minimum of three ligatures set at intervals of 1.25 cm are necessary. Dale et al. (1956) observed that the inferior vena cava of dogs was recanalized in 92 per cent of cases in 2 to 4 months when chromic catgut was used for ligation, but they added that recanalization does not occur if in addition the lumbar veins are ligated, with or without resection of a segment of the caval vein. However—and this is important—the new lumen does not attain the diameter of the original one. More or less marked stenosis results because of two opposing processes: recanalization of the occlusion, and its connective tissue organization.

Recanalization of venous thromboses following grafting was described in several experimental reports (DeWeese and Niguidula, 1960; Dale, 1960, 1961; Cerino et al., 1964; Waddell et al., 1964, 1967; Epfelbaum and Dimaria, 1965; Nay and Fitzpatrick, 1966; Steinman et al., 1966, 1969 Miller et al., 1969). (These authors used different techniques: one used homoplastic vein and another, a heteroplastic vessel (calf aorta). McLachlin et al. (1965) and Waddell et al. (1967) systematically produced thromboses in order to replace them with grafts. Several experiments were carried out on valved veins. The resulting valvular function has already been analyzed. The lumen remained more or less narrowed and irregular in all cases.

These authors state that occlusions are recanalized in approximately 50 to 75 per cent of cases. Thromboses following sclerosing injections, called "experimental phlebitis," yield approximately similar figures, but the number of experiments is too small to permit definitive conclusions. On the other hand, thrombosis produced by crushing of veins and temporary clamping (48 hours), "*experimental thrombosis*," is followed by recanalization in almost 100 per cent of cases, another confirmation of the frequency of recanalization of venous thrombosis.

Flanc (1968) demonstrated by exact measurements a 25 to 50 per cent renewed patency of the lumen following experimental thrombosis of the femoral vein after 5 to 12 weeks. A recanalization rate of 50 to 70 per cent of the lumen is less common. It is noteworthy that venous grafting with arteriovenous fistula is after thrombosis followed by little or no recanalization (Flanc et al., 1968; Levin et al., 1971). Yao et al. (1974) also observed the loss of fibrinolytic activity of veins transplanted on arteries and secondarily thrombosed.

In fact it is known that recanalization of a thrombosed vein grafted onto an artery never occurs in man. Cox (1963) confirmed this for dogs.

The *structure of recanalized veins* is likewise markedly changed. The veins are thicker. They show irregular walls and occasionally deposits of hemosiderin. Histologically, there are round cells in the adventitia and media, as well as increased vascularization. On the intima there are plaques and organized thrombi, covered by endothelium, and blood pigment in places. The valves contain capillaries, normally never seen, and reveal a markedly changed structure. If the process has continued for some time, the inflammatory picture disappears and some sclerosing of the venous wall is present.

Mechanism of recanalization. Two factors play a part: enzymatic dissolution of the thrombus (thrombolysis), and organization and vascularization. Time and again ingrowing vessels are seen in the interior of ancient thrombi. Finally, sinusoid spaces are formed that communicate with one another and open into the lumen at the margin of the occlusion. Thus a considerable lumen is created, always smaller than that before thrombosis, but adequate to cause involution of the now superfluous collateral circulation. Restitution of patency depends chiefly on fibrinolysis, which must take effect before the vascular connective tissue organizes and is transformed to connective tissue. With rapid lysis, complete restitution is almost the rule. Most cases of recanalization observed in the laboratory occur within 2 to 12 weeks. But no really exact data as regards time of recanalization of grafts are available. Repeated phlebography entails vascular irritation and is therefore not an ideal method of observation.

Nevertheless, Robertson et al. (1954) threw some light on the problem of speed of absorption. They introduced sterile clots into the portal vein of dogs via a branch of the splenic vein. The clots stuck in branches of the portal vein and thus could be studied. The thrombi began to fragment after 24 hours and became smaller. After 1 to 2 weeks they had become very small, and after 3 weeks they were completely absorbed or only minor remnants were present. Robertson et al. (1957) observed the same findings after introducing thrombi into the iliac vein of dogs.

Recanalization is certainly a commonplace process. It is astonishing only that it also occurs with homografts. Waddell et al. (1964) observed it in three of 11 thromboses. It was even observed here by Epfelbaum and Dimaria (1965) in heterografts of calf aorta implanted into the inferior vena cava. The latter experiments still require confirmation.

In our experience, thromboses are rare when ring anastomoses are used. We had very few failures and only when there were gross technical errors. When the rings tilt, though, the walls become adherent together.

Venous Neocollaterals

We have noted venous neocollaterals only with autografts so far. We do not have enough experience to claim that they are impossible with homografts. In fact, we have never observed them on human veins that were grafted into arteries.

When we first removed venous grafts from dead experimental animals, we occasionally observed a small strand coming from the vessel which on sectioning appeared to be a small vein. Precise studies showed that new collaterals had indeed formed (Fig. 2.23).

Following this, we systematically applied a black nonabsorbable ligature around the collaterals of a vein prior to grafting, in order to recognize them on removal. We intended to clarify whether the stump of the ligated collateral was the point of origin of a new collateral.

Our experiments showed that neocollaterals are frequently found in grafts of jugular, femoral and iliac veins. They are in fact new formations, for they were not found at the marked vascular stumps. They are frequently multiple and occupy the suture zone predominantly. Their diameter varies from the size of a pinpoint to 2 mm in width. The largest were seen in the segment of the graft lying between the sutures. Stenosis favors formation of collaterals. The largest collaterals were found in a graft whose distal portion was obliterated. So far we have not seen any neocollaterals at the inferior vena cava, but we have not specifically looked for them when opening the vessel in situ. Perhaps minute

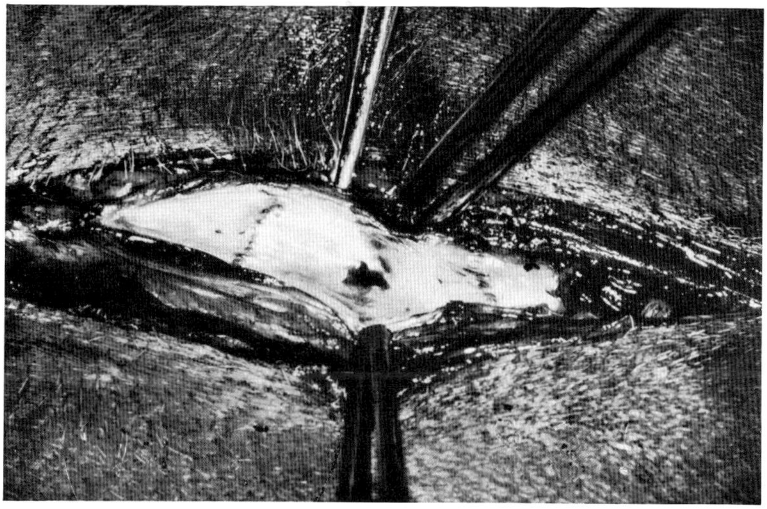

Fig. 2.23. Autoplastic venous graft, opened in situ. Hemorrhage from one neocollateral.

collaterals are present in the suture line. There are insufficient data to determine whether they occur at the superior vena cava, but we have seen some collaterals at long jugular-superior vena cava grafts (p. 53).

Formation of neocollaterals appears to be rather rapid. They are already visible in a phlebogram of a stenosed graft of the jugular vein 3 weeks after operation (Fig. 2.24). Their formation is possibly closely associated with the revascularization process of the wall of the graft. Vascular buds enter it and participate in the restoration of adventitia and media, which usually reveal signs of slight damage following grafting. But how does a junction form in the intima? In a slit or dehiscence?

It is conceivable that formation of the usually very small neocollaterals near the suture line is favored by partial fibrinolysis of small thrombi lying near the zone of union of the two vessels or at the stitch marks of the needle.

The general histologic structure of our venous grafts was examined by Jaulmes, and that of the

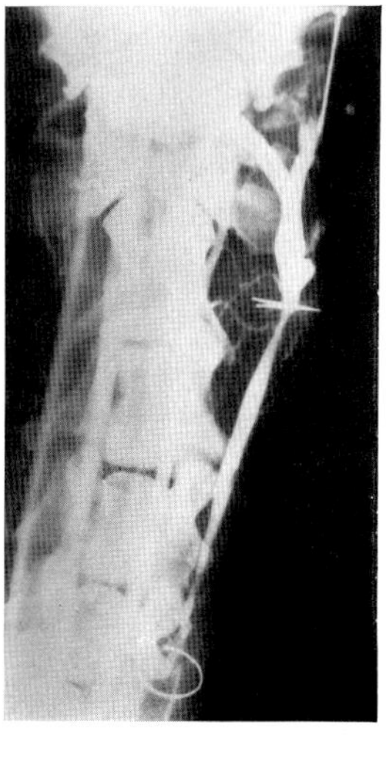

Fig. 2.24. Phlebogram of an autograft of the jugular vein 3 weeks after operation. The proximal ring has tilted and the anastomosis is stenosed; the graft remains patent owing to formation of new collaterals. (From Laude, M., Kunlin, J., Jaulmes, C.: Lille méd. 9 (1964) 933.)

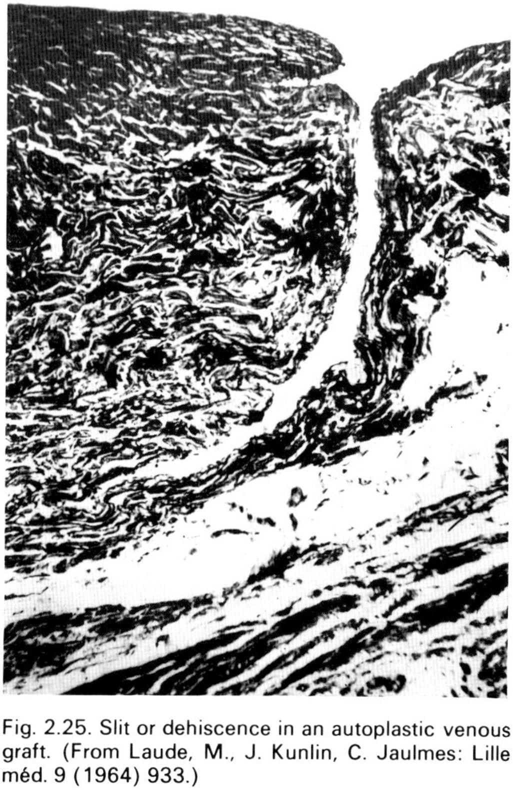

Fig. 2.25. Slit or dehiscence in an autoplastic venous graft. (From Laude, M., J. Kunlin, C. Jaulmes: Lille méd. 9 (1964) 933.)

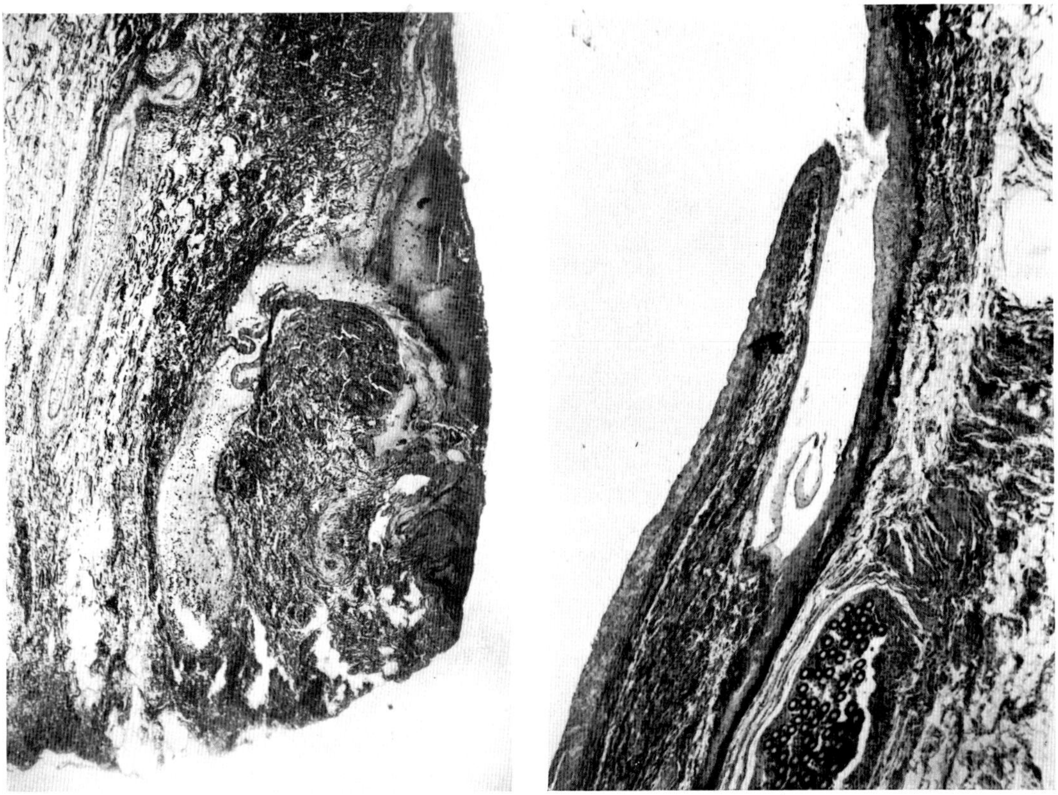

a b

Fig. 2.26. Pseudovalve formation in venous neocollaterals. (From Laude, M., J. Kunlin, C. Jaulmes: Lille méd. 9 (1964) 933.)

neocollaterals by Laude et al. (1964) and Mazabraud (Hôpital Foch, Paris-Suresnes).

Figure 2.25 shows an endothelial gap that could easily be the starting point and junction site of a new collateral. Unfortunately, most pictures show fully developed neocollaterals that have already adopted a characteristic structure. Up to now, we have not specially searched for primary stages of development. It would be a highly interesting task requiring much patience.

Two histologic aspects should be emphasized:

— Occasionally the neocollaterals are sinusoid, with tortuosities and dead ends, producing a pseudoangiomatous picture. Incidentally, this special configuration has much in common with the formation of genuine angiomas, which will be discussed later.
— Whiplike formations were observed in some neocollaterals. They resemble pseudovalves whose ends float in the lumen (Fig. 2.26).

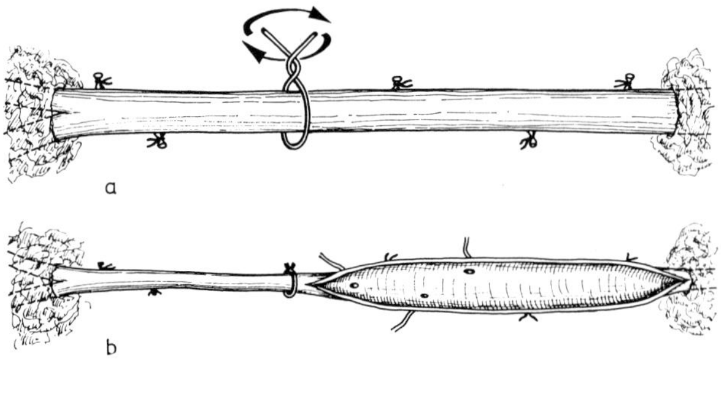

Fig. 2.27. Jugular vein, isolated in its entire length. The collaterals had been ligated and severed, producing stenosis (*a*); vein opened in situ several weeks later; neocollaterals have formed (*b*).

These are possibly only subendothelial abrasions due to decaying blood elements, but this explanation seems insufficient. Effectively the lobules are anchored by a continuous elastic band to the wall and are covered with endothelium on both sides.

We attempted to answer the question whether new collaterals form in a normal, nonsutured, nongrafted vein. Hence, we dissected the jugular vein of a dog in its whole extent (10 and 11 cm in a dog weighing 14 kg) and ligated all collaterals with a nonabsorbable thread. An incomplete ligature of Vitallium was applied between the distal and middle thirds, reducing the caliber of the vein to a quarter of its normal size and producing a relative hyperpressure distally. After several weeks the vessel was opened in situ. New collaterals had formed without connection with the previously ligated collaterals (Fig. 2.27).

Cavernous angioma. The junction of two collaterals with a graft of the femoral or jugular vein of a dog presents a sinusoid picture (Fig. 2.28). We found a cavernous angioma on a suture of a graft of the jugular vein which had formed in the interior and partly obstructed the lumen (Fig. 2.29).

But all these formations—neocollaterals, pseudovalves, angioma-type structures, and so forth—only show that the venous system possesses

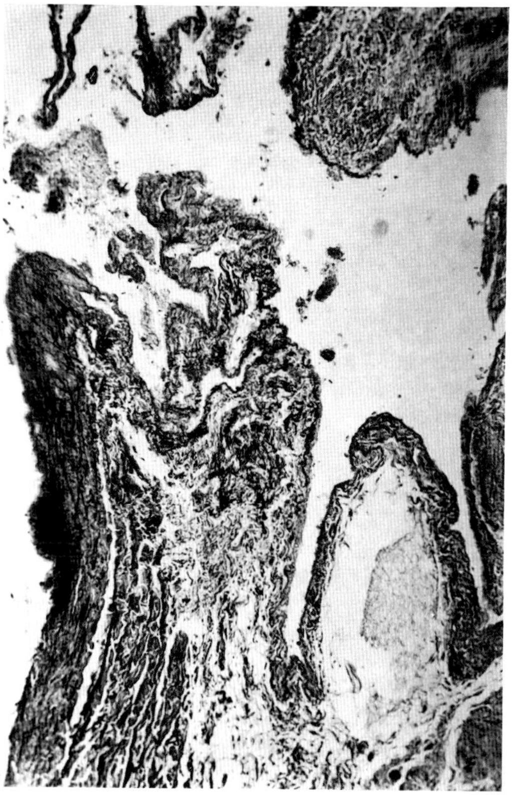

Fig. 2.28. Sinusoid picture of a venous neocollateral in a graft. (From Laude, M., J. Kunlin, C. Jaulmes: Lille méd. 9 (1964) 933.)

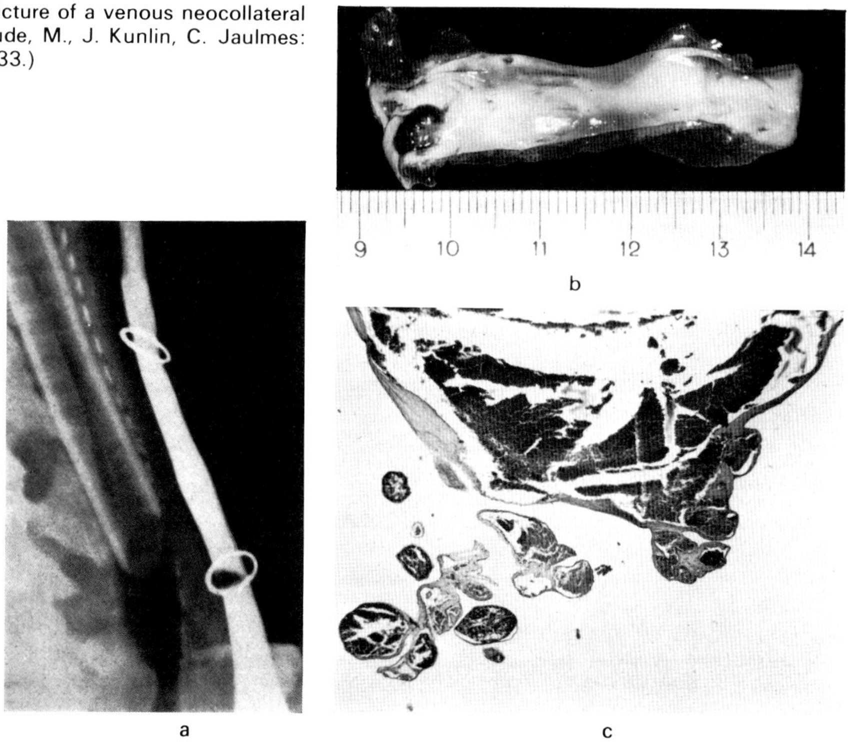

a c

Fig. 2.29. Graft of jugular vein after 12 months. (*a*) A cavernous angioma had formed at the proximal suture and produces stenosis. (From Kunlin, J.: J. Chir. (Paris) 85 (1963) 305.) (*b*) Cavernous angioma at the proximal anastomosis; (*c*) Microscopic view of *b*.

an enormous capacity to regenerate, which often overshoots the target. "L'homme peut fabriquer des veines de toutes pièces une fois sa croissance terminée." (R. Leriche). Nevertheless, effective valves cannot be newly formed.

Experimental Endophlebectomy

Thrombectomy in acute thrombosis is a frequent and proven method of intervention in man. Removal of obstructions from a vein that is involved in an inflammatory or neoplastic process is only occasionally successful, apparently only in the superior vena cava syndrome.

Studies and Experiments of Other Authors

O'Neill (1962) appears to have been the first to incise the superior vena cava in treating fibrosing mediastinitis and to free the lumen from obstructing fibrous tissue. Blondeau et al. (1959) restored the caliber of the same vein by removing metastatic neoplastic tissue. Templeton (1962) operated on two patients and Toty (1967) on one. Part of these procedures somewhat corresponds to thrombectomy. Templeton described having to use a knife to fragment the firm mass that filled the vein, and he stressed that it was difficult to find the correct layer. He eliminated the venous wall so that only a thin transparent layer remained. He called his intervention "*endvenectomy*."

Jackson et al. (1966) applied the same measure to the inferior vena cava once, and once each at the axillary vein and femoral vein. They called this "thrombointimectomy," and were of the opinion that this operation is not feasible in veins of smaller caliber than the axillary or femoral of man. This technique unites thrombectomy—removal of an organized thrombus—with intimectomy, which is incomplete, however. Anticoagulation was systematically maintained for a prolonged period (1 year). Apparently no phlebograms were obtained in the last cases.

Our Own Investigations

We examined a vein in 1950 that had been implanted for arterial occlusion and later thrombosed. It became clear that the wall could be separated in three parts (Kunlin, 1964), but separation of layers is much more difficult than with arterial occlusions. A fresh vein removed during surgery for varicosities, can also be cleaved in three layers.

With Pajot we have since 1958 successfully employed endophlebectomy on four veins that had been inserted as bypass in arterial occlusion. They showed stenosis of the proximal anastomosis and in the middle portion in one case.

Our Own Experiments

In 1967 we have done a series of experiments on removal of the venous intima of dogs (J. Kunlin, Testart, Derieux). The technique is rather difficult but, with patience, the goal can be achieved. After a longitudinal incision has been made, one or two small sutures are fastened to the edges of the vein. The intima, which is under tension from the pull of the threads, is nicked with the tip of a scalpel. The endovenous layer is pulled off after being lifted with fine anatomic forceps and is rolled away. The venous intima tears less easily than the arterial. Care should be taken to keep the nick and the forceps as superficial as possible. This method is relatively simple when used in the superior vena cava, especially in its juxtacardial portion where it is slightly thicker. The technique here resembles endarterectomy. Intimectomy is also comparatively easily done in the inferior vena cava, but it becomes really difficult in the jugular and femoral veins. The remaining wall is as thin as cigarette paper. The intima of the venous valve can also be stripped with great care. After intimectomy the wall is not as smooth and shiny as it appears on endarterectomy. It is matted, and this gives it a dull appearance (Fig. 2.30). But it is sufficiently resistant to permit suturing (with Tevdek gauge 7–0). After the clamps have been removed, the vein has a slightly smaller diameter, like any sutured vein of equal size. At times, tears require additional sutures, which can cause stenosis; these tears should be sutured transversely, so they produce less narrowing. We did not give anticoagulants.

We have performed endophlebectomies, between 0.5 and 4 cm in length, on the jugular and femoral veins and the inferior and superior venae cavae of the dog. Results were evaluated in 15 cases, either by phlebography or by removal. After observation for 2 to 12 months (average $5\frac{1}{2}$ months) the vessel was patent in 11 of the 15 controls (Figs. 2.31 and 2.32). Thrombosis occurred in four, in one case immediately in a dog that died the following night, probably as a result of the anesthesia.

Macroscopically, the endophlebectomized vein showed slight fibrosis of the wall, especially near the suture line. Otherwise it differed little from neighboring normal segments. When the vessel was opened, the new endovenous layer appeared whiter and thicker (Fig. 2.33). A few small strands were seen in smaller veins (jugular and

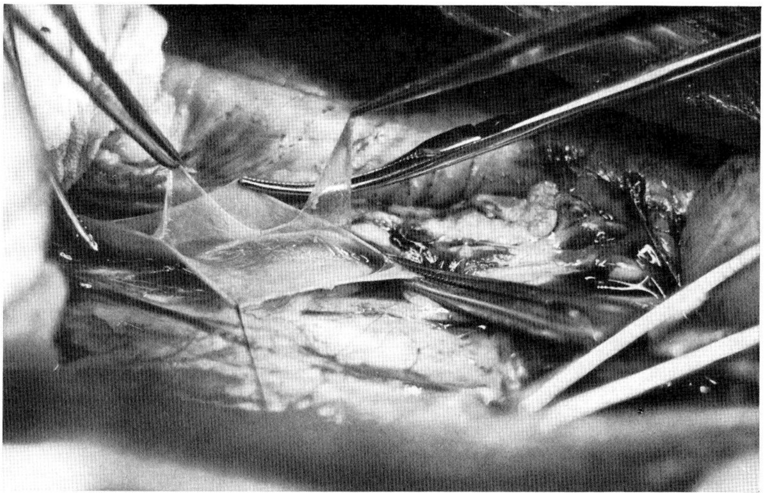

a

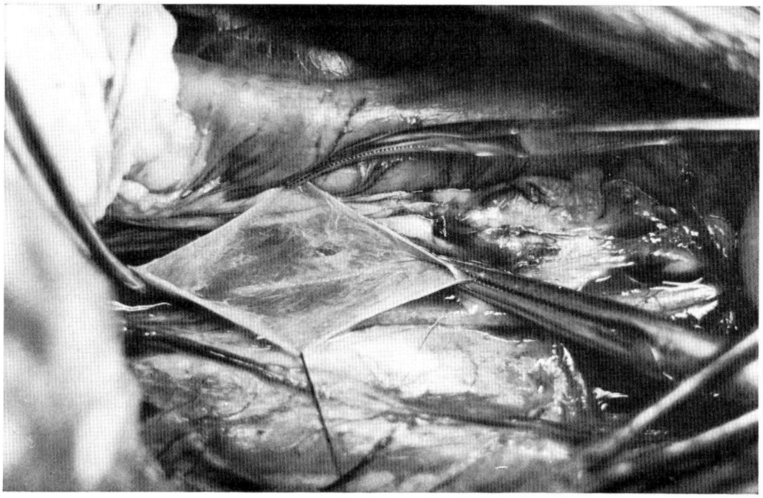

b

Fig. 2.30. Endophlebectomy of the inferior vena cava. (*a*) Very delicate and transparent intima lifted by two forceps; (*b*) After removal of the intima, the inner surface of the vein is not smooth, and it appears dull.

femoral). After removal of the clamps, the diameter of that vein was only 2.5 to 3 mm in the suture line owing to contraction. The dead animals had a small thrombus at the suture.

Histologic examination showed structural changes (Fig. 2.34). The elastic fibers were interspersed with collagen fibers, some hyaline fibers and fibers that were difficult to stain. No muscular structure was recognizable. The interior surface was covered by a layer of connective tissue on which endothelium was superimposed. Some macrophages and lymphocytes were found in the suture zone. Vessels were dilated in the adventitia (Mazabraud, Hôpital Foch, Paris-Suresnes).

Problems of Venous Plastic Surgery

The aim of our efforts is restitution not only of obstructed venous flow but also of the valves. The latter is surely the more difficult to attain. One should have no illusions and consider the following carefully: Even if one or more valve segments are successfully grafted onto large venous trunks, a satisfactory permanent result can

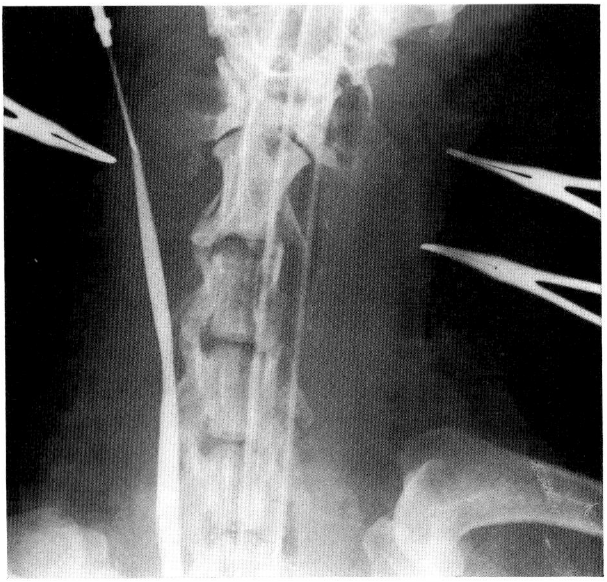

Fig. 2.31. Phlebogram of the right jugular vein of a dog 11 months after endophlebectomy.

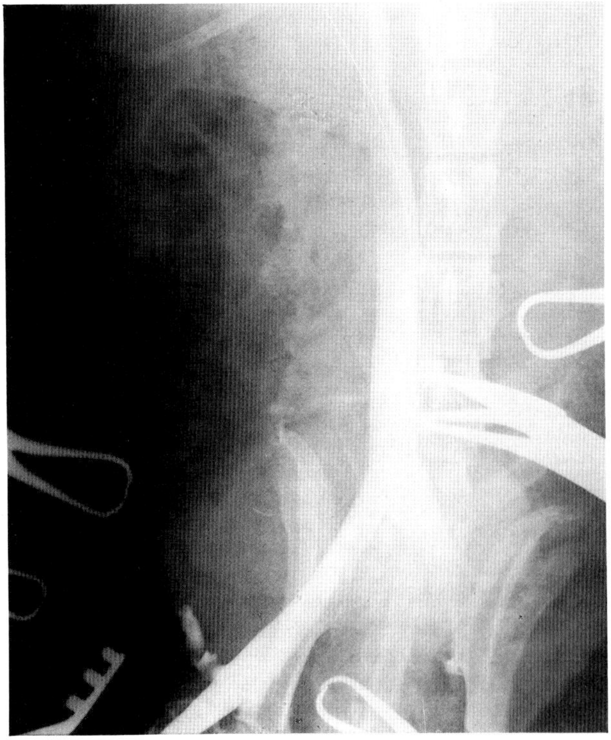

Fig. 2.32. Phlebogram of the inferior vena cava of a dog 5 months after endophlebectomy.

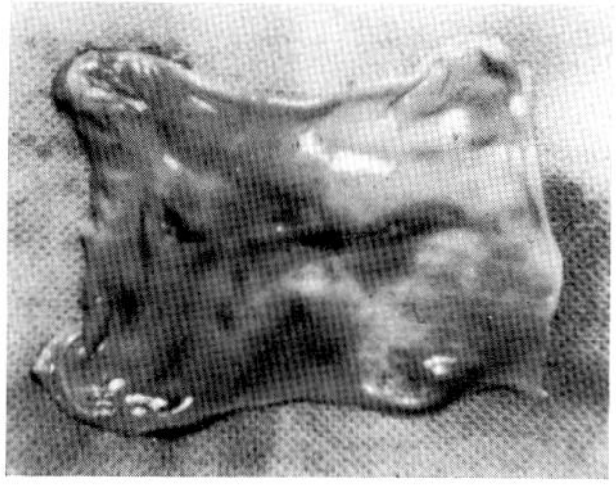

Fig. 2.33. Appearance of the inferior vena cava 4 months after endophlebectomy. The inner surface is smooth and shiny; the suture is seen in the center of the dark line.

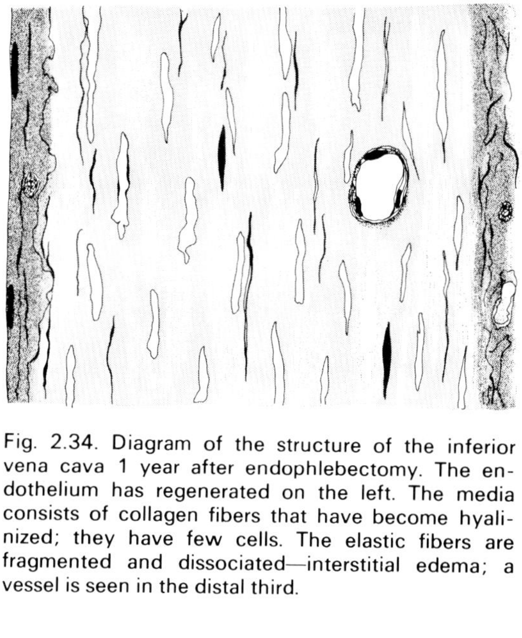

Fig. 2.34. Diagram of the structure of the inferior vena cava 1 year after endophlebectomy. The endothelium has regenerated on the left. The media consists of collagen fibers that have become hyalinized; they have few cells. The elastic fibers are fragmented and dissociated—interstitial edema; a vessel is seen in the distal third.

be expected only in the absence of valvular insufficiency of secondary veins. In other words, at least partial preservation of the peripheral venous pump is probably necessary. But our clinical and roentgenologic methods do not yet provide a complete and detailed picture of all venous areas in the limb. Again and again we are struck by the same conclusion: If these as yet unsolved problems are squarely faced, the urgent necessity of preventing late sequelae to thrombosis is clear. This is achieved only by prophylaxis and correct early therapy of thrombosis.

This includes systematic clearance of thrombi, and in addition to eliminating thrombi, it is equally important to free valves to which fibrin deposits adhere.

If spontaneous thrombolysis of vein grafts in the laboratory showed in individual cases that valvular function can be restored, it may be hoped that it might be possible by early measures to restore full venous function in man.

Addendum. Lately there have been clinical reports that the valves remain fully functional if fibrinolytic treatment is given early, within 2 or 3 days of occurrence of thrombosis. Let us hope that this will be confirmed.

Conclusions

The following conclusions may be drawn from experimental work in surgery of the veins:

— With improved atraumatic technique, especially with progressively finer suture materials and on small vessels with the aid of surgical microscopes, it will be possible to enhance results of experimental surgery of the veins quite considerably.
— Autoplastic grafts are superior to homoplastic, and far superior to heteroplastic grafts and prostheses.
—Teflon prostheses yield the best results, only for veins of large caliber.
— A certain rigidity of the vessel wall of the graft, as is naturally possessed by the aorta or can be achieved with prostheses or by use of rings to keep the graft patent, enhances results.
— Similarly, support of the suture by external rings (ring suture) is useful. But the rings used should be of no greater diameter than the vein. In mobile zones (neck, extremities), near muscle, the risk of tilting, and hence of stenosis, is great.
— Increase in venous pressure and flow in graft or prosthesis is also favorable, particularly that produced by an arteriovenous fistula, which provides better nutrition of the graft in addition. But nutrition seems not to be as important as increased flow velocity and raised outflow.

Attention to the following points is necessary for the success of grafting:

— wherever practical, use of fresh autografts;
— fine suturing as far as possible or use of a suspended suture with rings or preferably a mechanical one with clips;
— rinsing of the vein and surgical field with heparin-Ringer solution;
— applying an arteriovenous fistula close to the

graft for 2 to 4 weeks in animals, and longer (2 to 4 months) in man; and
— anticoagulants for 2 weeks (animal) or longer, depending on the size of the graft and the pathologic state (man).

If no autoplastic material is available, a Teflon prosthesis appears at present to be the most advantageous for large veins like the vena cava. The problem has not been solved for small veins with a diameter of 5 to 8 mm. Here, only autoplastic material can be expected to be successful. With Gore-tex the experience is still too brief.

It would be highly desirable to find a way of using organic homoplastic and heteroplastic grafts successfully.

For suppression of rejection by the body, two methods have been tried:

—Application of immunosuppressive substances, which as far as we know had not been done in this field before 1972, possibly because the vessels have a weak antigenic effect (Sautot et al., 1954, Schwartz, 1967).
Perloff et al. (1972) had 90 per cent permeability with homoplastic veins grafted on the canine femoral vein with azathioprine instead of only 37 per cent without immunosuppression. Long-term results, however, are absent. With azathioprine and prednisone Carpenter et al. (1973) could not avoid the antigenic reaction against arterial and venous homografts placed on the dog's carotid artery. Deltz et al. (1975) observed antigenicity with fresh venous homografts in rats. This reactivity was suppressed when the vessels were treated with formalin (Anders et al., 1976).
—Progressive adaptation of the graft to the recipient, a problem still studied in the early part of the twentieth century (Bode and Fabian). We started trials in 1968 but could not finish them. The heteroplastic vessel (human vein, obtained by saphenectomy) is drawn over a bland Silastic tube and implanted under the skin of the recipient or at the site of the intended application. Once the immunologic reaction has ceased, the vessel has adopted the character of the recipient and is tolerated in the future. It can now be implanted into the vessel, or only its ends mobilized, and then sutured into the neighboring vein or artery after removal of the tube. Such a graft is thinner after $3\frac{1}{2}$ months, whitish and fragile. The elastic tissue has largely disappeared. The inner surface is covered with an irregular layer of cuboid cells (Mazabraud, Hôpital Foch, Paris-Suresnes).

We also attempted to inject irritating, sclerosing substances into the vein before grafting to make it more resistant. Unfortunately these attempts had to be abandoned before acceptable results were obtained. We were successful only with patches on the inferior vena cava—but it is known that these are always successful no matter what material is used.

Hopefully experimenters will have better results in the future in preparing autologous fibrous organic tubes than Smith et al. (1975) had on veins and we had on arteries in unfinished trials (Kunlin 1953a).

Adhesive Rings

R. Gottlob and G. Blümel

The tendency of veins to shrink at the site of the anastomosis presents a particular problem. This problem also exists with "anastomosis by machine" with clip appliances. The ring anastomosis of Nakayama may indeed prevent stenosis, but there is the risk of snapping. A small shift of the ring causes snapping in the vein and thus the danger of obliteration. The problem of snapping may also play a part when the venous suture is suspended from resistant tissue near the anastomosis or from a metal ring around it, in order to relax the vessel, the method suggested by Kunlin (1953, 1959). To avoid these disadvantages and dangers, we applied to veins a technique of anastomosis that had proved successful with small arteries. It was necessary to modify the method slightly for use in veins, however. The original type of anastomosis is shown in Figure 2.35*a*. The end of the vessel to be anastomosed is glued to the inner surface of a conical ring. The cone is so applied that the lumen is widest at the site of the anastomosis. The vessel adheres to an area of the inner surface of the conical ring. Adherence is produced by inserting into the vessel a conical rod that moderately stretches the lumen near the anastomosis. The external surface of the vessel is glued to an area on the inner surface of the ring. Previous studies (Gottlob and Blümel, 1967a, 1967b, 1968) showed that application of adhesive to the adventitia is not well tolerated by veins. We think this is because the veins are nourished exclusively by the adventitia, without any contribution from the lumen. For this reason and because it was soon evident that the narrow site of the Teflon rings caused considerable stenosis with only slight shifting, we modified the method, as shown in Figure 2.35*b*. The rings are now away as far as possible from the anastomosis and adhesive is applied only to an everted

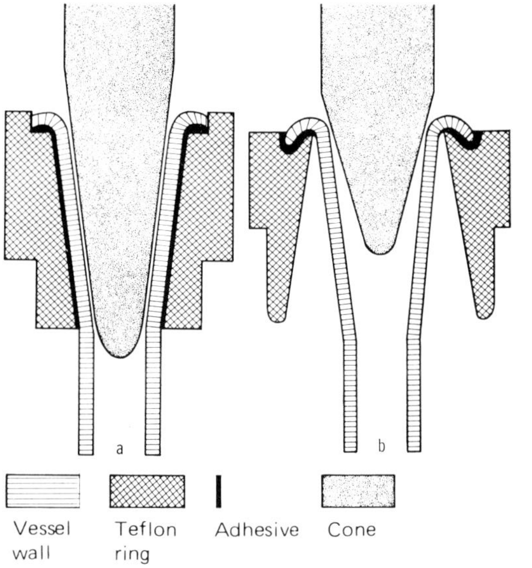

Fig. 2.35. Technique of anastomosis with adhesive rings. (*a*) Original anastomosis with adherence of the conical ring to the vessel wall; (*b*) modified type.

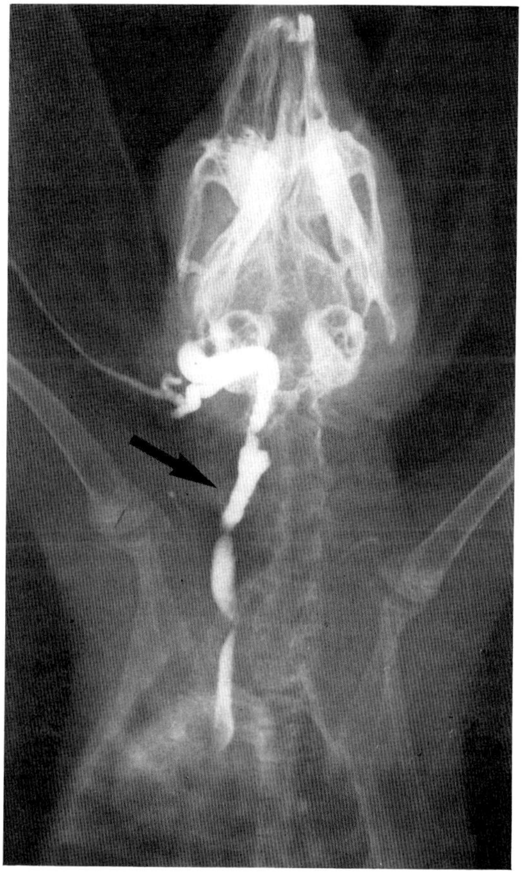

Fig. 2.37. Anastomosis of the right anterior facial vein of a rabbit. Angiogram 1 week postoperatively (→ site of anastomosis).

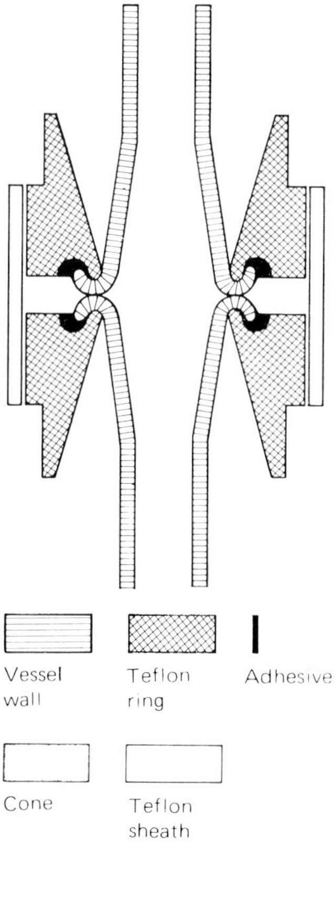

Fig. 2.36. Technique of anastomosis with adhesive rings. Cross-section of completed anastomosis.

portion of the vessel; this prevents lumen-forming segments of the veins from coming into contact with the adhesive. Figure 2.36 shows the completed anastomosis. It is easily seen from this drawing that the rings can make certain excursions without producing stenosis.

Procedure. The end of the vein to be anastomosed is pulled through the Teflon ring, and a conical rod of metal or plastic is introduced into the vessel. For easier introduction, the cone is lubricated (catheter purine). The edge of the vessel is gripped with fine clamps so that even tension is exerted. Once the cone is introduced, the Teflon ring is pushed forward to the end of the anastomosis so that the edge is closely applied to the vessel. Now an adhesive (butyl-2-cyanoacrylate) is applied in a notch of the ring near the anastomosis. The end of the vessel is pushed into this notch with a scalpel, and eversion results. After repeating the procedure at the other end, a Teflon sheath is placed over one of the Teflon rings. Now the second ring must be inserted into the sheath, and this completes the anastomosis. Air in the anastomosed segment of the vessel is removed by a saline-heparin solution before closure.

It proved necessary to slightly heparinize the animals for several days. In this way it is possible to maintain patency of the anastomoses for several weeks (Fig. 2.37). Long-term results of this technique of anastomosis are available with arteries of 2 mm diameter but not as yet with veins (Gottlob and Blümel 1968).

References

Abbe, R.: The surgery of the hand. N.Y. med. J. (1894)

Abramson, H. A.: Electrophoresis of the blood platelets of the horse with reference to their origin and to thrombus formation. J. exp. Med. 47 (1928) 677

Abramson, H. A.: Electrophoresis of Proteins and the Chemistry of Cell Surfaces. Reinhold Publishing Corp. 1942. Republished by Hafner, New York 1962

Acland, R.: A new needle for microvascular surgery. Surgery 71 (1972) 130

Acland, R.: Thrombus formation in microvascular surgery: an experimental study of the effects of surgical trauma. Surgery 73 (1973) 766

Adams, J. T., J. A. De Weese: Experimental and clinical evaluation of partial vein interruption in the prevention of pulmonary emboli. Surgery 57 (1965) 82–102

Alpert, J., Ch. Steinman, H. Haimovici: Suture plication of the inferior vena cava. A long term experimental evaluation of plication channels. Arch. Surg. 93 (1966) 388–391

Altschul, R.: Endothelium: Its development, morphology, function and pathology. MacMillan Comp.: New York 1954

Anders, A., A. Thiede: Der Wert formalinfixierter allogener Venen für den Gefäßersatz im Langzeitversuch. Chirurgiches Forum 1976. Arch. für Chir., Supplement 1976

Andersen, M. C., T. W. Schields: An evaluation of factors which influence the incidence and extent of venous thrombosis. Surgery 51 (1962) 347

Androsov, P. I.: New method of surgical treatment of blood vessel lesions. Arch. Surg. 73 (1956a) 902–910

Androsov, P. I.: Operations in case of aneurysms. Arch. Surg. 73 (1956b) 911–916

Anlyan, W. G., J. F. Schauble: Diskussionsbemerkungen in: Surgery 47 (1960) 132

Anlyan, W. G.: Discussion of Baird, R. J., et al.

Arnulf, G.: Documents expérimentaux sur les greffes veineuses (greffes sur tubes en inox). Lyon chir. 60 (1964) 734

Arnulf, G.: Re-establishment of the venous circulation by graft with an inox tube. Experimental study. J. cardiovasc. Surg. 6 (1965) 541

Arnulf, G.: Greffes de Coronaires. Données expérimentales. Chir. expér. 1 (1967) 92

Aschberg, S., T. Hindmarsh: Distal arterio-venous shunts in auto-transplantation of canine venous valves. Acta chir. Scand. 137 (1971) 503

Ashburn, F. S., W. H. Sewell, C. E. Huggins: Experimental replacement of the superior vena cava with homologous arteries and report of a case with malignant obstruction replaced with a heterologous artery. J. thorac. Surg. 31 (1956) 618–624

Ashton, F., R. Geddes, J. Fejar: Woven silicone rubber as a venous prosthesis. Brit. Med. J. 3 (1969) 409

Astrup, T., K. Buluk: Hemostatic mechanism in the animal arterial wall. Nature 185 (1960) 541

Aureggi, A.: Plastic substitution of the inferior vena cava. Policlinico (Chir.) 79 (1972) 49, according to Scherck, J. P., et al.

Baird, R. J., I. H. Lipton, R. T. Miyagishima, C. J. Labrosse: Replacement of the deep veins of the leg. Arch. Surg. 89 (1964) 797

De Bakey, M. E.: Diary of my trip to the U.S.S.R. 1958. Bull. Amer. Coll. Surg. 44 (1959) 505

Barcia, P. J., T. G. Nelson, T. J. Whelan: Importance of venous occlusion in arterial repair failure: an experimental study. Ann. Surg. 175 (1972) 223

Barnes, R. W. et al.: The use of low molecular weight Dextran in Superior Vena Caval replacement. Dis. Chest 53 (1968) 390

Batchelor, W. H.: Lipoproteins in arterial wall. Symposium on atherosclerosis. Nat. Acad. Sc. Public. 338 (1955) 212

Bauchhens, G. H.: Anastomosierung kleiner Venen. Maschinelle und Klebe-Anastomosen im Tierversuch. Chir. Praxis 12 (1968) 43

Baumann, G.: Segment replacement of the inferior vena cava in dogs with peritoneum. Dtsch. Mediz. Wochenschr. 97 (1972) 957

Baumgarten, V.: Entzündung, Thrombose und Embolie. Lehman, München 1925

Baxter, Th. J., B. M. C. O'Brien, P. N. Hendersen, R. C. Bennet: The histopathology of small vessels following microvascular repair. Brit. J. Surg. 59 (1972) 617

Beneke, R.: Die Ursachen der Thrombusorganisation. Beitr. path. Anat. 7 (1890) 95

Benjamin, R. B., C. E. Turbak, D. W. Hannon, N. E. Shumway, F. J. Lewis: Polyvinyl sponge in experimental surgery. Ann. Surg. 145 (1957) 509

Bergan, J. J., H. A. Kaupp, O. H. Trippel: Critical evaluation of vena cava plication. Prevention of pulmonary embolism. Arch. Surg. 88 (1964) 1016

Bhonslay, S.: Diskussionsbemerkungen in: Arch. Surg. 80 (1960) 119

Bischof, M., P. Donas, N. Pridun, R. Gottlob: Endothelschäden nach Venen Bypass. 6. Jahrestag. Österr. Gesellsch. f. Gefäßchir. Klagenfurt 1973, Karger Basel 1975

Blakemore, A. H., J. W. Lord: The technique of using Vitallium tubes in establishing porto-caval shunts for portal hypertension. Ann. Surg. 122 (1945a) 476–489

Blakemore, A. H., J. W. Lord: A non-suture method of blood vessel anastomosis. Experimental and clinical study. J. Amer. med. Ass. 127 (1945b) 685

Blocker, F. G.: Notes on a visit to the U.S.S.R. to observe surgical technics and research. Amer. J. Surg. 99 (1960) 615

Blondeau, Ph., C. Wapler, A. Piwnica, Ch. Dubost: Deux cas de syndrome de la veine cave supérieure traités: chirurgicalement avec succès, l'un par désobstruction, l'autre par greffe. Arch. Mal. Coeur 52 (1959) 504

Bode, Fabian: Transplantation konservierter Gefäße; Beiträge zur klinischen Chir. January 1910, 67

Bond, M. G., J. R. Hostetler, P. E. Karayannacos, J. C. Geer, J. S. Vasko: Intimal changes in arterio-venous bypass grafts, with varying the angle of implantation and with stenosis in the distal runoff artery. J. Thorac. Cardiovasc. Surg. 71 (1975) 907

Borst, Enderlen: La transplantation de vaisseaus et d'organes entiers. Dtsch. Z. Chir. 99 (1909) 54–164

Botham, R. J., Th. T. Dracopoulos, J. W. Gale: Superior vena caval replacement with Sponge Teflon prosthesis. J. thorac. cardiovasc. Surg. 39 (1960) 202

Bothezat, P. E.: Contribution à la chirurgie des artères. Thèse, Montpellier 1893–1894

Boutelier, P., C. Couinaud: Les anomalies dites primitives de la veine cave inférieure. J. Chir. (Paris) 82 (1962) 199

Bower, R. V., Federicci, J. M. Howard: Continuing studies of replacement of segments of the venous system. Surgery 47 (1960) 132–139

Bradham, R. R.: Relationship of the hind-limb lymphatic system to experimental femoral vein thrombosis. Surgery 58 (1965) 682–693

Brais, M., E. Bertranou, A. Brassard, P. Stanley, C. Chartrand: Effect of Dextran on patency of pericardiac tubular graft of the superior vena cava in the dog. J. Thorac. Cardiovasc. Surg. 65 (1973) 296

Brea, C. A.: Superior vena cava replacement with autogenous fascia. An experimental study. Amer. Surg. 31 (1965) 611–613

Breslau, R. C., S. I. Schwartz, D. W. Smith, Ch. G. Rob: Inferior vena cava replacement with bovine arterial heterografts. N.Y. St. J. Med. 65 (1965) 1967.

Bryant, M. F. Jr., W. D. Lazenby, J. M. Howard: Experimental replacement of short segments of veins. Arch. Surg. 76 (1958) 289–293
Bunke, H. J.: The suture repair of one-millimeter vessels. In: Micro-Vascular Surgery. R. M. P. Donaghy, M. G. Yasargil (eds.). Thieme, Stuttgart 1967
Büttner et al.: Fibrinolytic activity of the wall of veins. Vasa 1 (1972) 24
Calvert, M. H., M. H. Gough: The effect of antithrombotic drugs on prosthetic grafts in the canine inferior vena cava. Brit. J. Surg. 63 (1976) 910
Carabaloma, P., J. J. Picard, H. Baumel, J. B. Priotan, J. Vidal: Ischémie aiguë du membre inférieur par traumatismes fermés du genou. Mém. Acad. Chir. 88 (1962) 186–192
Carlson, H. A.: Obstruction of the superior vena cava. Arch. Surg. 29 (1934) 667
Carpenter, E. W., S. M. Lindenauer: Immunosuppression in arterial and venous allografts. Arch. Surg. 106 (1973) 75
Carrel, A.: La technique opératoire des anastomoses vasculaires et la transplantation des viscères. Lyon méd. 98 (1902) 859
Carrel, A., C. C. Guthrie: Uniterminal and biterminal venous transplantation. Surg. Gynec. Obstet. 2 (1906) 266
Carrel, A.: Results of transplantation of blood vessels, organs and limbs. J. Amer. med. Ass. 51 (1908) 1662
Carrel, A.: Technique and remote results of vascular anastomoses. Surg. Gynec. Obstet. 14 (1912) 246
Carter, P. D.: Suture and non-suture methods of small vein anastomosis. Arch. Surg. 84 (1962) 350–352
Carton, C. A., L. A. Kessler, B. Seidenberg, E. S. Hurwitt: Experimental studies in the surgery of small blood vessels. IV. Non-suture anastomosis of arteries and veins using flanged ring prosthesis and plastic adhesive. Surg. Forum 11 (1960a) 238
Carton, C. A., L. A. Kessler, B. Seidenberg, E. S. Hurwitt: A plastic adhesive method of small vessel surgery. Wld Neurosurg. 1 (1960b) 356
Cerino, M., J. Y. McGraw, J. G. Luke: Autogenous vein graft replacement of thrombosed deep veins. Experimental approach to the treatment of the postphlebitic syndrome. Surgery 55 (1964) 123–133
Chabal J., G. Esposito, D. Duffrene, F. M. Dogru: Action expérimentale de l'hypothermie modérée sur l'occlusion portale aiguë chez le chien. Lyon Chir. 59 (1963) 704
Chabal, J., D. Duffrene, A. Dogru: Mécanisme de la mort après obstruction portale aiguë. Etude expérimentale. Lyon Chir. 61 (1965) 194–211
Chakrabarti, R., P. Birks, E. Fearnley: Origin of blood fibrinolytic activity from veins and its bearing on the fate of venous thrombi. Lancet 1963, 147
Chvapil, M., M. Krajicek: Principle and construction of a highly porous collagen-fabric vascular graft. J. surg. Res. 3 (1963) 358–368
Clark, R. E., H. W. Margraf: Antibacterial vascular grafts with improved thromboresistance. Arch. Surg. 109 (1974) 159
Coccheris, Astrup: Thrombo-plastic and fibrinolytic activities of large human vessels. Proc. Soc. exp. Biol. 108 (1961) 369
Coenen: XVIIe Congrès Allemand de Chirurgie. Zbl. Chir. 15 (1913) 27
Collins, H. A., G. Burrus, M. E. De Bakey: Experimental evaluation of grafts in the canine inferior vena cava. Amer. J. Surg. 99 (1960) 40–43
Collins, R. E., F. M. Douglass: Small vein anastomosis with or without operative microscope. A comparative study. Arch. Surg. 88 (1964) 740–742
Courbier, R., Y. Baille, C. Juban, A. Goudard, H. Tramier: Conditions d'action des thrombolytiques dans les oblitérations artérielles. Ann. Chir. thor. cardiovasc. 7 (1968) 313
Csillag, I., H. Jellinek, I. Novak: New method of restoring defects in wall of great veins. Bull. Soc. Internat. Chir. 19 (1960) 320–328
Dale, W. A.: Thrombosis and recanalisation of veins used as venous grafts. Angiology 12 (1961) 603
Dale, W. A.: In discussion of Bower, R., V. Federicci, J. M. Howard: Continuing studies of replacement of segments of the venous system. Surgery 47 (1960) 132
Dale, W. A., Mahoney: Venous Autografts, Thomas, Springfield/Ill, 1959
Dale, W. A., H. W. Scott: Grafts of the venous system. Surgery 53 (1963) 52–74
Dale, W. A., M. R. Lewis: Modified bovine heterografts for arterial replacement. Ann. Surg. 169 (1969) 927
Daniel, W. W.: Bridging defects in canine portal and superior mesenteric veins with plastic tubes and vascular grafts. Preliminary report. Cancer 5 (1952) 1041–1048
Danis: Les causes d'insuccès dans la suture vasculaire. Presse méd. 71 (1912)
Darling, R. C., R. Linton, M. A. Razzuk: Saphenous vein bypass grafts for femoro-popliteal occlusive disease. A reappraisal. Surgery 61 (1967) 31
Dart, C. H., G. Johnson, R. M. Peters, N. A. Womack: Hemodynamic effects of femoral venous occlusion before and after an acute arterio-venous fistula. Ann. Surg. 164 (1966) 190
Dean, R. E., R. C. Read: Influence of increased blood flow on thrombosis in prosthetic grafts. Trans. Amer. Soc. artif. intern. Org. 9 (1963) 312
Dean, R. E., R. C. Read: The influence of increased blood flow on thrombosis in prosthetic grafts. Surg. 55 (1964) 581–584
Delbet, P.: Chirurgie des Artères et des Veines. XVe Congrès International de Médecine, Lisbonne. 1906 (p. 28)
Deltz, E., H. G. Sonntag, A. Thiede: Die humorale und zelluläre Immunantwort nach allogener Venentransplantation bei Ratten. Chir. Forum München 1975 Arch. für Chir. Supplement 1975
Demetz, A., L. L. Philips, D. V. Habif, J. H. Jacobson: Use of fibrinolysin in experimental inferior vena caval replacement. Arch. Surg. 83 (1961) 883–886
Deterling, R. A., S. B. Bhonslay: Use of vessel grafts and plastic prostheses for relief of superior vena cava obstruction. Surgery 38 (1955) 1008
Devin, R., H. Brandonne, F. Benady, J. Mignard, Y. Cure, B. Garabedian: Tentatives expérimentales de greffes veineuses valvulées avec anastomoses suspendues à des anneaux. Marseille chir. 16 (1964) 179
De Weese, J. A.: Dans Discussion de Darling, Linton et Razzuk: Saphenous vein by-pass grafts for femoro-popliteal occlusive disease. A reappraisal. Surgery 61 (1967) 31
De Weese, J. A., F. Niguidula: The replacement of short segments of veins with functional autogenous veins or grafts. Surg. Gynec. Obstet. 110 (1960) 303–308
De Weese, M. S., D. C. Hunter: A vena cava filter for the prevention of pulmonary embolism. Arch. Surg. 86 (1963) 852
Dimaria, G.: La Chirurgie restauratrice des gros troncs veineux. Thèse, Paris 1964
Dobrowolskaia, N. A.: Zur Technik der Nähte an Gefäßen kleinen Kalibers. Dtsch. Z. Chir. 119 (1912) 31
Dogru, A. M., T. Ertunc, G. Yakut: La réparation des pertes de substance de la veine cave inférieure susrénale. Recherche expérimentale. Lyon chir. 67 (1971) 461
Dos Santos, J. C.: Late results of reconstructive arterial surgery. Special issue VI Congress of the International Cardio-Vascular Society, Roma 1963, p. 445. Minerva Medica, Turin 1964
Dost, K.: Eine Methode zum plastischen Ersatz größerer Venen. Langenbecks Arch. klin. Chir. 313 (1965) 854
Dost, K.: Plastischer Ersatz der Vena Cava Inferior im Tierexperiment. Arch. Kreisl.-Forsch. 51 (1966) 191
Doyen, E.: 22e Congrès Français de Chirurgie, Paris (Oct. 1909). Procès-verbaux, Mémoires et Discussions, 181
Ducharme, J. C.: End-to-end venous anastomosis in small puppies. Technique, results, growth and some factors influencing thrombus formation. Ohio med. J. 57 (1961) 777
Eadie, D. G. A., G. De Takats: The early fate of autogenous grafts in the canine femoral vein. J. cardiovasc. Surg. 7 (1966) 148
Earle, A. S., J. S. Horsley, J. L. Villavicencio, R. Warren: Replacement of venous defects by venous autografts. Arch. Surg. 80 (1960) 119–124
East, W. M., W. H. Muller jr.: An experimental study of resection and replacement of the superior vena cava. Amer. J. Surg. 99 (1960) 6–12
Edwards, E. A., J. E. Edwards: The effect of thrombophlebitis on the venous valve. Surg. Gynec. Obstet. 65 (1937) 310
Egdahl, H., D. M. Hume, H. A. Schlang: Plastic venous prostheses. Surg. Forum 5 (1955) 235
Ehrly, A. M., B. Bapistella: Verbesserung der Fließeigenschaften des Blutes bei der Therapie mit Streptokinase und Arwin. 10. Jahrestagung der Deutsch. Gesellsch. für Angiologie, Frankfurt Oktober 1972, Hans Huber, Bern 1973
Enerson, D. E., N. Galante: The use of external supported aortic homografts in the superior vena cava. Amer. Coll. Surg. surg. Forum 8 (1957) 450.

Epfelbaum, R., G. Dimaria: La chirurgie restauratrice des gros troncs veineux. Etude expérimentale. J. Chir. (Paris) 89 (1965) 47–68

Eufinger, H.: Plastische und Wiederherstellungschirurgie an Venen. Langenbecks Arch. klin. Chir. 313 (1965) 771

Exner, A.: Einige Tierversuche uber Vereinigung und Transplantation von Blutgefäßen. Wiener klin. Wschr. 16 (1903) 273

Fadhli, H. A.: Endvenectomy and decompression in fibrosing mediastinitis causing obstruction of the superior vena cava. J. Thorac. Cardiovasc. Surg. 53 (1967) 881

Fallon, J. T., W. B. Stebens: Venous endothelium of experimental arterio-venous fistula in rabbits. Circulat. Res. 31 (1972) 546 abstract in Vasa 3 (1974) 97

Ferrero, R., C. Mairano: Venous stasis and thrombosis. Angiology 6 (1955) 462

Flanc, C.: An experimental study of the recanalization of arterial and venous thrombi. Brit. J. Surg. 55 (1968) 119

Fonkalsrud, E. W., L. M. Linde, W. P. Longmire: Portal hypertension from idiopathic superior vena caval obstruction. J. Amer. med. Ass. 196 (1966) 129

Fontaine, J.-L., et al.: Fibrinoylse et prothèses artérielles. Actualités Chirurgicales. 74 Congrès Français de Chir. Sept. 1972, Masson Cie 1973

Fontaine, J.-L., G. Foucher, J. C. Plot: Les microanastomoses vasculaires à l'aide d'appareils de suture mécanique. Etude comparative. J. Chir. (Paris) 101 (1971) 315

Fontaine R., Ch. Dubost: Les greffes vasculaires. 56e Congrès Français de Chirurgie, Paris, (4-9 Oct. 1954) Presses Universitaires de France, Paris 1954 (p. 129–205)

Fontaine, R., C. Bollack, M. Kim, R. Kieny: Les prothèses en matière plastique en chirurgie vasculaire. Etat actuel de la question. J. Chir. 75 (1957) 231–248

Fontaine, R., C. Bollack, B. Winnisdoerfer, E. Wolf, B. Briot: Des modifications structurales de l'endothélium veineux sous l'effet de diverses agressions. Lyon Chir. 52 (1956) 229

Forster, E., J. Kunlin, R. Schnoebelen, J. Coblentz, J. Muller: Anastomose porto-cave par greffe veineuse avec suture suspendue à des anneaux. Mém. Acad. Chir. 87 (1961) 797–801

Foster, J. H., P. C. Jolly, P. N. Symbas, W. L. Dively: Vein grafting in Portal Venous system. Arch. Surg. 91 (1965) 716–724

Fraser, R. E., W. L. Halseth, B. Johnson, B. C. Paton: Experimental replacement of the superior vena cava. Autologous veins, free inverted jejunal grafts, and dacron treated with graphite-benzalkonium-heparin. Arch. Surg. 96 (1968) 378

Fujiwara, Y., L. H. Cohn, D. Adams, J. J. Collins: Use of Goretex grafts for replacement of the superior and inferior venae cavae. J. Thorac. Cardiovasc. Surg. 67 (1974) 774

Gaylis, H.: Subcutaneous implantation of varicose veins for future arterial grafting. Surgery 63 (1968) 591

Gerbode, F., J. Yee, F. F. Rundle: Experimental anastomosis of vessels to the heart. Possible application to the superior vena caval obstruction. Surgery 25 (1949) 556–565

Gillot, C.: L'anastomose porto-auriculaire. 68e Congrès Français de Chirurgie. Presses Universitaires de France. Paris 1966 (p. 623)

Gillot, C., J. Mouiel, S. Touboul, Le Guillou: Une plastie polyvalente: le lambeau pédiculé tubulé cave.–69e Congrès Français de Chirurgie. Presses Universitaires de France, Paris 1967 (p. 478)

Gillot, C.: Der lange arterialisierte intervenöse by-pass beim Hund. 6. Jahrestagung Österr. Gesellsch. f. Gefäßchir., Klagenfurt Juni 1973, Karger, Basel 1975

Gillot, C.: Tubulärer Vena Cava Lappen. Studie am Hund. 6. Jahrestagung Österr. Gesellsch. f. Gefäßchir. Klagenfurt 1973, Karger, Basel 1975

Gillot, C., M. Baron, M. Sakka, S. Germa, J. M. Monnier, Vindrinet: Les longs pontages inter-veineux artérialisés chez le chien. Actualités Chirurgicales. 74. Congrès Français de Chirurgie Sept. 1972, I vol. Masson et Cie 1973

Gillot, C., S. Germa, M. Baron, P. Kehr: Les pontages veineux artérialisés. Premiers résultats expérimentaux et cliniques. Actualités Chirurgicales. 73. Congrès Français de Chirurgie Sept. 1971 I volume, Masson et Cie 1972

Gott, V. L., D. A. Koepke, R. L. Dagett, W. Zarnstoff, W. P. Young: The coating of intravascular plastic prostheses with colloidal graphite. Surgery 50 (1961) 382

Gott, V. L., R. I. Leininger, R. D. Falb, M. M. Ameli M. S. Viliathan: In vivo and in vitro evaluation of newer nongraphited heparinized surfaces. Surgery 63 (1968) 60

Gottlob, R., G. Blümel: Über Gefäßwandveränderungen nach Einwirken von Alkylcyanoakrylatklebern. Langenbecks Arch. klin. Chir. 317 (1967a) 160

Gottlob, R., G. Blümel: The toxic action of alkylcyanoacrylate adhesives on vessels. J. surg. Res. 7 (1967b) 362

Gottlob, R., G. Blümel: Anastomoses of small arteries and veins by means of bushings and adhesive. J. cardiovasc. Surg. 9 (1968) 337

Gottlob, R. et al.: 92. Kongreß Deutsch. Gesellsch. f. Chir.: Arch. f. Chir. 1975

Gottlob, R., P. Donas, B. El Nashef: Untersuchungen am Endothel arterialisierter Venen. Vasa 5 (1976) 313

Gottlob, R., G. Zinner: Treatment of venous thrombosis by continuous local infusions of Streptokinase: experimental investigations. J. int. Coll. Surg. 28 (1975) 575

Gottlob, R. G. Zinner: Regeneration geschädigter Endothelien nach hartem und weichem Trauma. Virchows Arch. path. Anat. 336 (1962) 16

Gravens, D. L., et al.: The antibacterial effect of treating sutures with Silver. Surgery 73 (1973) 122

Greenstein, A. J., J. A. Mannick: Comparison of Dacron and vein grafts under conditions of arterial outflow restriction. Amer. J. Surg. 113 (1967) 464

Grillo, H. C., J. Gross: Thermal reconstitution of collagen from solutions and the response to its heterologous implantation. J. surg. Res. 2 (1962) 69

Grode, G. A., S. J. Andersen, H. M. Grotta, R. D. Falb: Northrombotic materials via a simple coating process. Trans. Amer. Soc. Artif. Intern. Organs 15 (1969) 1

Gross, R. E., A. H. Bill, E. C. Peirce: Methods for preservation and transplantation of arterial grafts. Surg. Gynec. Obstet. 88 (1949) 689

Gruenagel, H. H., W. Bernauer, L. Schmidt: Strömungsmessungen bei spleno-renalen und spleno-pulmonalen Anastomosen im Tierexperiment. Langenbecks Arch. klin. Chir. 313 (1965) 939

Gruenagel, H. H., B. Dombres, V. Weber, S. Baumann: Spleno-Pulmonaler Shunt mit autologem Venentransplant beim Hund. Z. ges. exp. Med. 155 (1971) 128

Haering, R., G. Rotthoff, S. Grohme: Langzeitbeobachtungen und histologische Untersuchungen an Gefäß- und Herzwandtransplantaten aus Dünndarm. Langenbecks Arch. klin. Chir. 313 (1965) 664

Haimovici, H., P. W. Hoffert, N. Zinicola, C. Steinman: An experimental and clinical evaluation of grafts in the venous system. Surg. Gynecol. Obstet. 131 (1970) 1173

Haimovici, H., N. Zinicola, M. Noovani, P. W. Hoffert: Vein grafts in the venous system. Arch. Surg. 87 (1963) 542

Hales, M. R., J. H. Scatliff: Thrombosis of the Inferior Vena Cava and Hepatic veins (BUDD-CHIARI syndrome). Ann. intern. Med. 65 (1966) 768

Halpert, B., M. De Bakey, G. L. Jordan, W. S. Henley: The fate of homografts and prostheses of the human aorta. Surg. Gynec. Obstet. 111 (1960) 659

Hambraeus, G., M. A. Andersen: Experimental vena cava replacement with Teflon prosthesis. Arch. Surg. 2 (1962) 221–222

Hart, W., I. Klempa, D. Balser, K. H. Welsch, G. Parrisius: Tierexperimentelle Untersuchungen zum Cavaersatz durch ein gestieltes Dünndarmsegment; Arch. f. Klin. Chir. 325 (1969) 1186

Hasegawa, T., H. Matsumoto, M. Yamamoto, K. Fuse, A. Mizuno, M. Saigusa: Prosthetic replacement of superior vena cava. Anti-platelet-adhesive drug influence. Arch. Surg. 106 (1973) 848

Hasegawa, T., A. Mizuno, H. Matsumoto, K. Fukushima, K. Fuse, H. Saigusa, T. Takamatsu, E. Fukada: Use of copolymer graft developed to serve as venous prosthesis. Surgery 74 (1973) 696

Healy, J. E., R. L. Clark, H. S. Gallagher, P. O'Neill, K. S. Sheena: Nonsuture repair of blood vessels. Ann. Surg. 155 (1962) 817

Healy, J. E.: The use of liquid plastic adhesives in vascular repairs. In: Micro-Vascular Surgery, P. Donaghy, M. G. Yasargil; Thieme, Stuttgart 1967 (p. 63–167)

Hess, H.: Thrombolytische Therapie. Symposium der Deutschen Gesellschaft für Angiologie, München 27–28 Oct. 1966. Schattauer, Stuttgart 1967 (S. 67)

Hiemeyer: cit. in H. Hess 1967

Hobbs, J., J. Davies: Detection of venous thrombosis with ^{131}J labelled fibrinogen in the rabbit. Lancet 2 (1960) 134

Hobson, R. W., R. D. Croom, N. M. Rich: Influence of Heparin and low molecular weight Dextran on the patency of autogenous vein grafts in the venous system. Ann. Surg. 178 (1973) 773

Hobson, R. W., B. Wright: Peripheral side to side arteriovenous fistula. Hemodynamics and application in venous reconstruction. Amer. J. of Surg. 126 (1973) 411

Hoepfner: Langenbecks Archiv f. klin. Chir. 70 (1903) 417

Holt, M. H., F. J. Lewis: Experimental grafts of the superior vena cava with temporary arterio-venous shunts. J. thor. cardiovasc. Surg. 49 (1965) 818–823

Homans: zit. nach. E. A. Edwards, J. E. Edwards 1937

Hufnagel. Ch. A.: Discussion in: Surgery 63 (1968) 60

Humphries, A. W., W. A. Hawk, A. M. Cuthbertson: Arterial prosthesis of collagen-impregnated dacro-tulle. Surgery 50 (1961) 947

Inokuchi, K.: A new type of vessel suturing apparatus. Arch. Surg. 77 (1958) 954

Inokuchi, K.: Stapling device for end-to-side anastomosis of blood vessels. Arch. Surg. 82 (1961) 337–341

Inokuchi, K., A. Kasaba: Alternative device for vascular stapling anastomosis. J. Cardiovascul. Surg. 15 (1974) 458

Inokuchi, K., K. Ono: Experimental venous replacement by transplanted synthetic grafts. Surgery 60 (1966) 862–866

Inou, T., S. Mori, K. Mizuno, K. Ota: A new adhesive for vascular surgery. J. Int. Coll. Surg. 44 (1965) 241

Jaboulay, M., E. Briau: Recherches expérimentales sur la greffe artérielle. Lyon Méd. 81 (1896) 97

Jackson, B. B., S. Graves, J. E. Bryan: Thrombointimectomy for recent venous thrombosis. Surgery 60 (1966) 797–801

Jacobson, J. H.: The development of microsurgical technique. In: Micro-Vascular Surgery, hrsg.; von R. M. P. Donaghy, M. G. Yasargil: Thieme, Stuttgart 1967

Jacobson, J. H., H. T. Katsumura: Small vein reconstruction. J. cardiovasc. Surg. 6 (1965) 157

Jacobson, J. H., T. Reich: Applications of microsurgery in small vessel reconstruction. Special issue devoted to the VIIIth Congress of the Internat. Cardiovasc. Surgery, Vienna. J. cardiovasc. Surg. 10 (1967) 169

Jacobson, J. H., E. L. Suarez: Microsurgery in anastomosis of small vessels. Surg. Forum 11 (1960) 243

Jacobson, J. H., R. A. Moody, B. K. Kusserow, T. Reich, M. C. M. Wang: The tissue response to a plastic adhesive used in combination with microsurgical technic in reconstruction of small arteries. Surgery 60 (1966) 379

Jeger, E., W. Israel: Über Ersetzung eines Stückes der Vena Cava Inferior durch frei transplantierte Vena Jugularis Externa desselben Tieres. Arch. klin. Chir. 100 (1913) 1018 Jensen, G.: Über circuläre Gefäßsutur. Arch. klin. Chir. 69 (1903) 989

Jeger, E.: Die Chirurgie der Blutgefässe und des Herzens. Hirschwald, Berlin 1913. Reprint Springer-Verlag Berlin, Heidelberg, New-York 1973

Jensen, G.: Über circuläre Gefässutur. Arch. f. klin. Chir. 69 (1903) 989

Jiano, J.: Restauration de la veine fémorale par un lambeau saphénien. Analyse dans: J. Chir. 23 (1924) 500

Johns, T. N. P.: A comparison of suture and non suture methods for the anastomosis of veins. Surg. Gynec. Obstet. 84 (1947) 939

Johnson, V., B. Eiseman: Evaluation of arteriovenous shunt to maintain patency of venous autograft. Amer. J. Surg. 118 (1969) 915

Jones, T. W., J. K. Stevenson, J. E. Jesseph, H. N. Harkins: A critical evaluation of polyvinyl sponge (Ivalon) as a vascular and tissue substitute. Ann. Surg. 24 (1958) 401

Jouve, A., J. Vague: La circulation de retour. Masson, Paris 1940

Just-Viera, J. O., G. H. Yeager: Prevention of thrombosis in the inferior vena cava. Surg. Gynec. Obstet. 117 (1963) 271

Just-Viera, J. O., G. H. Yeager: Protection from thrombosis in large veins. Surg. Gynec. Obstet. 118 (1964) 354

Kay: zit. nach L. D. Maclean, C. M. Phibbs, R. S. Flom, J. B. Brainard 1959. Ann. Surg. 149 (1959) 549

Kayser, C.: Physiologie. Les grandes fonctions. Flammarion, Paris 1963

Kilman, J. W., J. A. Waldhusen, H. B. Shumaker: Effects of low molecular weight dextran on peripheral blood flow with controlled cardiac output. Ann. Surg. 166 (1967) 190–194

Klassen, K. P., Andrews, Curtis: Diagnosis and treatment of superior vena cava obstruction. Arch. Surg. 63 (1951) 311–325

Krajicek, M., V. Zastava, M. Chvapil: Collagen-fabric vascular prostheses. Biological and morphological experience. J. surg. Res. 4 (1964) 290–296

Kunlin, J.: Les greffes veineuses. 15e Congrès de la Société Internationale de Chirurgie, Lisbonne, 14–20 Sept. 1953 Edition Société Internationale de Chirurgie, Brüssel 1953a (p. 875–907)

Kunlin, J.: Le rétablissement de la circulation veineuse par greffe en cas d'oblitération traumatique ou thrombophlébitique. Greffe de 18 cm entre la veine saphène interne et la veine iliaque externe. Thrombose après trois semaines de perméabilité. Présenté par R. Leriche. Mém. Acad. Chir. 79 (1953b) 109–110

Kunlin, J.: Techniques de la suture veineuse suspendue (anastomoses ou greffes). Presse méd. 69 (1961) 1917

Kunlin, J.: Long-term results of restorative arterial surgery for arteritis obliterans. Venous grafts. Prostheses. Endarterectomy. Attempts to graft on the tibial arteries with suspended suture. J. cardiovasc. Surg. 5 (1964) 568

Kunlin, J., A. C. Benitte, S. Richard: La suspension de la suture veineuse. Etude expérimentale. Réunion commune de la Soc. Internal. de Chir. et de la Internat. Cardio-Vasc. Society, München 19–20 Sept. 1959. Bull. Soc. int. Chir. 19 (1960) 336–338

Kunlin, J., A. C. Benitte, S. Richard, B. Adam: Sur une nouvelle méthode de suture veineuse. Présentée a la séance du 14 avril 1959 de la Société de Pathologie Comparée. Rev. Path. Gén. 711 (1959) 1061–1064

Kunlin, J., A. Kunlin, S. Richard, T. Trégouet: Le remplacement et l'anastomose latéro-latérale des veines par greffon avec suture suspendue à anneau. Etude expérimentale. J. Chir. 85 (1963) 305-337

Kunlin, J., F. Lengua, S. Richard, T. Trégouet, A. Mourton: Grafting of valvulated veins: an experimental study. J. cardiovasc. Surg. 7 (1966) 520

Kunlin, J., A. Pajot, R. Cohen, R. Caballero, M. Merlat-Guitard, F. Lengua: Greffe de veine cave inférieure avec suture suspendue à un anneau. IIe Congrès Soc. Europ. Chir. Expér., Louvain, Avril 1967. L'Expansion, Paris 1967

Kunlin, J., C. Bitry-Boely, F. Roth, J. Volnie, A. Mandicas, E. Beaudry, J. D. Martinet: Expériences de perfusions supradiaphragmatiques et de circulation extracorporéale totale chez le chien. Rev. Chir. 1952, 237

Kwaan, H., T. Astrup: Fibrinolytic activity in thrombosed veins. Circulat. Res. 17 (1965) 477

Laude, M., J. Kunlin, C. Jaulmes: Les néo-collatérales sur les greffons veineux autoplastiques. Anatomie expérimentale. Lille méd. 9 (1964) 933

Lawler, M. R., J. H. Foster, H. W. Scott: Evaluation of canine intestinal submucosa as a vascular substitute. Amer. J. Surg. 122 (1971) 517

Lazzarini-Robertson, A. A.: Hemodynamic principles and end-to-side vascular anastomoses. Arch. Surg. 82 (1961) 384–386

Leger, L., J. C. Patel, C. Boury: Dérivation veine splénique – vaisseaux pulmonaires par syndrome de Budd-Chiari. Presse méd. 74 (1966) 2017

Leger, L., M. Cachin, J. Auvert, B. Cazes, J.-L. Chevrier, P. Marion, R. Roy-Camille: Symposium sur les indications et les résultats de la chirurgie de l'hypertension portale. J. Chir. 76 (1958) 695–701

Leininger, R. I., M. M. Epstein, R. D. Falb, G. A. Grode, C. W. Cooper: Preparation of non thrombogenic plastic surfaces. Trans. Amer. Soc. artif. intern. Org. 12 (1966) 151

Lejars: Chirurgie des gros troncs veineux. Congrès Français de Chirurgie, Octobre 1906.

Leriche, R.: La vie tissulaire des veines. Presse Médicale 1944 p.243

Leriche, R., A. Jung: Recherches expérimentales sur les oedèmes chirurgicaux des membres d'origine phlébitique. J. Chir. (Paris) 37 (1931) 481

Leshnower, A. C., H. B. Shumacker, A. N. Shariatzadeh: Experimental studies with synthetic venous bypass grafts including a new experimental model. Amer. J. Surg. 128 (1974) 392

Levin, P. M., N. M. Rich, J. E. Hutton, W. F. Barker, J. A. Zeller: Role of arterio-venous shunts in venous reconstruction. Amer. J. Surg. 122 (1971) 183

Lewis, F. J.: High defects of the atrial septum. J. thorac. Surg. 36 (1958) 1–11

Lexer, E.: XVIIe Congrès Allemand de Chirurgie. In: Zbl. Chir. 15 (1913a) 27

3 Anesthesia for Venous Surgery

W. Purtscheller

In the last 11 years we have administered anesthesia to roughly 10,000 patients operated on by May in our hospital for mostly *chronic venous diseases*: varicosities of the lower extremities, and chronic venous occlusion in the pelvis. All these operations were carried out on *inpatients* and under *general anesthesia*.

Conditions for the anesthesiologist are virtually ideal in these cases. As a rule, the patients are middle-aged and usually are not suffering from other serious diseases. Electrolyte imbalances are not anticipated because fasting is brief. The operations are elective, and all preliminary examinations can be completed without pressure.

Normal Procedure

Preliminary Examination

We believe strongly that the preliminary examination should be done by the anesthesiologist himself. In our experience, important information relative to anesthesia is usually incomplete or absent from case histories. Hence, we attempt to get an impression of the general and mental state of the patient by answering the following questions:

—Previous disease: Has the patient ever suffered an unpleasant effect due to an anesthetic?
—Is the patient active in athletics? What is his general capacity?
—Does the patient over use alcohol or nicotine? Does he tolerate alcohol?
—Is he allergic to drugs?
—Does he suffer from insomnia?
—Has the patient taken antihypertensives for some time?
—Has he been treated with corticosteroids?

While these questions are being asked, the clinical examination is begun; the following points are particularly looked for:

—general state (color of skin, edema);
—eyes (glaucoma);
—teeth (prosthesis, loose teeth);
—lungs (bronchial asthma, emphysema, bronchitis);
—heart (limits of heart, rate, rhythm);
—circulation (blood pressure, amplitude);
—abdomen (liver, palpable tumor); and
—extremities (note the extent of varicosities in order to estimate duration of operation).

It is thus possible within a short time to obtain the information required for the performance of an individual anesthetic procedure. Any further investigations can now be requested and therapeutic measures ordered.

Most patients are more apprehensive of the anesthesia than of the operation. It is necessary therefore to relieve their anxiety in order to secure induction without complications and optimal anesthesia. Frequently, brief explanation of the procedure on the day of operation will suffice to eliminate apprehension and to create essential confidence. *Drugs are only adjuvants.*

Preparation

The aim of preparation is to reduce reflex excitability by both psychologic and drug treatment. Whereas the former is initiated by the examination of the anesthesiologist, the latter follows oral administration of a sedative *on the eve of the operation.*

Numerous drugs are available. It must be judged from the history, especially the sleeping habits, of the patient, which drug is the most suitable and what dose will be needed.

In any event, the dose must be adequate for the patient to sleep properly.

We employ two sedatives chiefly, which are given singly or in combination:

—pentobarbital, 100 to 200 mg; and
—chlordiazepoxide, 20 to 40 mg.

Fasting

On the eve of the operation, the patient receives a

light meal of fluids and remains fasting till operation. This 8 to 12 hour fast largely excludes risks and creates optimal conditions for the patient.

Premedication

The patient receives the specific premedication on the day of operation. It must be adapted in composition to his state and to the anesthetic to be used. It consists of an analgesic with sedative action and a parasympatholytic.

Analgesics

Since we employ anesthetics with little analgesic effect, pain reduction is included in the premedication.

Morphine and its derivatives continue to be the most used drugs. The marked analgesic and sedative effect contrasts with the most unpleasant side effects—nausea and vomiting, especially in women.

Morphine:
- —duration of effect, 4 to 6 hours;
- —analgesic peak, $1\frac{1}{2}$ hours after subcutaneous injection, 20 minutes after intravenous;
- —dose, 10 to 20 mg.

Vilan (morphine derivative):
- —duration of effect, 6 to 8 hours;
- —analgesic peak, 30 minutes after subcutaneous injection, 5 minutes after intravenous;
- —better tolerated than morphine, especially by women;
- —dose, 10 to 20 mg.

Both preparations may trigger colic by increasing the tone of the biliary passages in patients with cholelithiasis and should be avoided in those with this history. In their place, the antispasmodic meperidine, 50 to 100 mg, is employed; it is effective for 2 hours.

Parasympatholytic

Most anesthetics have a marked parasympathomimetic effect. Sudden strong vagal stimulation may cause cardiac arrest or ventricular fibrillation owing to interruption of conduction. The views on the necessity of applying a sedative or analgesic for premedication are divided, *but a parasympatholytic must be given.*

We use

Atropine:
- —0.1 mg/kg body weight;
- —depresses cardiac and pulmonary vagus;
- —reduces salivation and mucous secretion;
- —is generally antispasmodic.

Only in patients with increased intraocular pressure is administration of atropine contraindicated.

Time

Morphine and its derivatives cause depression of the respiratory center, which is barely noticeable with small analgesic doses but may cause death by paralysis of the respiratory center when an overdose is given. The peak of the respiration-depressing effect of morphine preparations is reached considerably sooner than that of full analgesia. Since the anesthesia should always begin between the full analgesic phase and already declining respiration-depressing phase of premedication, the injection must be given 90 minutes before anesthesia is induced.

The atropine effect lasts only 2 hours. In order to achieve a reliable effect at the onset of anesthesia, we have in the last few years been injecting atropine intravenously immediately before beginning anesthesia. Thus, atropine cover is safeguarded during the whole operation and the unpleasant dryness of the mouth experienced by many patients with this drug is eliminated.

Drugs of long-lasting or potentiating effect are intentionally avoided for premedication.

Procedure

Among the many possibilities of combinations for up-to-date anesthesia, the method described below has worked well in our hands for some time. It is an attempt to unite simple technique with low toxicity under easy control. There are no unpleasant side effects, and the patient is able to leave his bed soon after surgery for varices (2 hours postoperatively), as we believe to be so important.

Drugs

Following premedication described above, we inject *propanidid*, 250 to 300 mg, within a few seconds intravenously (3 to 7 mg/kg body weight). As soon as hyperventilation due to propanidid sets in, the patient is made to inhale a previously prepared mixture of nitrous oxide and oxygen (2:1) with the addition of initially 3 vol per cent halothane and a total flow of 6 to 8 liters per minute for maintenance.

When the hyperventilation wears off, artificial ventilation is applied. The primary halothane

concentration is retained for a maximum of 3 minutes and slowly reduced to a maintenance dose of approximately 1 vol per cent halothane and a total flow of 3 to 4 liters per minute.
In order to keep the anesthesia as superficial as feasible, the required muscle relaxation is obtained with Curarin-Asta, d-tubocurarine, tubocurarine chloride (15 to 20 mg) or alcuronium chloride (10 to 15 mg), which is injected after hyperventilation has ceased.
In this manner, correct depth of the anesthesia is achieved after a short period, reinjection of propanidid or analgesics is not necessary and, with some experience, the adjusted halothane concentration can be left till the end of the operation.
After discontinuance of halothane and artificial ventilation, spontaneous breathing usually follows quickly and decurarization (with neostigmine and atropine in the usual manner) is only rarely required.

Side Effects

Propanidid. The rapid injection we prefer is always followed by a slight drop in blood pressure and erratic increase of the pulse rate.
Both alterations are transient and last up to 2 minutes. Increased heart minute volume and decreased stroke volume produced by this augmented rate likewise return to normal within this period.
Local vascular tolerance is satisfactory; we have not seen allergic or anaphylactic reactions on repeated anesthesia of the same patient.

Halothane. Halothane-induced hypotension and bradycardia certainly depend on concentration. Opinions about the cause vary. All pathways (effect on peripheral vascular musculature, on ganglia of the autonomic nervous system and on myocardium) were tested and confirmed. However, it is of practical significance that the drop in blood pressure can immediately be stopped by reduction or interruption of the halothane supply. Vasopressors were never required.

Ventilation

We use a semiclosed system with carbon dioxide absorption and apply intermittent positive-pressure respiration manually. Normally, intubation is not necessary for surgery on varices; free air passages are practically always attainable by means of a gag.
Conditions differ with surgery for occlusions in the pelvis, in which case intubation is indicated because of the longer duration of the operation.

Infusion

In our experience, intraoperative infusions are required only for operations on veins in the pelvic region.

Surveillance

Repeated checks of blood pressure and close clinical observation of the patient during anesthesia suffice for surveillance in this type of surgery.

Position

Surgery on the *great saphenous vein* and the *Palma operation* are carried out with the patient recumbent with slight abduction of the limb to be operated on and do not present any problems in positioning.
Surgery on the *small saphenous*, however, is performed with the patient prone. Firm bolsters of suitable size placed under both clavicles facilitate respiratory excursions and allow the head to be turned to permit fitting of the breathing mask. Any pressure on the eye must be avoided since occlusion of the central artery of the retina may be followed by blindness. The upper extremities should be in such a position that the forearms are in pronation with the elbows bent and rest on padded splints at the side of the patient.

Aftertreatment

On termination of the operation, the patient is generally fully responsive and able to actively help when transferred to his bed. He should get up 2 hours after surgery for varices and walk about aided by a nurse. After surgery on veins in the pelvis, bed rest is required for a few days. Analgesic tablets or suppositories are adequate; alkaloids are superfluous. The patient begins a liquid diet on the evening of the operation.

Anesthesia for Venothrombectomy

For the anesthesiologist, the main problem in local and general anesthesia for thrombectomy is the risk of preoperative pulmonary embolism.

We have considered this problem in detail and exchanged views with Brunner and Nachbur during a symposium (see May, 1971).
The view we expressed there was: "Many surgeons are of opinion that removal of a thrombus is considerably facilitated by raising the pressure in the vena cava, and in many cases, without that, removal would not be feasible at all. Active cooperation of the patient during this operation is essential and it should therefore be carried out only under local anesthesia.
"We have seen curves in which pressure in the vena cava had markedly been raised by pressing.
"In our experience, difficulties are repeatedly encountered in convincing patients of the suitability of local anesthesia; they insist on general anesthesia."
What are the options open to the anesthesiologist in the course of general anesthesia in order to attain an effective increase of pressure in the area of the vena cava? It is understandable that such an increase requires changes of pressure in the respiratory system. First, it must be considered that for the hemodynamic effect of artificial ventilation, it is not positive-pressure respiration that is decisive, but the mean intrapulmonary pressure or, since this is not always measurable, mean positive-pressure respiration.
We have made these measurements in a great number of patients. The great saphenous vein was dissected during surgery for varices under local anesthesia, a catheter was introduced into the vena cava under radiologic control and the patient was requested to press (Fig. 3.1, B). Anesthesia was then induced intravenously and the patient was intubated. The anesthesia was continued with a mixture of nitrous oxide–oxygen–halothane. Artificial ventilation was automatically performed with a Blease-Pulmoflat. Initially, artificial ventilation was carried out during anesthesia with normal values between +10 and −5 cm H_2O (Fig. 3.1, C).
As the operation proceeded, the positive-pressure respiration was augmented to maximal values, between +30 to +50 cm H_2O. Pressure thus rose in the vena cava (Fig. 3.1, D).
When respiratory pressure was reduced to maximally negative values, between −5 and −10 cm H_2O, the pressure in the vena cava dropped (Fig. 3.1, E).
It is clear that these maximal pressure amplitudes of the respiratory system are permitted only in young patients with healthy lungs and only for a brief period. Another way of producing an effective but uncoordinated pressure increase for a short time is by manipulating the endotracheal tube under superficial anesthesia, thus causing activation of the cough reflex and pressing by the patient (Fig. 3.1, F).
Thus, the rise in pressure is markedly greater than that produced by maximally increasing positive-pressure respiration, but considerably lower than that achieved with active participation of the patient.
The statement of Brunner during the symposium mentioned earlier should be cited: "Some measurements confirm the chief argument of the protagonists of local anesthesia, namely, that under Valsalva conditions the pressure in the superior cava and the pelvic veins rises approximately five times more than it does under high-pressure respiration with raised terminal expiratory pressure (+15 cm H_2O). Thus, a maximal pressure gradient as compared with

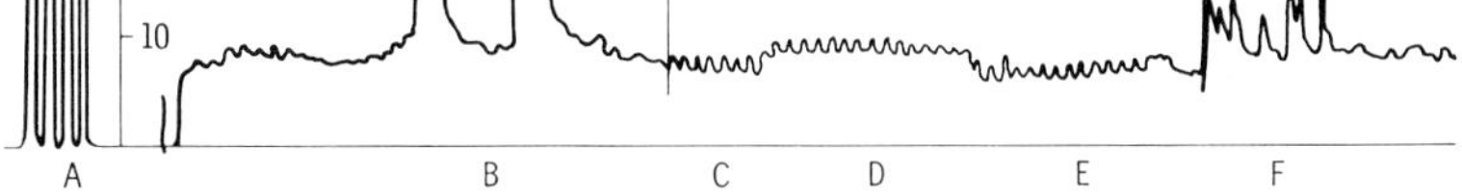

Fig. 3.1 Measurement of pressure in the vena cava. The catheter was pushed into the cava via the saphenous vein.

A Calibration deflections
B Patient carries out Valsalva maneuver under local anesthesia twice
C Patient under general anesthesia receiving normal artifical ventilation via a tracheal tube
D With respiratory pressure raised to maximal values, venous pressure rises by 2 mm Hg
E With respiratory pressure reduced to maximally negative values, venous pressure drops by 1 mm Hg as compared with normal artificial ventilation
F Manipulations of the tracheal tube cause activation of the cough reflex and pressing in the patient, and pressure in the vena cava is thus raised

atmospheric pressure obtains at the moment of active pressing in the venous system opened by subinguinal venotomy; this ought to prevent a thrombus from being washed centrally and help to wash it outward. This procedure naturally requires cooperation by the patient, which is not always guaranteed in emergencies. However, we noticed on repeated probing with the extraction balloon that the patient was rapidly exhausted under local anesthesia and pressed increasingly insufficiently. After discontinuing abdominal pressure, we demonstrated, on deep inspiration, a brief pressure gradient from the periphery toward the center, which in practice could suck in a thrombus to the center."

On the other hand, in general anesthesia the patient is spared unpleasant and frequently painful sensations of surgery that may occur under local anesthesia. Dissection of a scarred vein from its gelatinous surrounding is time-consuming, and a single probing with the extraction catheter is usually inadequate for complete clearance of pelvic veins. The rise in venous pressure under high-pressure respiration is indeed lower but it can be applied in exact amounts for some time and can be reduced slowly without the risk of suction.

In the anti-Trendelenburg position, a hydrostatic pressure of approximately 10 cm H_2O is added to the venous pressure produced by the Valsalva maneuver and high-pressure respiration. This hydrostatic pressure rise is especially important in view of the minor pressure rise due to end-expiratory high-pressure respiration. The sum of the end-expiratory high-pressure and the hydrostatic pressure is in our opinion sufficient to prevent pulmonary embolism.

Pulmonary embolism is less damaging to the circulation during general anesthesia than under local anesthesia because of the depression of vegetative functions.

The combination of anti-Trendelenburg position and raised end-expiratory pressure may affect the circulation unfavorably (decrease of minute volume). If hypovolemia is superimposed, the blood flow may be endangered. Therefore, the circulation must be strictly controlled under these conditions of anesthesia, and hypovolemia avoided at any price.

From comparison of the advantages and disadvantages, we are convinced that intubation anesthesia under high-pressure respiration in the anti-Trendelenburg position during the critical moments of extraction is an adequate method of anesthesia for thrombectomy.

Nachbur, discussing the thrombectomy procedure used at the highly expert clinic of Senn in Bern, expressed a different opinion at the above-mentioned symposium: "In order to banish the danger of propagating clots into the lesser circulation during manipulation with the balloon catheter, it is desirable or even necessary to produce a 'backflow' if possible. In this manner, it is hoped that the loosened clot will be washed not toward the heart but retrogradely to the venotomy. On the one hand, throttling and slowing of venous return is produced by raising the hydrostatic pressure and tilting the operating table into a steep anti-Trendelenburg position. Another considerable increase of venous pressure or 'backflow' follows application of active abdominal pressure. For this reason, local anesthesia is preferred for iliofemoral thrombectomy, since, with active cooperation of the patient, a notably higher rise in pressure can be attained than when insufflation anesthesia by overinflating the lungs is used, as will be shown."

It is evident, therefore, that many roads lead to Rome, even if they run in opposite directions. We agree with the view of Widmer (1971), who says that the curves are naturally correct but that the Valsalva maneuver can be maintained for only a few seconds, whereas the critical phase of operation lasts about 10 minutes. Hence, we now perform *thrombectomy under general anesthesia*.

Two further aspects appear to us of particular importance:

—The risk of preoperative pulmonary embolism should not be forgotten. For this reason, we intubate on principle.

—Replacement of blood is essential since blood loss may amount to 600 ml, according to our own studies.

Anesthesia in Pulmonary Embolism

If pulmonary embolism is suspected, the anesthesiologist must act as if this diagnosis were established. In the first, usually dramatic moment, exact diagnosis is often not available. Primary requirements are *immediate intubation* and artificial ventilation with oxygen. The responsible physician is then in a position to decide whether confirmation of the diagnosis by angiography is necessary. In our hospital, the patient is transferred under artificial ventilation to the operating room immediately and, conditions permitting, streptokinase is infused, without laboratory tests. If the patient does not recover within 1 hour, a Trendelenburg operation is carried out.

The anesthesiologist must be prepared to treat

cardiac arrest, and should have a defibrillator with external and internal electrodes, metaproterenol sulfate, calcium and digitalis at hand. However, application of these measures is appropriate and promising only after complete removal of the embolus.

Once cerebral circulation is sufficiently stabilized that consciousness and pain sensation return during the operation, a mixture of nitrous oxide and oxygen, possibly with relaxation, suffices for thoracic closure. But management of the postoperative course requires great care. The main problems are *metabolic acidosis* due to shock or cardiac arrest, renal shutdown and respiratory insufficiency.

Tracheotomy and prolonged artificial ventilation for avoidance of postoperative hypoventilation considerably aid the function of the heart damaged by hypoxia. Tris buffer solutions for elimination of the metabolic acidosis can be given during artificial ventilation without risk of respiratory depression.

References

Brunner, U.: Hämodynamische Vergleiche zwischen Preßatmung (Valsalva) und Überdruckbeatmung. In: Meßmethoden in der Venenchirurgie. R. May (ed.). Huber, Bern 1971 (S. 174)

May, R.: Meßmethoden in der Venenchirurgie. Huber, Bern 1971

Nachbur, B.: Druckmessungen in den Beckenvenen. In: Meßmethoden in der Venenchirurgie. R. May (ed.). Huber, Bern 1971

Purtscheller, W.: Druckmessungen in den Beckenvenen. In: Meßmethoden in der Venenchirurgie. R. May (ed.). Huber, Bern 1971

Widmer, L.: Diskussion Part VI. In: Meßmethoden in der Venenchirurgie. R. May (ed.). Huber, Bern 1971

4 Varicose Veins

R. May

In this chapter only the surgery of primary, essential, constitutional varicose veins will be dealt with. For surgery of secondary varicose veins, varicose veins concomitant with damaged deep veins see page 139f, 144f.

Sclerotherapy or Operation, Definition

We operate only for marked actual incompetence of the great or small saphenous vein. If solely individual perforating veins are incompetent, these are ligated separately. We apply strict criteria and reject so-called prophylactic operation for commencing or slight incompetence of the veins since the great and small saphenous veins have become so important for bypass operations in the reconstruction of leg and coronary arteries that a not strictly indicated removal of these veins may be a great disservice to the patient.

Indications for Operation

1. Patient's complaints, especially sensation of heaviness. But: If the patient complains of serious discomfort, we always have a thorough orthopedic examination carried out, particularly of the vertebral column. Varicose veins do not cause much trouble and never cause calf cramps at night.
2. Cosmetic indication.
3. Complications of varicose veins: rupture, hemorrhage, thrombophlebitis, varicose eczema, periphlebitic infiltration, particularly in the distal portion of the leg, leg ulcers. Also, recent thrombophlebitis of varicose veins is *no* contraindication!

Contraindications to Operation

1. General diseases: The question of operability of a patient with hypertension, diabetes, cardiac disease, etc, should in each case be considered only after consultation with the attending physician.
2. Chronic occlusion of arteries: Before every operation for varicosities it is established whether the arterial circulation of the limb is normal; this is recorded in the patient's case history. Chronic arterial occlusion is a contraindication to surgery. Complaints thus produced are attributed by the patient to incidentally existing varicose veins. Furthermore, wound healing is at risk.
3. Edema: The cause of edema must be elicited before operation in every case. In principle, all patients with a tendency to edema of the lower extremities are examined by phlebography of the deep leg and pelvic veins, even if the history does not reveal any thrombosis. In addition to post-thrombotic injuries, e.g. venous valves may congenitally be absent. Uncomplicated primary varicosities and large incompetent perforating veins in the distal portion of the leg never lead to edema. In the case of entirely normal deep veins, chronic inflammation of subcutaneous tissues in the presence of incompetent perforating veins causes only local swelling. If the phlebogram shows that the deep veins are normal, the swellings are eliminated by pressure: large pads of foam rubber are applied over the infiltration and retained by bandages. Bed rest is not required. This treatment frequently lasts for many months. We consider it important to operate only after the inflammation has fully subsided.
4. Lymphedema: Attention is paid, especially in younger patients, during the preliminary examination to a slight, frequently unilateral swelling of the forefoot. It may be a sign of a commencing primary lymphedema. For clarification, staining of the lymphatics with patent blue is undertaken in these cases on principle: 0.5 ml of a 2.5% or 11% solution of patent blue is injected subcutaneously proximal to the 1st and 2nd interdigital web. If a commencing lymphedema is present, a blue

spot soon develops. If the lymphatics are normal, one to three blue lymphatic vessels become distinct on the dorsum of the foot after 30 minutes. Any lymphedema deteriorates considerably following operation for varices. The impression is gained that a just compensated congenital lymphedema regularly goes wrong irreparably due to surgery.

5. Age: By and large, age, even above 70 years, is no contraindication if the patient is still physically active.
6. Pregnancy: In the first few months, pregnancy presents no objective contraindication to surgery of varicose veins. According to our experience, cosmetic results, and particularly scars, are not satisfactory during pregnancy. Therefore, we prefer to wait till four months after delivery, on principle. Only for varicose ulcers, local ligatures of the perforating veins are performed under local anesthesia. Ruptured, bleeding varicose veins in pregnancy are locally sclerosed.
7. Obesity: Even considerable overweight does not promote formation of varices and would thus not present an objection to surgery. Nevertheless, preoperative weight reduction is prescribed, as a rule. Postoperative discomfort will be less.
8. Menstruation: The operation is performed also during menstruation.
9. The "pill": Discontinuation of the "pill" prior to operation does not appear to us to be necessary.
10. Infections: All febrile diseases should have subsided for at least one month before surgery. All suppurative foci, e.g., furuncles, should be healed at least two months before surgery.

Operation Technique

Every operation for varicose veins is based on the fact that the superficial and the deep venous system are separated by the fascia as by a wall that does not permit any communication by collateral routes. The only possible junction is via the perforating veins whose valvular arrangement allows blood flow from surface to depth only. Wherever these perforating veins are incompetent and the blood flows in the opposite direction, that is from deep to superficial, pressure waves from the deep veins are transmitted to the superficial venous system. Hence, all these sites have to be interrupted by ligature, flush to the deep vein. Any incompetent great or small saphenous vein is practically only an incompetent perforating vein.

Therefore, as Cockett repeatedly stressed with justification, every operation consists of two sections.

1. Flush ligature of every incompetent perforating or incompetent great saphenous vein.
2. Resection of superficial veins = stripping of main trunks in addition to extraction of varicose branches.

A varicose relapse in the first postoperative years means: the above two conditions have not been carried out exactly at some point.

We hold saphenous ligature by itself with subsequent obliteration of varices to be a completely insufficient method.

We perform a separate preoperative phlebography of the superficial veins as a routine measure, independent of the radiography of the deep veins, even if this examination is not necessary in many cases. The intact deep venous system has previously been elucidated by roentgenograms when necessary. The technique of the radiologic examination is described below in the chapter "Ligature of Perforating Veins". As soon as the radiographs have been taken, and while still in the radiology department, the varicosities are marked on the standing patient by the surgeon together with the radiologist and the perforating veins indicated by small circles.

Marking Solution

Pyrogallic acid	2.5
Acetone	25.0
Ferric chloride solution 50%	20.0
Alcohol	ad 50.0

Ligation of the Great Saphenous Vein in the Groin

Position: The patient is supine, the limb is slightly flexed in hip and knee joint and slightly everted.

The skin incision: In principle, the skin incision is aimed at providing optimal approach. In addition, location and direction should produce a cosmetically acceptable scar. A third factor is essential during the incision: the lymphatics must be damaged as little as possible. The prefascial bundle of the lymphatic vessels is always at risk during the stripping of the great saphenous vein.

Grave lymphedema due to surgery for varicosities is rare. But we have carried out very careful checkups following operations for varicose veins! Time and again, mild swelling of the leg was found even years after the operation. This slight swelling, as demonstrated by staining of lymphatics, is almost exclusively caused by damage to lymphatic vessels. Formerly, about one per cent of patients developed erysipelas years after operation. These also are due to surgical injury of the lymphatics. The *ventromedial prefascial bundle of the lymphatic vessels* is a main drain of lymph. Brunner showed that this bundle accompanies the great saphenous vein like a sheaf. Above all, it is important that these collecting tubules are gathered in groin and medial area of the knee joint, whereas they unfold in leg and thigh. See Fig. 4.1.

Even sharp dissection of the long saphenous vein in the groin or a large skin incision around the knee joint may cause permanent damage to lymphatic drainage. In regions where the lymphatics course wider apart, injuries are less serious. Here, the bundle itself may compensate, or drainage follows via the dorsolateral bundle, as Brunner showed.

Thus, the skin incision in the groin must be so directed that the bottleneck of the lymphatics in the groin is largely left undamaged.

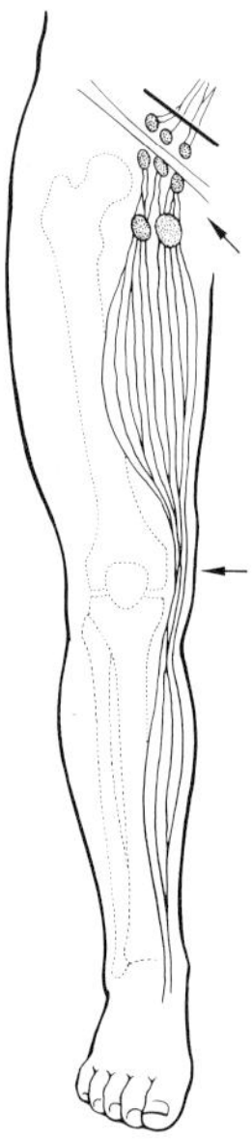

Fig. 4.1. The ventromedial prefascial bundle of the lymphatic vessels with the two bottlenecks at the level of the knee joint and the groin, after Brunner. Skin incision of Brunner.

Therefore, we recommend incising the skin according to Brunner one fingerbreadth *proximal* to the groin. The index finger of the left hand rests on the pulsating artery. That is, the incision runs parallel with the groin. It is usually 5–6 cm in length. A small incision of 2–3 cm does not permit a clear view and may thus be dangerous. A very large incision of 8 and 10 cm is generally superfluous. But the beginner is well advised to make his incision rather too large. It is no accident that many well experienced vascular surgeons revert to large incisions in the course of years. In the case of very obese patients, the incision is made directly in the groin. The skin and subcutaneous tissues are divided and two blunt hooks are inserted. The superficial fascia is split. The assistant pulls strongly at the distal hook. The surgeon displaces the tissues under the fascia distally with a small gauze swab. As soon as the first vein is exposed, dissection continues along this vein with a blunt curved clamp. It is followed up to its junction with the femoral vein. As soon as this is visualized, it is exposed ventrally and medially; all venous branches are thus automatically exposed. Frequently, the external pudendal artery courses above these just short of the union with the great saphenous vein. It is carefully dissected, divided, and ligated. The great saphenous vein must be double ligated on principle. Stump bleeding, which might become highly dangerous, is then impossible. I advise every surgeon to inject 0.3 ml 2.5% or 11% solution of patent blue between 1st and 2nd and 2nd and 3rd toes proximal to the interdigital fold.

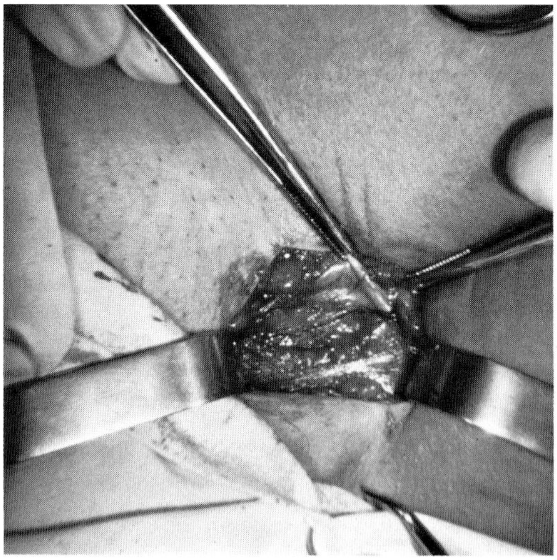

Fig. 4.2. The great saphenous vein has been drawn aside with a clamp just below the junction. The underlying stained lymphatic is visible.

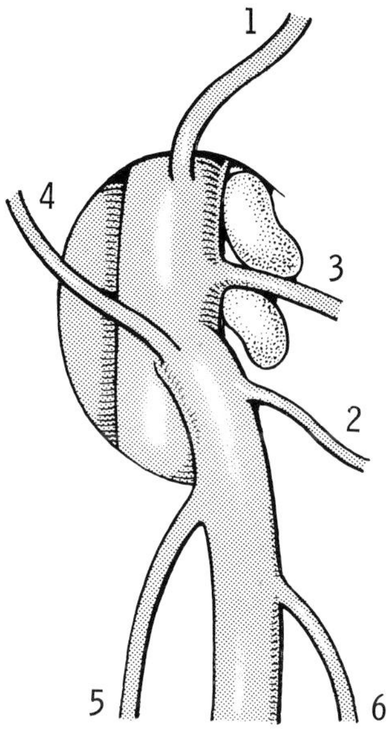

Fig. 4.3. Diagram of the normal ramification of the great saphenous vein and its branches at its union with the femoral vein.
1. Superficial epigastric vein
2. Superficial external pudendal vein
3. Deep external pudendal vein
4. Superficial circumflex iliac vein
5. Lateral superficial femoral vein = lateral accessory saphenous vein
6. Medial superficial femoral vein

The lymphatics alongside the great saphenous vein will be stained by the time of the operation.

The surgeon receives an impressive object lesson why he is to dissect bluntly and how close to the great saphenous vein the lymphatics lie.

The figure shows the normal ramification of the great saphenous vein and its branches. This normal type hardly occurs in practice. Hilty published a monograph on the variations of the branches. The great saphenous vein may also occur double or triple. In addition: The femoral artery may lie subcutaneously. We have encountered the artery medial to the femoral vein. The femoral vein may apparently be twofold due to high junction with the profunda femoris vein. This explains repeated reports of injury to the artery, erroneous ligature of the femoral vein, but it does not excuse them. We advise the precept: After exposure, the great saphenous vein and its branches may only be ligated

1. if the pulsating artery has been palpated beyond doubt;
2. once the anterior and medial aspect of the femoral vein is clearly visualized. Circular dissection of the vein is superfluous and dangerous.

Once the anterior and medial aspect of the deep vein is exposed, not only every small branch of the great saphenous vein is visualized but also those branches that leave the femoral vein directly. Any branch of the great saphenous vein can flow straight into the femoral vein; particularly the superficial circumflex iliac and the epigastric veins. The deep external pudendal vein almost regularly joins the femoral vein medially and is repeatedly overlooked not only by beginners. If even one small branch remains, ugly relapses occur. The branches are not simply ligated, but are dissected as far as feasible, drawn forward, and ligated. Small branches are avulsed. Many surgeons ease their task of searching for the great saphenous vein by introducing a stripper into it in the ankle region and sliding it toward the groin. But I should like to warn of an anatomic variant: the low termination of the great saphenous a handbreadth distal to the fossa ovalis (see Fig. 1.13).

In this case, the stripper slides into the femoral vein at the area of operation. The surgeon sees the branches which ramify from the femoral vein at the typical site and ties the femoral vein erroneously. We also advise against introducing the stripper before ligature of the great saphenous vein in the groin is concluded for another reason. Particularly following phlebography, fresh thrombi repeatedly form in the great saphenous vein and these may be propelled into the pelvic veins. Ligation of the great saphenous must always be the first act.

The great saphenous vein is tied flush at the femoral vein. No strong pull is to be exerted at the great saphenous since constriction of the deep veins may ensue.

It may happen even to an experienced surgeon that a small tear occurs in the very thin-walled femoral vein during this preparation. This is recognized at once by very dark, almost black blood oozing from this vein. It is a grave error to try to stop the hemorrhage with a clamp for gross injuries not only of the deep vein but also of the artery follow. The assistant applies pressure to the tear. The surgeon should enlarge the incision and order a vessel suture. The assistant prepares the vein with a broad hook. As soon as the assistant releases the pressure, the blood is aspirated. The surgeon can then easily repair the tear with a fine U-suture without using forceps or even clamp. If one follows the suggestion of Fischer of slightly revolving the stump of the great saphenous beforehand, the suture has a better chance of success.

Distal Exposure of the Great Saphenous Vein

Contrary to the habit of most surgeons, we do not expose the great saphenous vein at the medial side of the internal malleolus but 3 cm *distal* to it on the inner aspect of the dorsum according to Fischer. The cosmetic result is better. It makes no difference whether the incision is transverse or longitudinal.

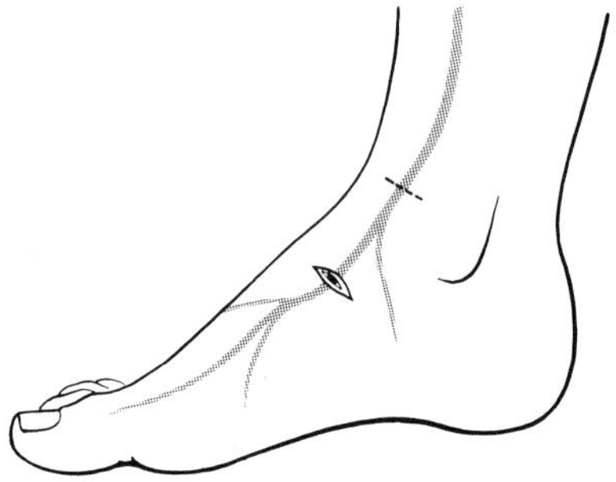

Fig. 4.4. Incision for exposure of the distal end of the great saphenous vein, after Fischer.

Stripping

Among the various strippers, no manufacturer can be given preference. It is not the stripper that is decisive but the surgeon. The only important point is that the cable of the stripper must not be too rigid. It ought to be flexible and elastic, and should revert to its normal shape automatically after use. Many strippers do not fulfill this important requirement. A series of strippers with exchangeable heads of different shapes should be available to the surgeon. The shape itself is not very important nor do we consider a disposable stripper a great improvement.

Direction of stripping: Lately, publications have become available that prove that cutaneous nerves and lymphatics are better preserved on stripping from proximal to distal. This is correct. Therefore, we also extract from proximal to distal. We always introduce the stripper distally. If it is carefully pushed forward and constantly revolved, it can mostly be brought into the groin. A head is now screwed on in place of the guide tip, and the vein is tied to the stripper. The suture remains long. The vein is then extracted from proximal to distal. If, despite cautious turning, the stripper cannot be extracted proximalward in its whole length, we prefer to make a counter-incision. These counter-incisions should be only large enough to just permit passage of the stripper head.

Important:

1. The head of the stripper must not be too large, otherwise subcutaneous fat will also be removed. This is a mistake, as lymphatic vessels and cutaneous nerves are certainly contained in this fat.
2. The head must not be too small, otherwise the vein will be slit and venous tissue remains. Since these venous residues may be connected with branches and incompetent perforating veins, relapses will follow. Removal of these residues requires additional incisions that may be kept extremely small. Pierced veins can also be removed with an *external ring stripper*. If at all practical, additional incisions in the knee region should be avoided.

Extract with caution and slowly. The left index should continually follow the head of the stripper during extraction. If a branch is noticed to be tense, it is not torn away. A minute stab incision of 2–3 mm is made over the tensed vein with a fine, pointed scalpel, and this branch is caught. It is followed up with a long, narrow, slightly curved clamp and extracted. In this way, hematomas are kept to a minimum.

Removal of Branches

Branches have been marked preoperatively. They must be carefully removed by operation. Only very small branches are sclerosed later. Branches are exposed by minute stab incisions with a small, pointed scalpel. These incisions ought not to exceed 4 mm even for larger varices. Mostly, 3 mm is adequate. The vein is caught with a delicate clamp. The vein is followed with a long, slightly curved clamp till a new incision is required. If the incision is kept very small by using delicate instruments, the number of incisions need not be considered as they become practically invisible later. In any case, blind burrowing in subcutaneous tissues with coarse instruments from large incisions is to be avoided as lymphatics and nerves are unnecessarily destroyed in this way and the cosmetic result will be poor.

Ligation of the Lesser Saphenous Vein

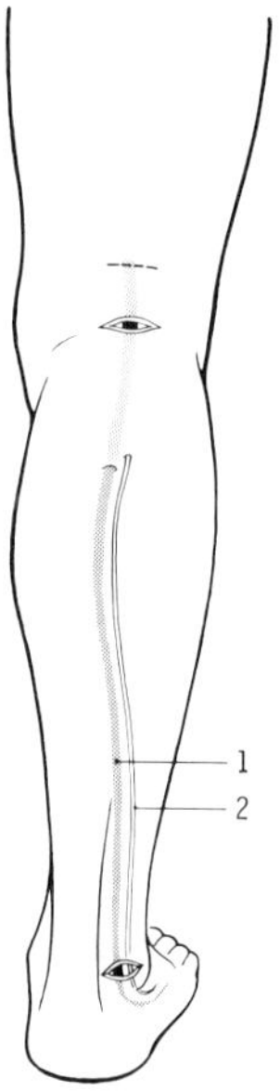

Fig. 4.5. Incisions for exposure and stripping of the lesser saphenous vein.

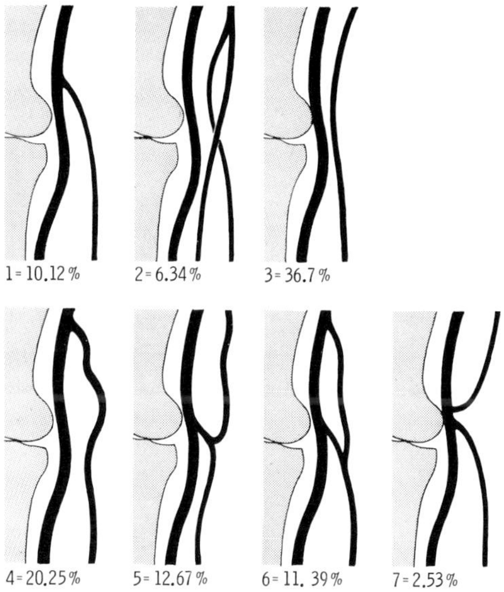

Fig. 4.6. Diagram of the seven typical variants of the lesser saphenous vein.

Position: The patient lies prone, the limb is rotated slightly inward, the foot end of the operating table is slightly raised.

Ligature of the lesser saphenous vein is performed on the same principles as for the greater saphenous vein; namely, close to the popliteal or the deep vein into which it flows. We refer to the diagram of variants of the lesser saphenous junction, and Figs. 1.23, 1.24 and 1.25.

If feasible, preoperative phlebography should establish which of the seven possible variants is present; particularly important is the fact that the lesser saphenous does not always flow into the popliteal vein. Roentgenograms of the junction of the lesser saphenous is generally successful if the radiologist injects the contrast medium into a branch of the lesser saphenous vein, with the table slightly tilted, taking the pictures under television control. Nevertheless, it is possible that the junction of the lesser saphenous vein may not be exactly demonstrated.

In particular, the junction of the femoropopliteal with the lesser saphenous vein should be visualized on the x-ray film. If this is not clear, we apply radiography to the lesser saphenous junction during the operation according to Gillot. After exposure of the lesser saphenous vein in the popliteal fossa, a catheter is introduced into the vein for 1 cm and 20 ml contrast medium are injected. The plate lies under knee joint and thigh. The picture is taken when almost all of

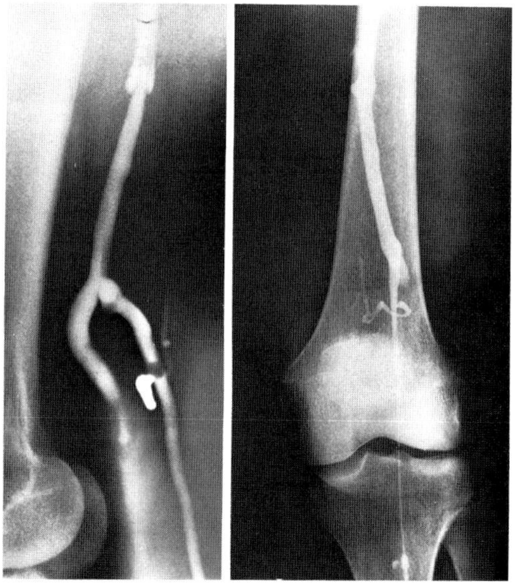

Fig. 4.7. High junction of the lesser saphenous vein, type IV
Left: ascending phlebography
Right: intraoperative phlebography after Gillot.

the contrast medium has been injected. This prolongs the operation only a little and permits exact ligature of the lesser saphenous and femoropopliteal veins from small, cosmetically unobjectionable incisions.

Technique of Ligation of the Lesser Saphenous Vein

The course of the vein has been marked on the standing patient preoperatively. A transverse incision, 2–3 cm in length, is made exactly in the flexion fold of the popliteal fossa. After division of the subcutaneous fat, the fascia is exposed. It is split bluntly and transversely in the direction of the fibers, and can thus later be closed by a single suture. The lesser saphenous vein is now exposed. It is dissected free and clamps are applied. The seven variants of junction require three variations of operation:

1. The radiograph shows that the lesser saphenous flows into the popliteal slightly proximal to the skin incision. In this case, the vein is dissected as far as the popliteal vein and is ligated close to the deep vein. Care should be taken that the ligature is proximal to the junction with the femoropopliteal. The femoropopliteal vein is caught separately and dissected proximally as far as practicable, and then ligated.
2. See Fig. 4.7. The radiograph reveals a high junction of the lesser saphenous with the popliteal vein. Nevertheless, the first incision is always level with the popliteal fold. Here, the suture becomes practically invisible later. The vein is taken up from this incision and divided between two clamps. If a pull is exerted at the proximal clamp, the second proximal skin incision can be kept quite small, although at this site the vein lies very deep under a thick layer of fat and the fascia. This is important since otherwise this incision leaves an ugly scar.
3. The radiograph shows that the lesser saphenous does not flow into the popliteal vein. A stripper is introduced into the lumen of the vein and pushed proximally. The tip of the stripper is palpated subcutaneously, and the vein can be exposed directly at the junction with the great saphenous vein, tied, and removed together with the stripper. If the femoropopliteal vein is very varicose, it is similarly followed up as far as possible and extracted.

Stripping of the Lesser Saphenous Vein

If the radiograph has shown that a marked *gastrocnemius point,* an incompetent perforating vein between the lesser saphenous and gastrocnemius vein exists, this is also visible on the erect patient as a globular protuberance of the vein. This is first exposed by a small skin incision and the perforating vein is caught and ligated immediately at the entry into the musculature by oversewing.

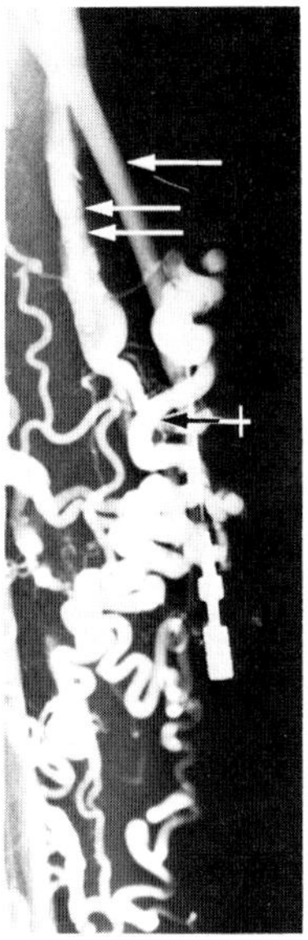

Fig. 4.8. The varicose convolution drains equally into the incompetent lesser saphenous vein ⟶ and gastrocnemius vein ⇉ The communication with the gastrocnemius vein must also be ligated ⟶+⟶

Stripping of the lesser saphenous vein is frequently complicated by injury to the sural nerve. The sequel is a troublesome, irreversible paresthesia at the lateral margin of the foot. The sural nerve is in close contact with the vein only in the region of the lateral malleolus. There are two possibilities of avoiding damage to it. A longitudinal incision of 3 cm is made at the distal end of the lesser saphenous between lateral malleolus and Achilles tendon, and the vein is freed carefully from the closely apposed nerve prior to stripping. This is the safest method. But a longitudinal incision of 3 cm is not always cosmetically acceptable.
Our procedure: We expose the vein by a small transverse incision between Achilles tendon and external malleolus. The vein is caught between two clamps and ligated distally. A pull is exerted at the proximal clamp and the nerve stump is

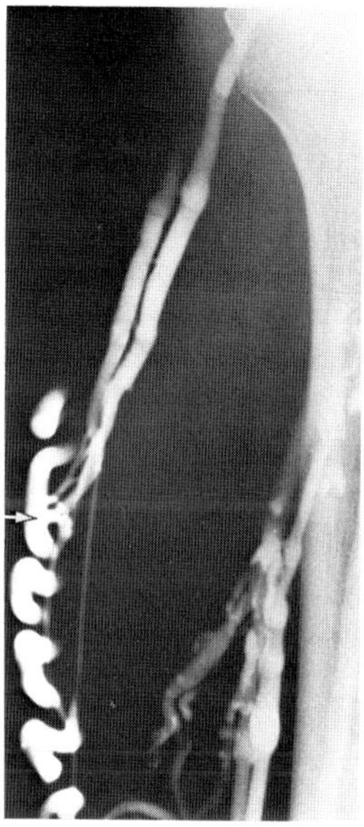

Fig. 4.9. Gastrocnemius point: the varices drain exclusively into the gastrocnemius veins.

cautiously pushed away as far as the incision allows. The vein is then extracted according to the principle from proximal to distal with the smallest stripper head. The extraction must be performed particularly slowly and carefully. Frequently, strong, varicose communicating veins to the greater saphenous become tense. They are not torn off but exposed by minute stab incisions and followed up to the greater saphenous vein.

Ligation of Perforating Veins

Skin Incision—Direction of Incision

The plastic surgeon knows the maxim: "Turn your knife seven times before you cut the Langer lines." This is not quite correct. Important are not the tension lines described by Langer in 1864 but the skin creases described by Pinkers in 1924, relaxed skin tension lines. Plastic surgeons actually mean these lines and pay attention to them, even if they incorrectly speak of Langer lines.
However, for ligation of perforating veins and exposure of large varicose branches we do not adhere to these lines. The skin incisions for **exposure of the greater saphenous vein have** already been discussed. The most correct incisions for exposure of perforators and large varicose convolutions are longitudinal incisions. However, comparative examinations have shown that transverse incisions yield just as satisfactory cosmetic results and hardly injure lymphatics if one proceeds with very fine instruments and avoids any necrosis of the wound margins. Even large perforating veins can be exposed by a skin incision of 1 cm. An exception are Cockett's perforating veins if the whole ankle region is altered by chronic inflammation. Even after preparation with foam rubber pads and compression bandages for months, a tough induration remains that makes small incisions impossible.

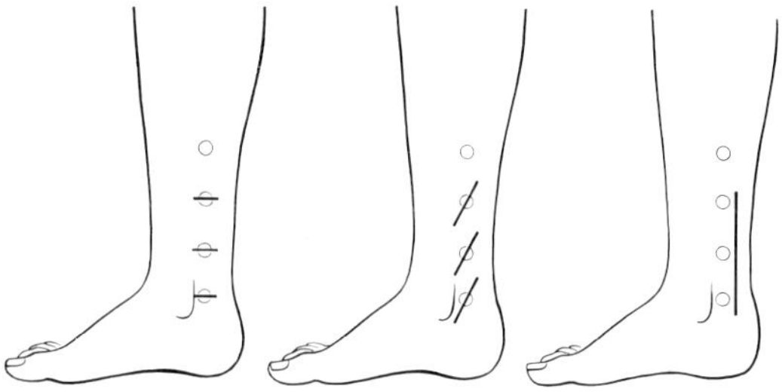

Fig. 4.10. Skin incisions for exposure of the perforating veins at the internal malleolus.

If this region has become horny, the perforating veins are exposed by oblique incisions 2–3 cm in length. Only in cases of very severe changes due to scars do we perform the longitudinal incision of Cockett. But the incision ought to be carried deep into the region of the ankle. Cockett's perforating vein I may otherwise be missed. The incision runs parallel with the Achilles tendon and 1 cm away from it.
The fascia is divided at once and the perforating veins are subfascially ligated primarily. The otherwise typical exposure of fascia and fascial gaps is impossible in the presence of chronic inflammation.
The skin can be closed with an intracutaneous suture, but this is not absolutely necessary. The cosmetic result depends in the first instance on the small size of the incision and the skin edges being undamaged as far as possible. In cosmetically important cases, the sutures are removed on the third day and Steristrip dressings are applied. The state of the scar is considerably improved if baths are prohibited for six weeks, and by correct bandaging for six weeks. Uniform pressure on the scar for weeks is the most important factor. We no longer use cortisone ointments, to promote healing.

Locating the Incompetent Perforating Veins

The most important perforating veins are seen in the following diagram. For details we refer to the chapter Anatomy of Perforating Veins.

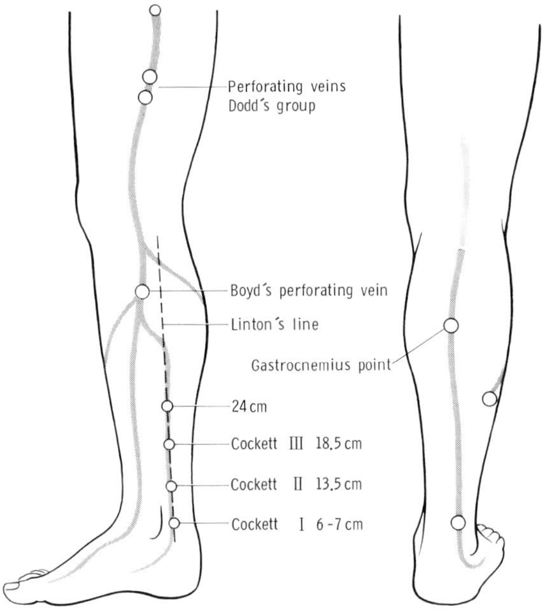

Fig. 4.11. Diagram of the most important perforating veins.

Large incompetent perforating veins are located on the standing patient by searching fascial gaps with the index finger at the sites of predilection. At the same time, a globular protuberance of the vein, Dow's sign, is frequently encountered. But even the experienced will overlook important perforatoring veins on purely clinical examination. Especially the incompetent perforating veins of the thigh — Dodd's group, Boyd's perforating vein and Cockett's perforating vein I are difficult to palpate and are frequently missed. Therefore, we suggest routine demonstration of perforating veins by the radiologist. As is known, the deep venous system is demonstrated by injecting the contrast medium into a vein of the dorsum of the foot of the standing but somewhat inclined, patient. The special examination of superficial veins, and particularly of perforating veins, is completely different. The patient lies on a table that is only slightly tilted at the foot end. The radiologist injects gradually from distal to proximal 5–7 ml contrast medium into each varix near the suspected perforating veins. Five to seven injections are required for examining a leg. The table is tilted after each injection so that the foot end is slightly above the horizontal. The flow of the contrast medium is observed on the screen and is photographed. Simultaneously, the perforating vein is marked under the screen. At the end of the examination, varicose veins and incompetent perforating veins are drawn using the x-ray pictures as a guide.

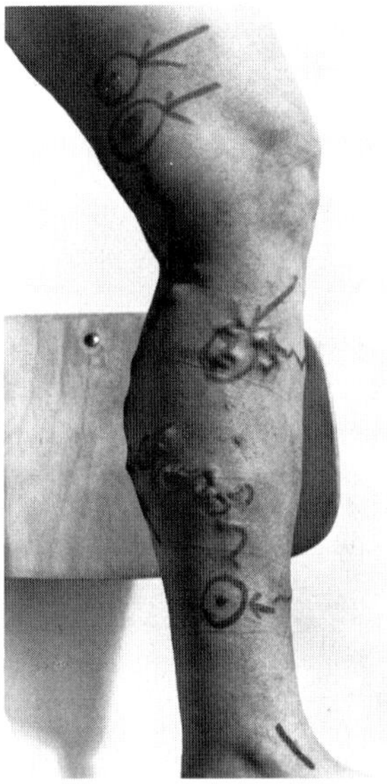

Fig. 4.12. The varices and most important perforators have been labeled preoperatively with marking ink.

We urgently recommend that the surgeon is present during the roentgen examination as this will enable him to operate more exactly. The radiologic examination is performed on principle on the afternoon prior to operation. Local thrombophlebitis frequently follows direct injection of contrast medium into the varices and interferes when there is a long interval between radiography and operation.

Which Incompetent Perforating Veins are Ligated

Ligation of incompetent perforating veins is necessary since stripping of superficial veins does not include many perforating veins or damages them so that new varicosities form in them after a

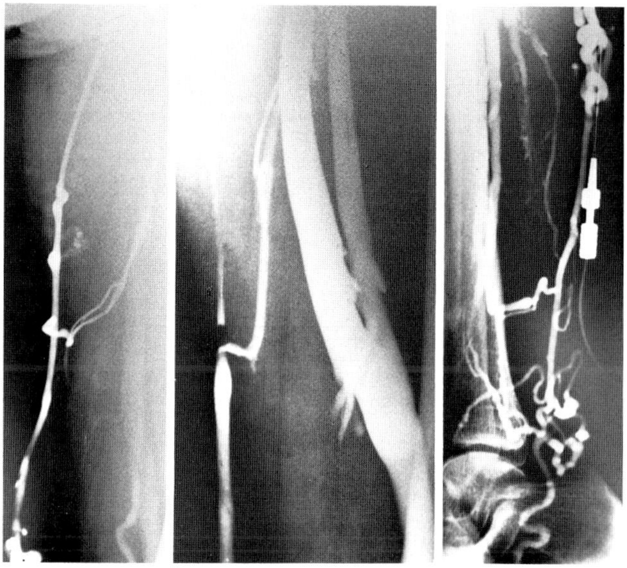

a b c

Fig. 4.13. Incompetent perforating veins
a—incompetent perforating vein in the thigh. Ligation not required.
b—incompetent perforating vein in the thigh. Ligation required, since the greater saphenous vein becomes incompetent only from this perforating vein onward.
c—perforating veins at the lateral malleolus and lesser saphenous vein. The distal perforating vein must be ligated. The proximal one is not ligated, but the perforating vein is recorded in the patient's case history.

few months. Remaining perforating veins lead to grave relapses.

Nevertheless, we do not ligate every radiologically incompetent perforating vein. Radiologically incompetent is every perforating vein that is not as thin as a thread and no longer reveals any valves. Exaggerated precision is not needed. We simply record in a sketch perforating veins that were not all ligated. We tell the patient that a minor operation may later be required if the perforating vein enlarges. It will be ligated under local anesthesia in the outpatient department.

Technique of Ligating Perforating Veins

If the perforating vein is exactly marked, a small skin incision suffices. The vein is dissected, caught with a clamp and the fascial gap through which the vein runs, is properly exposed. See also Ligation of Incompetent Perforating Vein in chapter 6, p. 147 and Fig. 6.28.

The perforating vein is drawn forward as far as possible and ligated as deep as feasible. The fascial gap is carefully closed by suture.

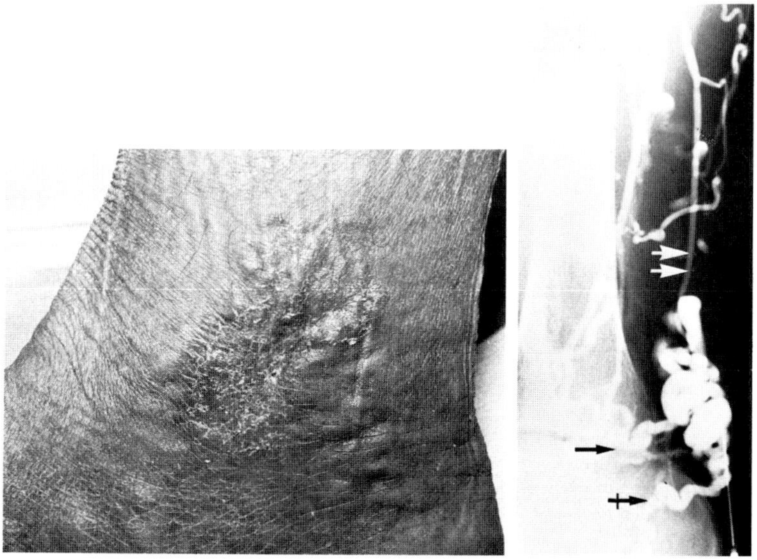

a b

Fig. 4.14a. Healed ulcer at the internal malleolus.
Fig. 4.14b. Phlebography reveals a varicosity under the ulcer scar.
Its sources are:
1. Incompetent perforating vein Cockett I ——→
2. Incompetent lesser saphenous vein ═══→
3. A superficial vein running toward the medial margin of the foot +—→

Termination of the Operation

At the end of the operation all hematomas are expressed before applying skin sutures. If bleeding is severe, pressure is first applied for a few minutes. We have never considered operation in a bloodless field necessary but proper removal of hematomas prior to wound closure facilitates aftertreatment. On completion of the skin sutures, the wounds are covered with sterile gauze on which large pads of foam rubber are placed. Exact bandaging from the toes to a handbreadth below the groin follows. The limb is well elevated in bed. Four hours after the operation the patient, now in care of the ward staff, is walking about. The bandages are loosened over night but not removed. The next morning, foam rubber pads and bandages are again firmly applied. The patient should be out of bed for half the day. The staff checks that the patient walks at intervals.

Operation for varicose veins can be performed in the outpatient department without difficulty. Four hours afterward, a further check is made that no bleeding has occurred, and the patient is sent home by ambulance. A relative is instructed about correct bandaging. The patient is informed in writing that absolute bed rest is forbidden, that he has to walk about regularly, and that in case of doubt he must telephone the duty surgeon without delay. He is asked to appear for checkup and removal of sutures on the 7th day.

We give all patients 0.5 g acetylsalicylic acid three times a day routinely. Prophylaxis of thrombosis and the light analgesic effect are thus combined. On principle, we reject combination of operation for varicose veins with other, nonurgent surgery, e.g. operation for hernia, during the same stay in hospital.

Aftertreatment

Every patient learns from the ward staff how to apply the bandages. He will be told that this is especially important for satisfactory formation of scars. Basically, the patient should apply the bandages till any edema and infiltration have disappeared. In the interest of optimal scar formation bandages should never be applied for less than six weeks.

Complications

Afterbleeding

Bleeding may occur in the groin. It is almost always of venous origin. Hemorrhage from an injured external pudendal artery is rare.

Hemorrhage from a stump of the great saphenous vein is impossible if the vein has been double ligated. Bleeding in the groin is stopped by applying pressure with a sandbag. Nevertheless, we advise opening the sutures and clearing the hematoma as the postoperative course will be more satisfactory.

Postoperative Thromboses

These have been infrequent among our patients. Mild infarction of the lungs was observed in 1 : 3000. One fatal pulmonary embolism occurred in 30000 operations.

Postoperative Swelling

This is practically never post-thrombotic, but rather due to impaired lymphatic drainage. Treatment: the patient must apply his bandages carefully, even if for many months, until any ankle swelling has disappeared even in the evening. He must continue to keep his legs elevated during the night. Systematic swimming and gymnastics are recommended also. This is the only way of preventing the swelling from becoming irreversible.

Lymphatic Cysts

These are occasionally seen, especially after operation for recurrence in the groin. They are aspirated once or twice. A few days rest are advised. Lymphatic cysts around small incisions were observed by us only four times. They have to be removed, including their capsule.

Nerve Lesions

Slight damage to cutaneous nerves can hardly ever be avoided. Therapy consists in explaining to the patient the unavoidability and harmlessness of the impairment. He will soon forget it.

Injury of Arteries and Deep Veins

Arterial injuries are corrected according to the rules of vascular surgery. It is important to recognize them promptly and, in particular, it is important that the less experienced operator does not attempt to perform the generally technically difficult repair, but transfers the patient to a vascular surgeon as an urgent case. The same applies to lesions of deep veins unless they can be repaired immediately by a small suture.

Recurrence

Recurrence in the Groin

This occurs when a small branch that flows directly into the femoral vein is overlooked, when the stump of the great saphenous vein is left too long, or a branch of a double great saphenous vein is missed. The sequel is a gross varicose convolution in the groin. Phlebography is mostly of little help and hence redundant.

The corrective operation can be technically difficult because of scarring and the large, easily damaged varicosities. Injuries of the deep veins or artery are described time and time again in connection with this procedure. The attempt at dissecting a varix is completely erroneous.

The leading thought has to be: Do not regard the varix initially at all, but expose the femoral artery first. Continue dissection medially and expose the femoral vein.

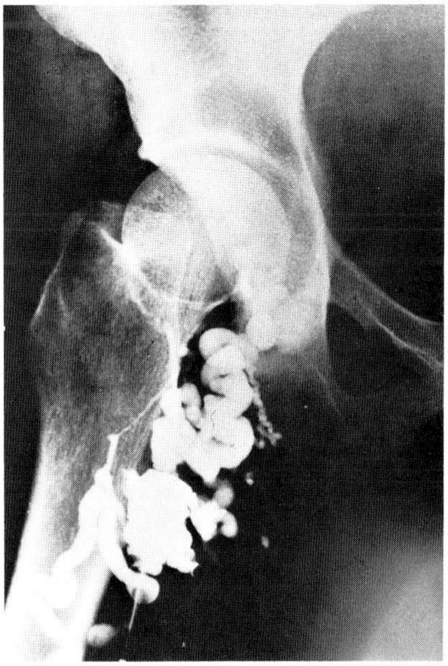

Fig. 4.15. Recurrent varicosity in the groin, originating from a saphenous stump.

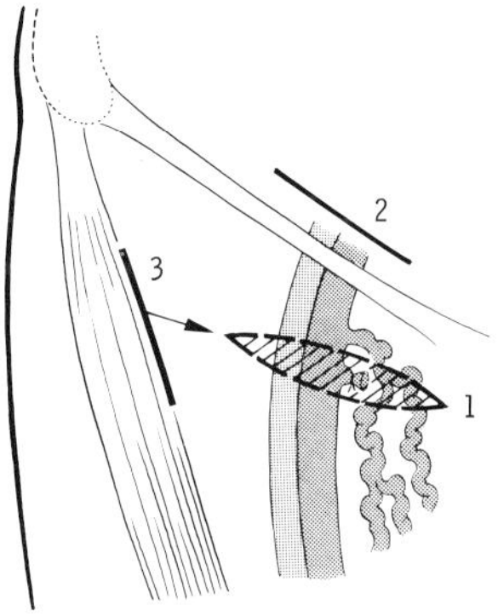

Fig. 4.16. Recurrent varicosity in the groin:
1. Approach of Li
2. Approach of Luke
3. Approach of Junod

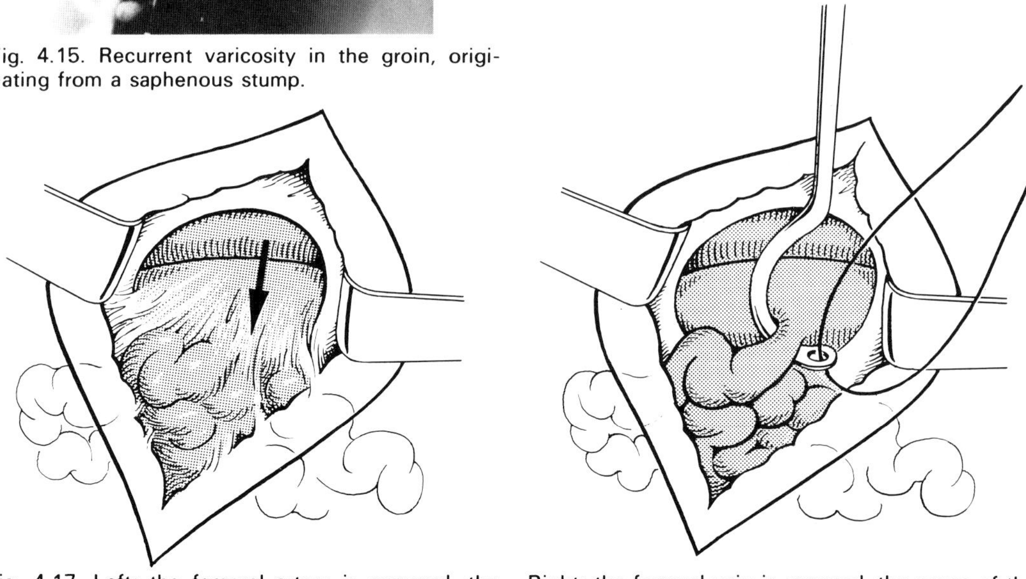

Fig. 4.17. Left: the femoral artery is exposed, the femoral vein can now be dissected. Right: the femoral vein is exposed, the cause of the relapse is an external pudendal vein. It is ligated and transected.

Technical Variants

1. Direct Approach of A.K.C. Li Feel the pulse of the femoral artery in the groin and make an incision in the groin itself about 8 cm in length. Any previous scars are excised. In any case, the skin incision must extend laterally beyond the palpable artery. Commence dissecting at the lateral angle of the incision. The artery is exposed for about 5 cm longitudinally after incising the vascular sheath. Continue dissecting medially.

The femoral vein is thus exposed without effort and the venous stump or branch which is the cause of the relapse is visualized. This stump is undermined with a curved clamp and ligated close to the vein. The wide mesh of the varicosity collapses at once. It is oversewn or excised together with the old scar.

However, extensive damage to the lymphatic vessels is practically the rule with this procedure. Therefore we prefer

2. The Technique of Luke The skin is incised more proximally, above the inguinal fold. Dissection proceeds then in normal tissues from proximal to distal. Here also, the artery is first exposed, followed by the deep vein. Disadvantage: The method is more difficult since little room is available due to the old scar. Nevertheless, we prefer this approach.

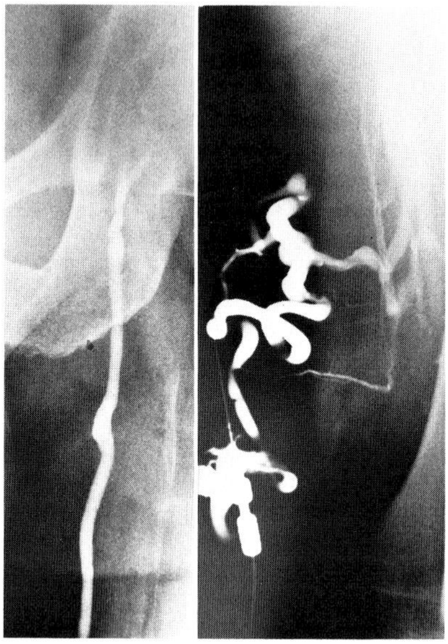

Fig. 4.19. Phlebography reveals that the relapse has two origins.
1. A vein originating in the groin: the external pudendal vein remained.
2. Incompetent perforating vein at the level of the adductor canal.
Dodd's group.
Therapy: Repair of the groin, liguature of the incompetent perforating vein, sclerosing of remaining varices.

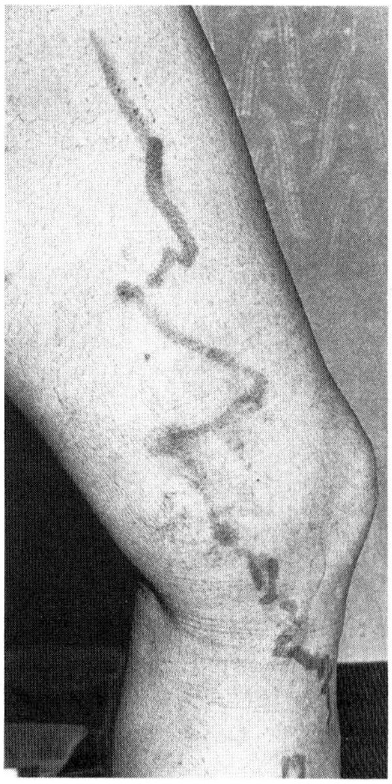

Fig. 4.18. Recurrent varicosity 5a after stripping operation.

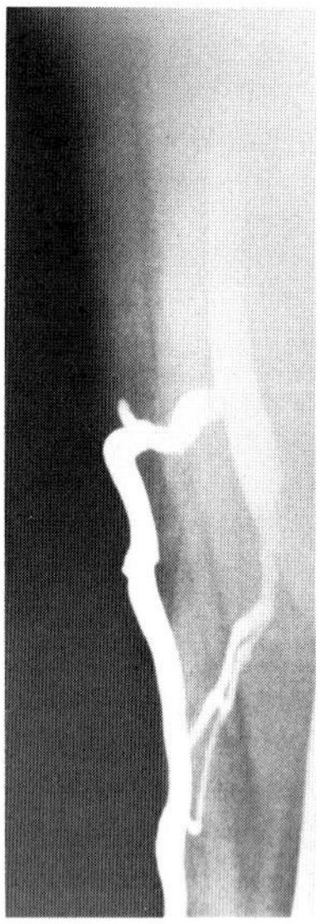

Fig. 4.20. Recurrence 4a after stripping of the great saphenous vein. The recurrence originates from a thick residual perforating vein at the level of the adductor canal.

3. Technique of Junod Incision of skin and fascia over the medial margin of the sartorius muscle in one longitudinal movement. Again, the artery is exposed first, then the femoral vein. The lymphatic vessels receive the least damage using this procedure. Disadvantage: The perpendicular incision may be cosmetically objectionable.

Recurrent varices: Every patient is called back three to four months after the operation. Residual varices are sclerosed percutaneously. All patients are advised to appear for checkup every second year and after every childbirth. Relapses in the groin are always corrected surgically. Remaining perforating veins which have enlarged, and lesser saphenous veins which in the meantime have become varicose are removed surgically in the outpatient department. Only then will residual varicosities be sclerosed.

References

Brunner, U.: Das Lymphödem der unteren Extremitäten. H. Huber, Bern 1969

Brunner, U.: Zur Vermeidung von secundären Lymphödemen nach Varicenoperation Phleb. u. Prokt. 4: 266, 1975

Dodd, H., F. B. Cockett, The Pathology and Surgery of the Veins of the Lower Limb. E. & S. Livingstone Limited, 2nd ed., Edinburgh and London, 1976

Fischer, R.: Die chirurgische Behandlung der Varicen. H. Huber, Bern 1976

Gillot, C.: Die intraoperative Phlebographie der V. saphena parva in Die Kniekehle by U. Brunner. Huber, Bern 1975, pp. 92–105

Hilty, H.: Die makroskop. Gefäßvariabilität im Mündungsgebiet der V. saphena magna des Menschen. B. Schwabe, Basel 1955

Junod, I. M.: Varices et leur complications, traitement chirurgical des cas difficiles, Helv. Chir. Acta: 167–170, 1971

Li, A. K. C.: A Technique for Re-exploration of the Saphenofemoral Junction for Recurrent Varicose Veins. Br. J. Surg. Vol 62: 745–746, 1975

Luke, J. C.: The Management of Recurrent Varicose Veins. Surgery 35: 40–44, 1954

May, R, R. Nissl: Die Phlebographie der unteren Extremität, 2nd ed., Thieme, Stuttgart 1975

5 Acute Thrombosis

R. Nissl

Roentgenologic Aspects

Early clinical diagnosis of recent thrombosis of the deep leg veins is unfortunately fraught with error, and phlebography is required for confirmation.

Schwartz (1965) published a list of questionable clinical diagnoses of thrombosis. In 595 cases of death due to pulmonary embolism, the diagnosis of the causative peripheral thrombosis had been made in only 10.6 per cent of the patients. Roentgenologic verification of clinical signs and symptoms revealed that local muscular tension and pain had been accurate indications of thrombosis in 41 per cent and false-positive signs in 11 per cent. Skin changes (coloration, temperature differences) were indicative in 50 per cent and false-positives in none. Superficial venous dilatations were indicative in 25 per cent of cases but false in 11 per cent. Homans' sign, pain on dorsiflexion of the foot, which is generally considered significant with an expected reliability of 40 per cent, revealed 8 per cent positive and 6 per cent false-positive results. Lowenberg's test (pain on application of a sphygmomanometer cuff to the calf), and its modification by May (1955) (unilateral pain on symmetric inflation of cuffs on both calves), gave false-negative results in 22 per cent and false-positive results in 26 per cent of cases. Laboratory tests for hypercoagulability and assessment of the prethrombotic stage also failed as a rule.

Swelling of the ankle, but only on the left, was indicative in 83 per cent of cases. This is understandable since this is no longer regarded as early sign, as Piulachs (1956) emphasized.

According to Piulachs, the first sequel to thrombosis is subfascial edema. It pervades the deep musculature and causes pain on pressure (Fig. 5.1). But deep tenderness is a very vague sign.

Ankle swelling does not occur with subfascial edema. Not until later, when superficial epifascial edema is present does clearly visible ankle and leg swelling appear (Fig. 5.2). At present there is no clinical possibility of recognizing a completely silent thrombus in good time. Whether a patient's vague symptoms of slight restlessness, minor unexplained rise of pulse rate, and indefinable complaints in the leg should really be interpreted as thrombosis poses a question that can be answered only with uncertainty, and the prescription of anticoagulants over several weeks is justifiable. It is easy to see why anyone who has disregarded these vague symptoms and lost a patient due to pulmonary embolism will in the future consider all patients with vague complaints as having thrombosis, accepting the possibility of superfluous treatment of some. This is the only explanation for the fact that four to six patients are seen every month who claim to have been treated in the hospital for some time but in whom roentgenography reveals a completely intact deep venous system.

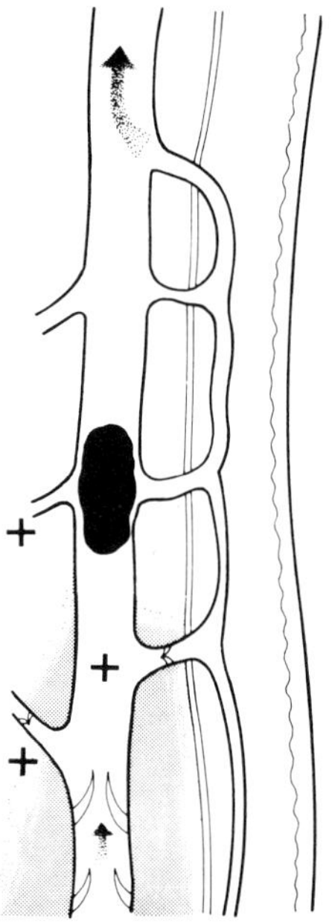

Fig. 5.1. Subfascial edema.

On the basis of our own experience, of observation of patients referred to us and of reports in the literature, we believe wrong clinical diagnoses of early thrombosis are made, both positively and negatively, about 25 to 30 per cent of the time.

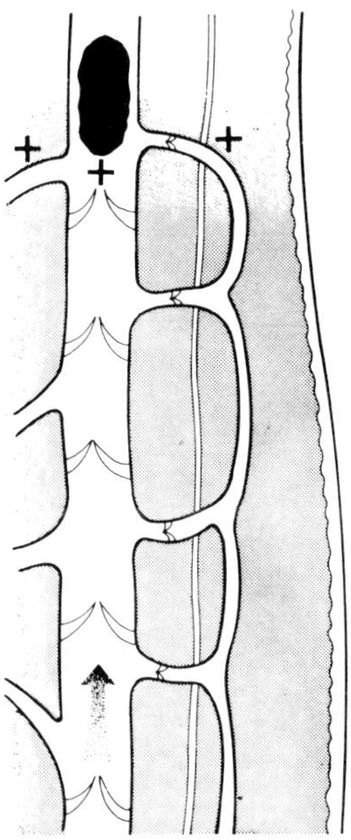

Fig. 5.2. Epifascial edema.

This means that about one quarter of patients suspected of having thrombosis do not; and one quarter of those with vague complaints in whom thrombosis is excluded clinically do have it. This uncertainty is mainly due to the fact that many thromboses originate not in the calf veins, as assumed hitherto, but primarily in the femoral vein.

It is known today that Rössle's statement (1937), apparently first confirmed phlebographically by Bauer (1961), that at least 80 per cent of thromboses originate in the calf veins is no longer tenable.

More recent careful studies, especially by McLachlin et al. (1962), revealed quite different facts. Painstaking autopsies of 1000 cadavers revealed thrombosis in 34 cases (Table 5.1).

Table 5.1. Incidence of Thrombosis at Postmortem Examination in Different Venous Segments of 34 cases

Pelvic veins only	2
Thigh and pelvic veins	1
Thigh veins only	17
Thigh and leg veins	10
Leg veins only	4

The femoral vein was the primary seat of thrombosis in 64 per cent of cases (Table 5.2) (Sevitt and Gallagher, 1961).

Table 5.2. Distribution of 76 Thrombi in 34 Cases of Thrombosis Found at Postmortem Examination

Pelvic veins	6
Thigh veins	49
Leg veins	21

The findings of the pathologists are supported by similar results of phlebographic examinations (Table 5.3).

Table 5.3. Primary Site of Thrombosis in 100 Patients Examined Roentgenologically

Iliac vein, predominantly the left	7%
Femoral vein	43%
Popliteal vein	12%
Calf veins	38%

These figures were largely confirmed by x-ray examinations of 420 cases of recent thrombosis by Servelle (1944). Schwartz (1965) therefore proposed the most exact method, scintillation scanning with ^{131}I-labeled fibrinogen. As convincing as his results are, general and routine application of the procedure will remain restricted to a few centers. We attempt to exclude all uncertainty and employ phlebography in all questionable cases. Phlebograms are taken only in doubtful early cases — that is, unfortunately, almost every case initially; they are dispensed with in clinically manifest thrombosis.

The fear that injection of contrast media is risky in recent thrombosis has not been borne out in practice. Detailed experiments by Borgström and Greitz (1965) and by Williams and Carey (1954) showed that the expected intimal damage is not seen when heparin is given simultaneously. More important, embolism is not caused by appropriate careful examination and transport following heparin administration.

We ourselves, as well as Fontaine (personal communication, 1969), DeWeese and Rogoff (1963), Servelle (1964) and Vanderhoeft (1961), have performed these examinations and never experienced the complication of embolism.

We apply 5000 units of heparin intravenously before radiography, and continue anticoagulant therapy if the findings are positive. No accidents resulting from this technique are known to us. The classic description of thrombosis was given by Bauer (1940).

Diagnosis of thrombosis that is just beginning is difficult. It should be emphasized time and again that absence of a venous segment does not in itself necessarily mean thrombosis. The surest

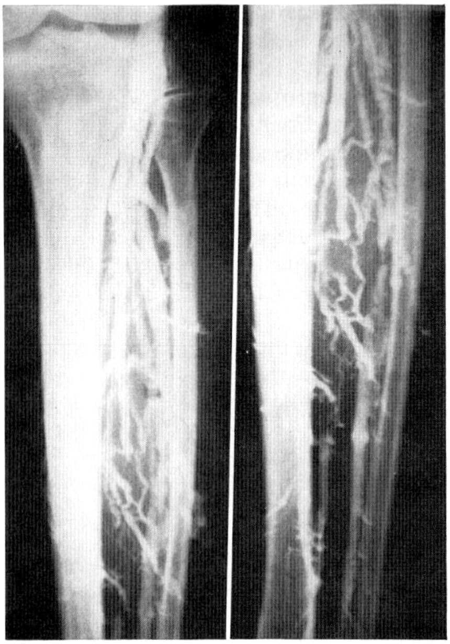

a b

Fig. 5.7. Two-week-old thrombosis. Peroneal veins segmentally interrupted; eraser phenomenon; collateral circulation (*a,b*).

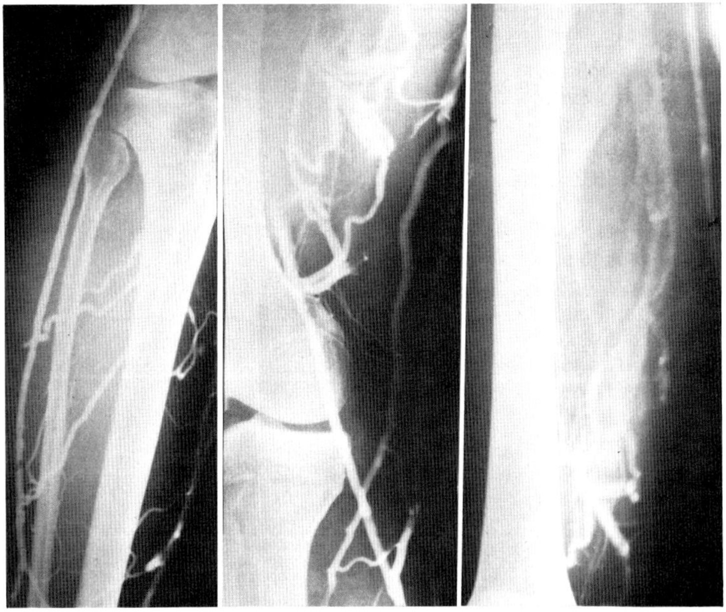

a b c

Fig. 5.8. Ten-day-old thrombosis. Eraser phenomenon in leg and popliteal region (*a,b*); dome sign in femoral vein (*c*); collateral circulation.

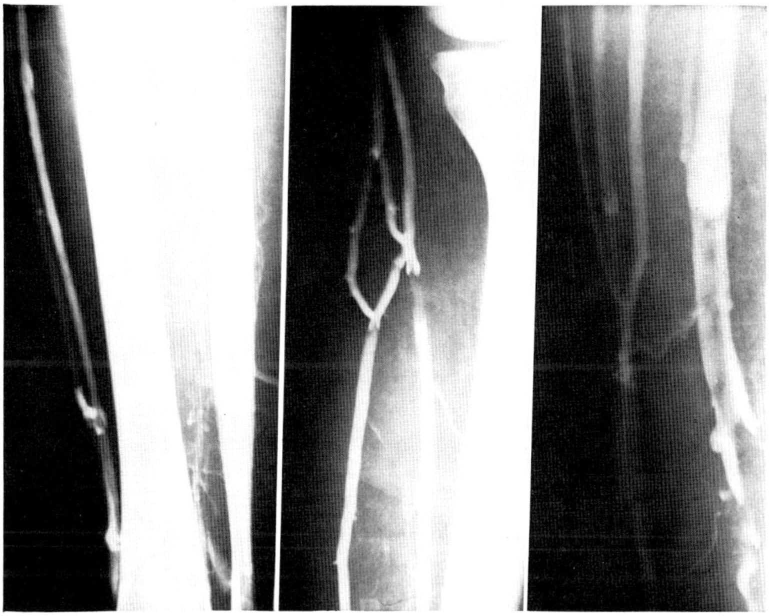

a b c

Fig. 5.9. Three-week-old thrombosis. Eraser phenomenon in leg and popliteal region (*a,b*); dome sign in femoral vein (*c*); collateral circulation. Clinically, the patient had only slight indefinite symptoms at this time.

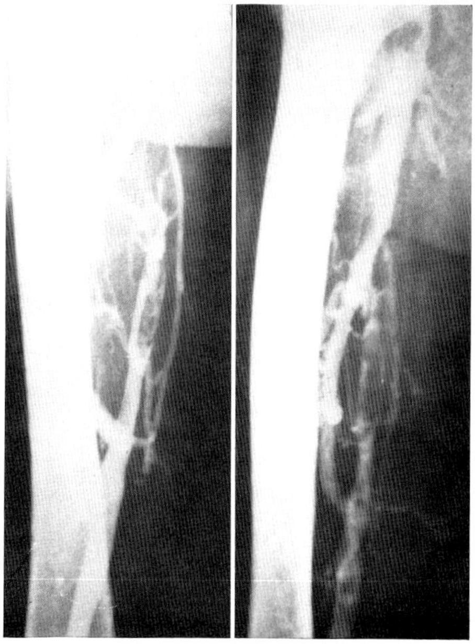

a b

Fig. 5.10. Fresh thrombus in the femoral vein, identical on two exposures.

repeated, with two or three exposures of the site in question. The source of error, a central translucency due to greater blood flow velocity in the center of the vessel (Fig. 5.11), can usually be excluded by an additional film of the same segment.

Interpretation of a film may be made difficult by the inflow phenomenon, when a vein without contrast medium drains into one carrying it. Eysholt (1945) pointed out how easily the so-called "inflow phenomenon" may simulate a thrombus. A translucency in the dense shadow of the main trunk at the junction points like a finger into the central direction of the main trunk,

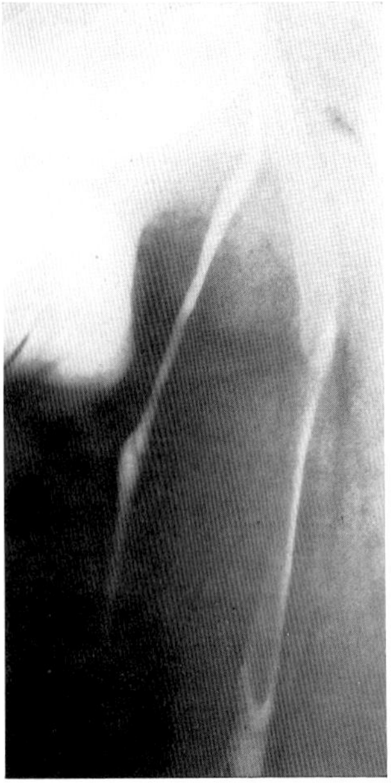

Fig. 5.11. Central translucency in the femoral vein produced by faster blood flow in the center of the vessel.

occasionally crossing the lumen obliquely to the opposite wall. Then it turns centrally to disappear slowly in a central zone of dilution. The same effect is observed in nature where a clear brook flows into a muddy stream. This phenomenon is of little importance for the deep leg veins and occurs mainly in the area of the popliteal and femoral veins (Fig. 5.12), that is, in segments where larger veins, such as gastrocnemial, small saphenous and large perforating veins, enter the deep venous system. A thrombus always has clear contours; the inflow phenomenon is hazy. Here also, an additional film clarifies the issue. Filling defects that develop at boundaries with the valves rarely cause difficulties in interpreting a film.

Of the three false-positive signs of thrombosis, the pseudothrombosis of Almén and Nylander (1964), the first two are important. The third type is caused by pathologic states of the stream due to superficial varices and plays no part in recognition of thrombosis of the deep leg veins. Pseudothrombosis is caused by stream conditions due to contraction of muscle toward the end of the examination, never at the beginning. In the first type, there are filling defects of differing lengths in the deep veins when the blood is expressed from them by muscular contraction. If muscular tension eases, the deep veins are normal. In the second type, the deep veins are apparently avalvular and the venous wall is irregular, as seen in recanalized thrombosis. This picture arises when muscular contractions press large quantities of unmixed blood into the deep veins, the widely open valves being apposed to the venous wall and thus escaping demonstration. Furthermore, the blood from the muscles mixes only poorly with blood containing contrast medium, and simulates filling

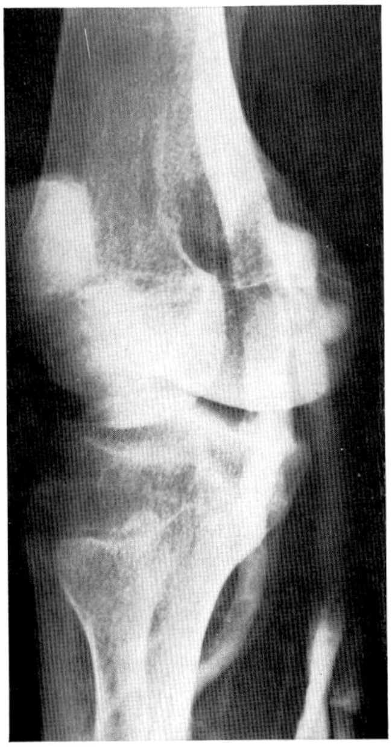

a

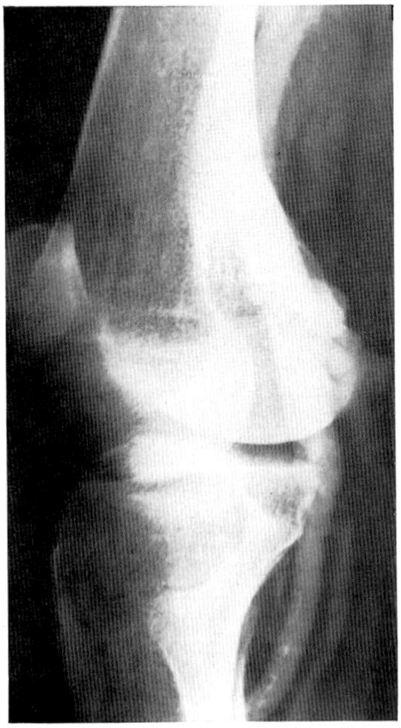

b

Fig. 5.12. Inflow phenomenon in the popliteal vein near the small saphenous junction (*a*), no longer demonstrable (*b*).

defects in the deep veins. The second type actually corresponds to the "inflow phenomenon." But none of these appearances can mislead if the old rule is observed: a filling defect can be considered due to thrombosis only when it is identical on two pictures.

Recent thrombosis of the pelvic veins should be briefly discussed. The pelvic veins ought to be demonstrable up to the vena cava on ascending intravenous phlebography of the leg, and this procedure alone suffices to exclude thrombosis. With negative findings, the films are clear-cut. The contrast medium flows unimpeded through the external and common iliac veins as a smooth, broad band. With positive findings, collateral circulation to the opposite side occurs: films of the pelvis after ascending intravenous phlebography may be indistinct and unsatisfactory, and pelvic phlebography may be required for clarification of details. Since direct pelvic phlebography involving puncture at the level of the inguinal canal is rather risky because of floating thrombi, intraosseous pelvic phlebography through the greater trochanter, including serial films, is preferred.

The basis of intraosseous demonstration was described in detail by Guilhem and Baux (1954), Chambraud (1940)and Dimtza (1951).The sites of injection are shown in Figure 5.13. May has for some time preferred injection into the greater trochanter (May and Nissl, 1959). The patient lies flat with his legs extended. The greater trochanter is palpated under light general anesthesia, and a small stab incision is made through the skin with the scalpel. A Ballade needle (Fig. 5.14), used for intraosseous injection into the calcaneus, is pushed as far as the bone, the spike is driven into it with a hammer until it is firmly in place, and then it is fixed by a few turns. The skin is swabbed with antiseptic, and sterile wraps and gloves must be used. When the stylet is removed, blood containing marrow flows from the needle. If a test injection with saline takes effort, the needle rests too superficially. Forty millilitres of 45 per cent contrast medium is then injected in exactly 10 seconds. The plate lies under the patient's pelvis. The first exposure is made after 3 seconds, and the next two immediately afterward—the second at the end of the injection and the third 10 seconds later. After injection, 0.5 ml heparin in 10 ml saline is introduced, the needle is removed by gentle turning and the skin is sutured.

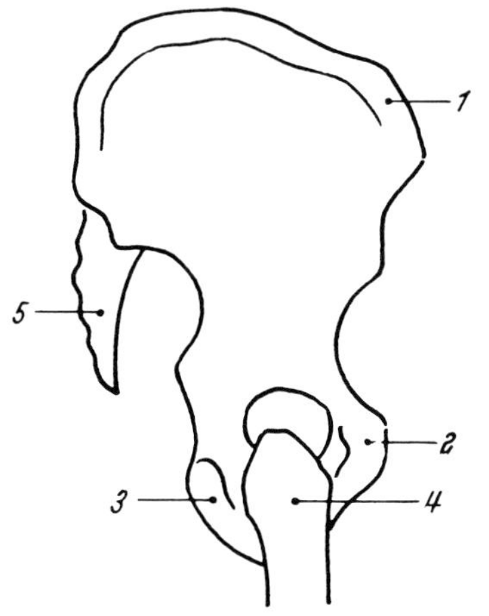

Fig. 5.13. Sites of injection for intraosseous demonstration of veins. (Figs. 5.13 to 5.15 from May, R., and R. Nissl: Die Phlebographie der unteren Extremität. Thieme, Stuttgart, 1959.)

1 Iliac crest
2 Pubic bone
3 Ischial tuberosity
4 Greater trochanter
5 Sacrum

Guilhem and Baux (1945) drew particular attention to the difference of venous flow on the two sides because of anatomic variation.

Right-sided drainage is direct from the obturator and internal iliac vein to the common iliac and inferior cava veins, without any demonstration of collaterals, but drainage on the left is always more complicated. The physiologic impression is that the right common iliac artery, which lies on the common iliac vein, interferes with the flow, thus necessitating drainage via collaterals (Fig. 5.15).

We consider *phlebography* essential *in acute thrombosis*

—if diagnosis is in doubt in early cases,

—if surgical intervention is intended. (Several American authors currently perform thrombectomy without x-ray confirmation. We have grave doubts about this practice. It is only too easy to overlook clinically silent thrombosis, particularly in the pelvis. Roentgen examination of pelvic veins should always be carried out bilaterally in these cases. In addition, it is important to have exact details of the upper limits of the thrombus if surgery is to be done.)

—before and after fibrinolysis. (Purely clinically, it cannot be judged whether fibrinolysis produces the desired results. Time and again it is seen that bed rest and elevation cause detumescence of the limb simulating therapeutic success, but the deep veins remain completely closed. Roentgen examination is essential since the chance exists of correcting the result by surgery.)

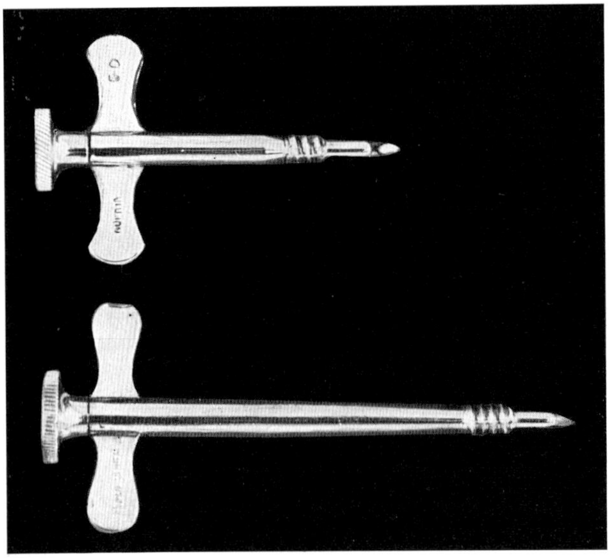

Fig. 5.14. Ballade's needles.

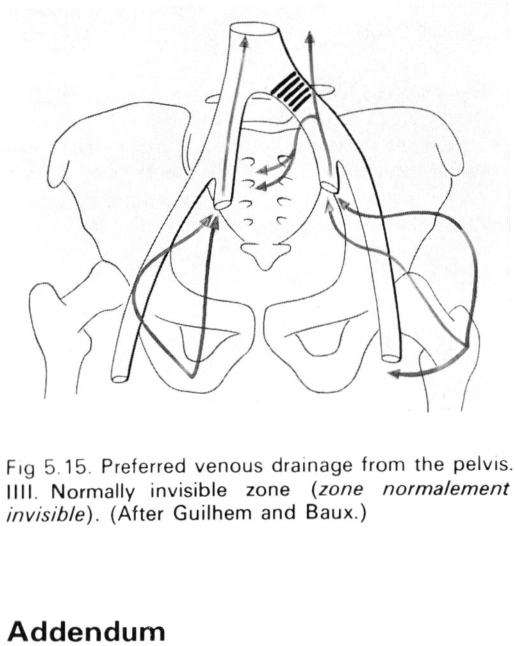

Fig 5.15. Preferred venous drainage from the pelvis. IIII. Normally invisible zone (*zone normalement invisible*). (After Guilhem and Baux.)

Addendum

Recently we have radically changed our *technique* in *fresh pelvic thrombosis*.
Fresh pelvic thrombosis demands an active procedure, either fibrinolysis or thrombectomy.
In both cases, precise demonstration of the thrombus, especially of its proximal limits, is imperative. Intraosseous injection into the trochanter does not always produce ideal films, in addition to making subsequent fibrinolysis risky. Hence, we developed the technique of encirclement.

Encirclement Technique

Ascending phlebography from the ankle, with the patient lying obliquely, is an obvious requirement; it should be monitored by an image intensifier.
The patient is placed flat on the table, the pelvis over the serial filmer.

1. We inject the contrast medium as rapidly as possible into the long saphenous vein in the region of the slightly raised ankle of the recumbent patient or, better, at the level of the knee. No tourniquet is used. This produces marked concentration of the contrast medium just proximal to the inguinal ligament and good demonstration of the deep veins.
2. Almost always in fresh iliofemoral thromboses, a dermal vein is obvious on the lateral aspect of the left flank or inguinal region that can be punctured.
3. Finally, we always inject into the femoral vein in the groin of the healthy side.

We expose four films with the serial attachment in slow succession when half the contrast medium has been injected. Each of these techniques performed on its own may cause considerable misinterpretation. Only comparison of all films permits precise diagnosis. Thus, we use intraosseous injection of the trochanter only exceptionally. Another advantage of the encirclement technique is that general anesthesia, which is practically indispensable for intraosseous injection, is not necessary.

Surgery of Acute Femoroiliac Phlebothrombosis*

U. Brunner

The surgical measures for acute forms of femoroiliac phlebothrombosis (Figs. 5.16 to 5.18 on Plate 1) are:

—thrombectomy as therapy of thrombosis; and
—fasciotomy as palliative therapy of compressive edema.

Thrombectomy

Purpose

Surgical removal of fresh clots from the deep venous system has a threefold aim:

—prophylaxis of fatal *pulmonary embolism* by clearing the main trunks.

Eighty per cent of fatal pulmonary emboli originate from thrombosis in the leg or the femoroiliac segment of the deep venous system (Encke et al., 1966; Gibbs, 1967; Kakkar et al., 1969; Mavor and Galloway, 1967, 1969; Nicolaides, 1971).

—easing *acute edema* by removing obstruction from the venous system, thus causing decompression of arterial blood flow.

Every leg swollen because of acute thrombosis of the deep main veins decreases noticeably in size after elevation, hot packs, and anticoagulant treatment in 2 to 4 days. The femoropopliteal segment contains two or three long intermuscular collaterals in 80 per cent of cases (Mavor and Galloway, 1969) (Fig. 5.19). These collaterals act vicariously but are not visualized on phlebograms of normal venous flow. Elimination of the swelling alone does not require surgery, but the thrombosis is only locally restricted by conservative measures. Pulmonary embolism and late sequelae are not prevented. The only thrombosis-induced type of swelling necessitating rapid relief for circulatory reasons is phlegmasia cerulea dolens with threatening "venous" gangrene.

—prophylaxis of the post-thrombotic syndrome by preservation of vessel walls and valves.

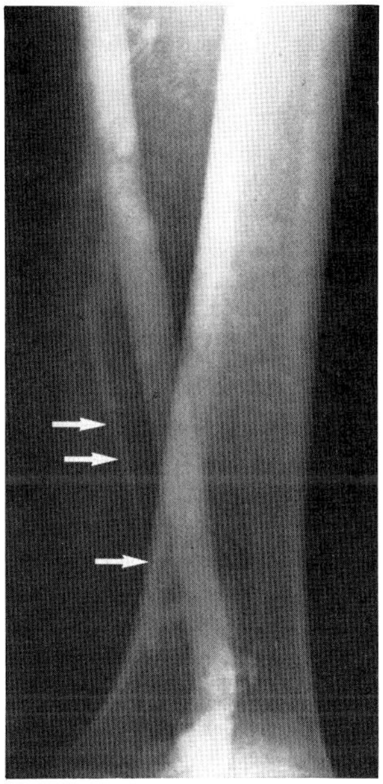

Fig. 5.19. Extended axis collaterals of the femoropopliteal segment (⟶).

Apart from obstructing venous lumens, thrombosis causes scarring of venous walls and adhesion of valvular cusps. Up to ninety per cent of segments of the deep venous system occluded by thrombosis become recanalized in the course of 2 years (Maranta and Wirth, 1968; Wirth et al., 1971), but this spontaneous recanalization leaves an insufficient system with rudimentary valves, diminished elasticity due to a wall thickened by scars, and increased permeability of the wall (Elliot et al., 1976; Thomas and Mc Allister, 1971). The post-thrombotic syndrome ensues. Clinically, swelling due to acute femoroiliac phlebothrombosis continues as chronic thickening without interval. The final picture of chronic venous insufficiency—bursting pain, secondary varices, trophic disturbances and leg ulcers—develops within an average of 2 years (1 to 10 years according to Halse, 1954). For the working person, the post-thrombotic syndrome means reduced earning power, producing perhaps 60 per cent total disability. Older people tolerate the post-thrombotic syndrome more easily by adaptation of their habits.

Besides these local changes, recurrence of thrombosis with corresponding renewed risk of embolism is frequent (Coon and Willis, 1973). (cf Chronic femoroiliac venous thrombosis with acute exacerbation, p. 124).

Procedure of Thrombectomy Using the Fogarty Balloon Catheter

Thrombectomy was first performed in Germany and France in the late thirties (Laewen, 1937;

---

* The phlebograms in this contribution are from the Röntgendiagnostisches Zentralinstitut of the Universitätsspital Zürich (Dir. Prof. J. Wellauer).

PLATE I

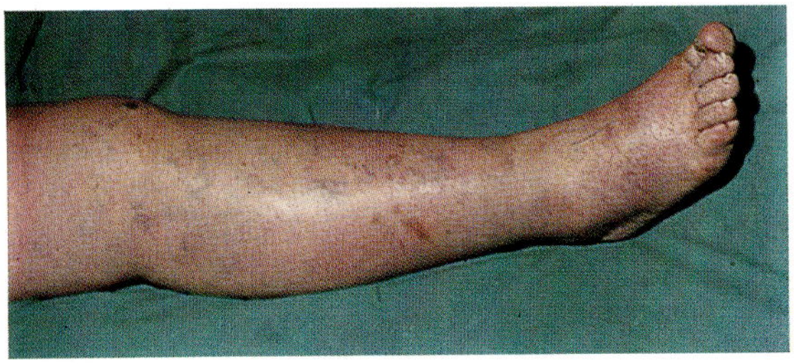

Fig. 5.16. Phlegmasia alba dolens (man aged 70 years).

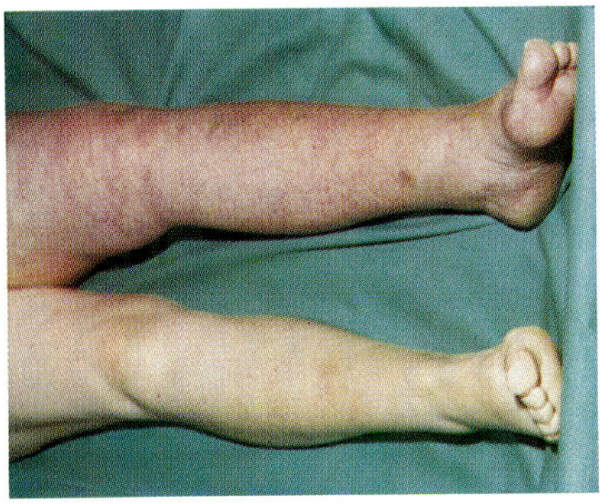

Fig. 5.17. Phlegmasia cerulea dolens (woman aged 34).

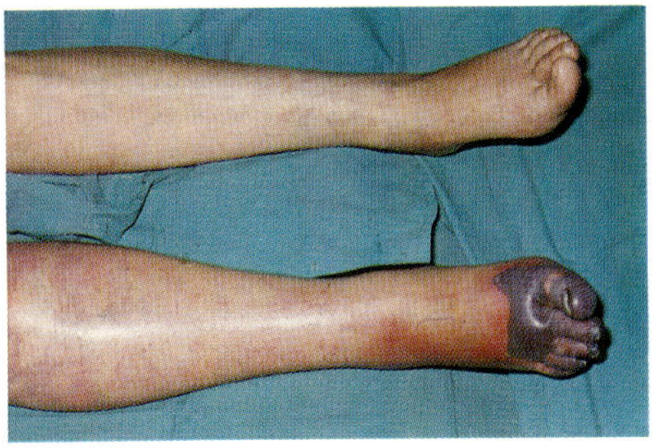

Fig. 5.18. Phlegmasia cerulea dolens with "venous" gangrene (woman aged 39 years).

Leriche and Geisendorf, 1939) but was discontinued for a prolonged period because of misadventures and technical problems.

The hemodynamic, biologic and technical problems of direct plastic venous surgery apply also to surgery for acute femoroiliac phlebothrombosis. Intervention in the venous system produces two elements of Virchow's triad, which are especially important in florid thrombosis: changes in flow conditions due to removal of the vein from its investment, and damage to the venous wall due to venotomy or suture. Hence, the technique of thrombectomy is, apart from elimination of clots, directed toward prevention of early occlusion and avoidance of intraoperative and postoperative pulmonary embolism.

Unlike the case in arterial occlusion, in which the sequelae are always local, thrombosis of the deep veins threatens the patient's life.

Intervention for unilateral thrombosis in limb and pelvis without caval thrombosis comprises:

—history and clinical and phlebographic examination to determine etiology, age and location of the thrombosis (Figs. 5.20 to 5.24);

—preparatory measures—

indwelling catheter in the bladder, availability of 2 to 3 liters of cross-matched blood for transfusion, antisepsis and wrapping with sterile towels, with the possibility of the necessity of an eventual Trendelenburg operation kept in mind (Fig. 5.25 on Plate II);

—measures for the prevention of intraoperative pulmonary embolism—

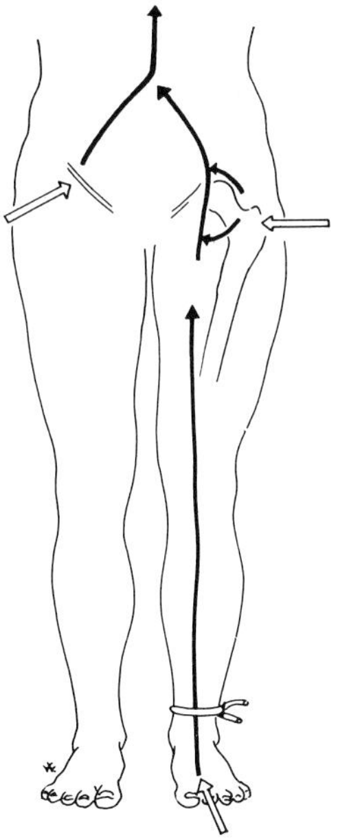

Fig. 5.20. Three-step combination phlebography for preoperative localization of a femoroiliac venous thrombosis. (From Wirth, W., J. Weber and U. Brunner: Radiologia clin. et biol. 40 [1971] 360.)

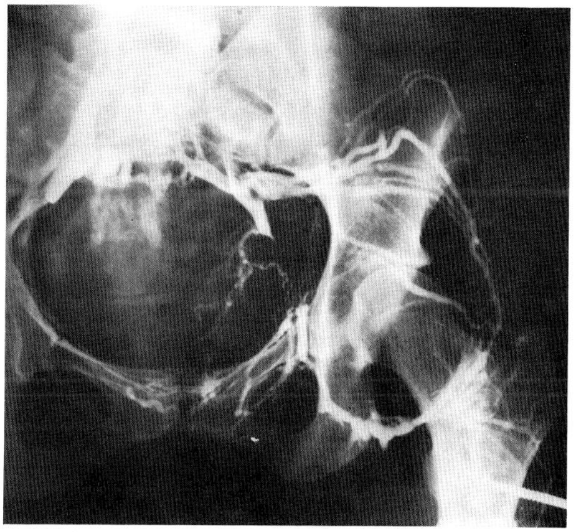

a

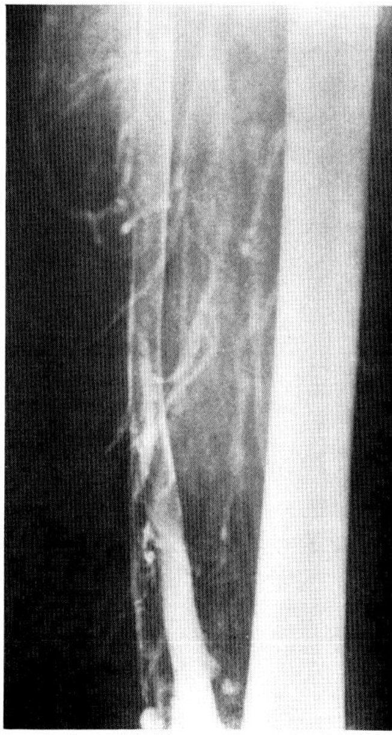

b

Fig. 5.21. Chronic pelvic thrombosis, recognizable by the site of occlusion and collateral veins (*a*), with acute exacerbation in the superficial femoral vein, recognizable by the floating thrombus, which is surrounded by an edge of contrast medium (*b*).

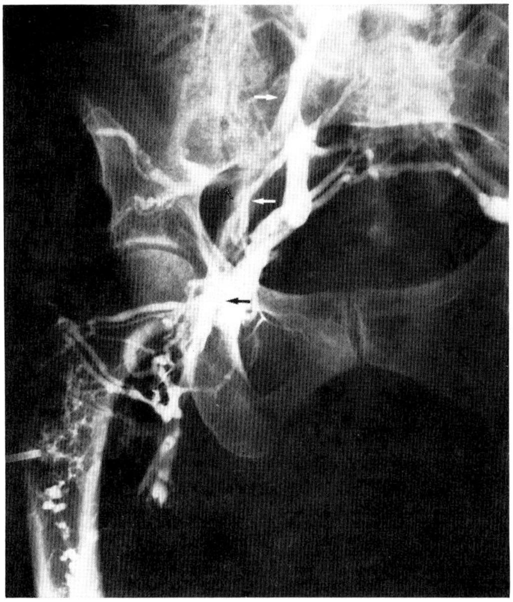

a

possibly retroperitoneal dissection of the inferior vena cava by right-sided lumbar gridiron incision for guidance of the balloon catheter,
introduction of a balloon catheter for temporary blockade of the inferior vena cava from the healthy side (Fig. 5.26 and Fig. 5.27 on Plate II), which has largely become superfluous because of end-expiratory high-pressure respiration, however (see Anesthesia, p. 79 f),
introduction of a balloon catheter into the common iliac or inferior cava vein from the thrombosed side (Fig. 5.26 and Fig. 5.28 on Plate II),

—thrombectomy proper—

reverse Trendelenburg position, high-pressure respiration, retrograde thrombectomy of the pelvic veins with balloon catheters (Fig. 5.26 and Fig. 5.29 on Plate II),
thrombectomy of the deep femoral vein and disobstruction of all neighboring affluents (Fig. 5.37),
anterograde thrombectomy of the main leg and thigh veins by external measures or balloon

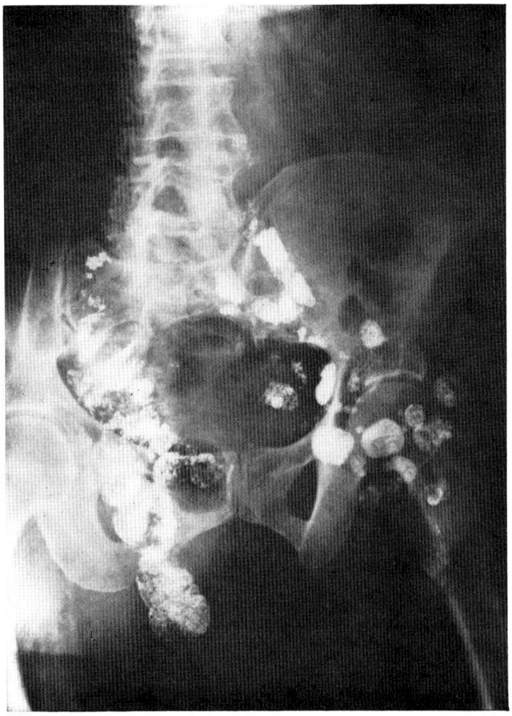

b

Fig. 5.22. Acute femoroiliac thrombosis due to compression (⟵) of the external iliac and common femoral veins by a giant follicular lymphoblastoma (Brill-Symmers disease) (*a*); corresponding lymphangiogram (*b*) (woman aged 74).

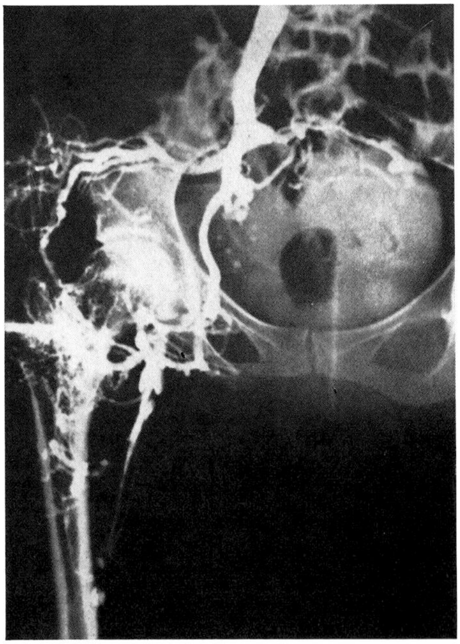

Fig. 5.23. Occlusion of the external iliac vein due to compression by pelvic metastases of a bronchial carcinoma. In contrast to the hyperacute signs of the occlusion, good drainage via the obturator and superior gluteal veins shows that the obstruction is slowly progressive (woman aged 57). (Figs. 5.23, 5.26 to 5.30, 5.34 and 5.39*a* from Brunner, U.: Act. Chir. 3 [1968] 298–365.)

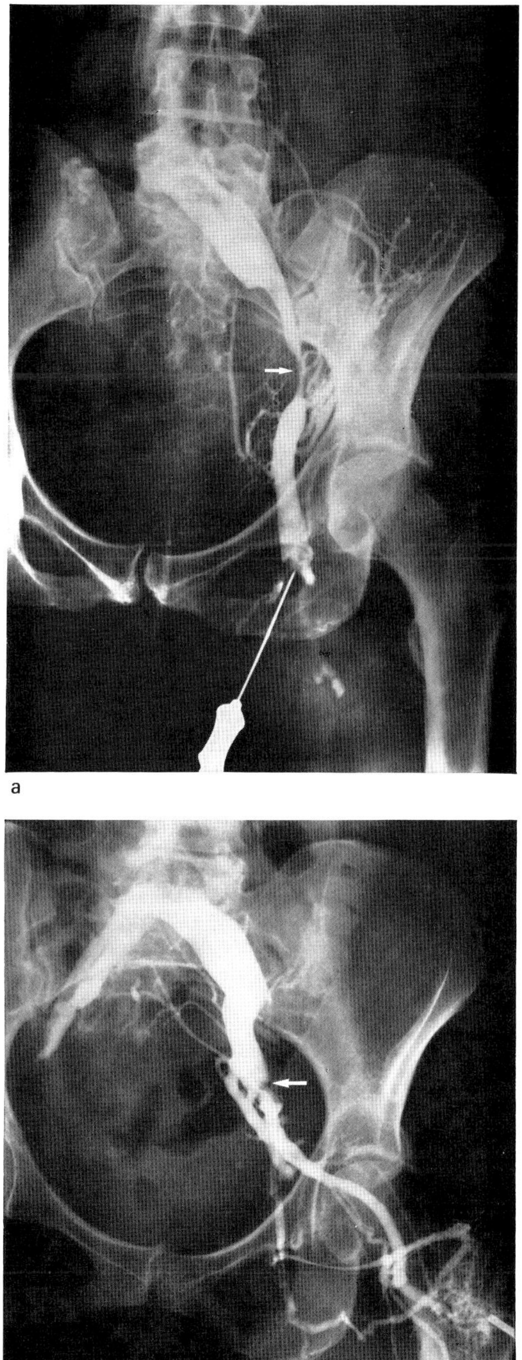

Fig. 5.24. Filiform stenosis of the common iliac vein (*a*) by lymph node metastases from a uterine carcinoma; total occlusion at this site 1½ months later (*b*) (woman aged 43).

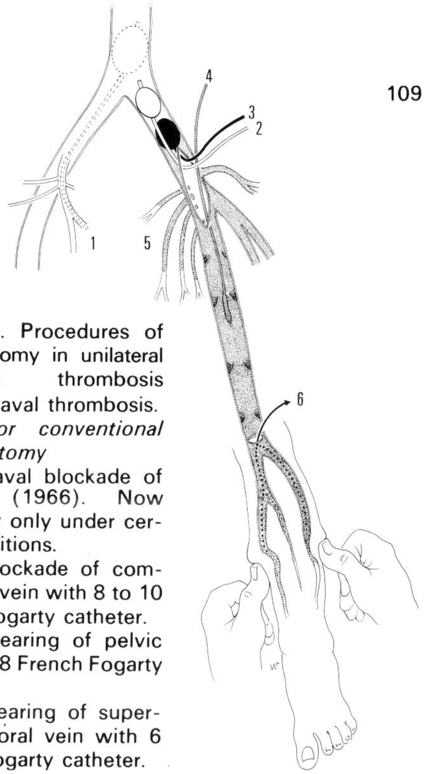

Fig. 5.26. Procedures of thrombectomy in unilateral leg-pelvis thrombosis without caval thrombosis.
Simple or conventional thrombectomy
No. 1 Caval blockade of Fogarty (1966). Now necessary only under certain conditions.
No. 2 Blockade of common iliac vein with 8 to 10 French Fogarty catheter.
No. 3 Clearing of pelvic vein with 8 French Fogarty catheter.
No. 4 Clearing of superficial femoral vein with 6 French Fogarty catheter.
Measures for the improvement of postoperative flow
No. 5 Clearing of all inguinal branches (cf Fig. 5.37).
No. 6 Clearing of leg veins and popliteal vein (cf Fig. 5.38).

catheters (Figs. 5.26 and 5.30) from the groin and by systematic opening of the popliteal vein in thrombosis of the distal popliteal and main leg veins (Fig. 5.38);
—establishing a temporary arteriovenous fistula in the case of residual obstruction in the pelvic axis;
—heparinization of obliterated pelvic veins by direct flushing through subinguinal infusion catheter (Fig. 5.31);

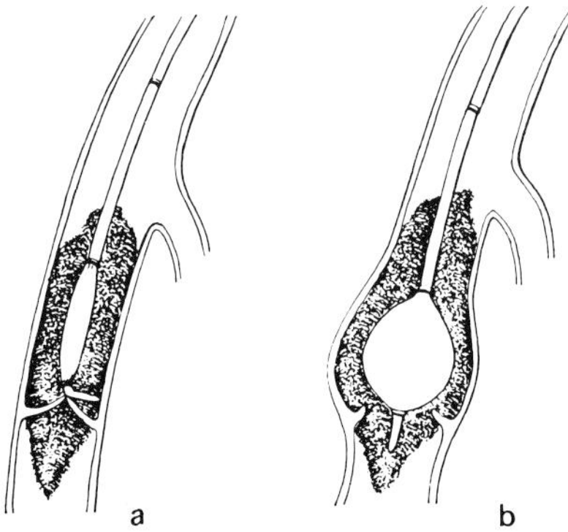

Fig. 5.30. If the flexible tip of the catheter is caught in valve pockets during distal probing (*a*), the check valve can be extended by inflating the balloon (*b*). (After Fogarty et al., 1966.)

Recently it is performed also under lumbar anesthesia (Senn and Nachbur, 1976). Our experience has shown that an adequate expulsive effect is obtained under insufflation anesthesia with high-pressure respiration and elevation of the head of the operating table (anti-Trendelenburg position).

Our measurements made in conjunction with the local Institut für Anästhesiologie (Brunner et al., 1971) confirm the main argument of the protagonists of local anesthesia, namely that under Valsalva conditions the pressure in the superior vena cava and the pelvic veins rises approximately five times as much as under high-pressure respiration with raised end-expiratory pressure (+ 15 cm H_2O). Thus, at the moment of active pressing, a maximal pressure gradient was obtained in the venous system opened by subinguinal phlebotomy as compared with atmospheric pressure, which worked to prevent thrombi from being washed centrally and facilitate their being washed out. This method obviously requires active cooperation by the patient, which is not always possible in emergency cases. However, we found that on repeated probing with the extraction balloon the patient became exhausted under local anesthesia, and his ability to press gradually diminished. On deep inspiration, after discontinuation of the abdominal pressure, we demonstrated moreover a brief pressure gradient from the periphery centrally, which in practice could suck a floating thrombus toward the heart.
With general anesthesia, the patient is spared the unpleasant and frequently painful sensations of surgery under local anesthesia. Dissection of an edematous vein from its gelatinous surroundings is time-consuming, and a single probing with the extraction catheter is usually not enough for complete clearance of the pelvic veins. Admittedly, the rise in venous pressure with high-pressure respiration is smaller, but it can be controlled for a prolonged period and can be reduced slowly without the risk of suction. In the reverse Trendelenburg position, a hydrostatic pressure of approximately 30 cm H_2O is superimposed on the venous pressure produced by the Valsalva maneuver or high-pressure respiration. This hydrostatic pressure rise is particularly helpful when the lower pressure rise due to end-expiratory high-pressure respiration is decided on. The sum of the end-expiratory overpressure and the hydrostatic pressure sufficed to prevent pulmonary embolism among our patients.
Furthermore, pulmonary embolism has a more deleterious effect on the circulation under local anesthesia than under general anesthesia, because of its vegetative depression.
The combination of the anti-Trendelenburg position and a raised end-expiratory pressure may be unfavorable to the circulation (decreased minute column). If hypovolemia supervenes, the circulation is at risk. Therefore, the circulation must be monitored under these conditions of anesthesia, and hypovolemia must be avoided at all costs.

After comparison of the advantages and disadvantages, insufflation anesthesia with high-pressure respiration in the anti-Trendelenburg position proved an adequate anesthetic method for thrombectomy during the critical moments of extraction.

Protection against Embolism (Temporary Intravenous Caval Block)

According to Fogarty's description, the first catheter, 8 to 10 French, is introduced on the healthy side via one of the collateral veins that join just before the saphenous junction (known from radical operations on varices), through the long saphenous and into the femoral (see Fig. 5.26 No. 1 and Fig. 5.27 on Plate II). This spares the long saphenous itself. If a vacuum is produced in the balloon before introduction of the catheter, it lies tightly against the shaft and is more easily introduced into the selected collateral. The long saphenous is used only if these tributaries are too small; it is ligated near the junction before the end of the operation.
After the balloon has been pushed to the inferior vena cava, it is inflated during dissection of the thrombosed vein and retracted to the bifurcation. Sudden total occlusion of the vena cava is occasionally followed by a drop in blood pressure, particularly in hypovolemia. Hence, to protect the circulation caval blockade must be restricted to a minimum length of time. In our experience, the original 8 to 10 French Fogarty catheter proved insufficient. Hence, we used a bladder catheter for cava blockade and lately one of the new occlusion catheters of Fogarty, 14 or 22 French.
But even without this precautionary measure, among our patients no embolic accident occurred during the probing and extraction phases in insufflation anesthesia under end-expiratory high pressure. That is why the caval blockade has been drawn as a dotted line only in Fig. 5.26 No. 1. The sole intraoperative pulmonary embolism among our own operations occurred after removal of the Fogarty caval blockade *without* high-pressure respiration. The patient was saved due to immediate Trendelenburg embolectomy from the pulmonary arteries.

Venotomy

The femoral bifurcation (union of the superficial and deep femoral with the common femoral) is exposed by a subinguinal longitudinal incision on the affected side. In the presence of femoroiliac thrombosis, the three main trunks at this junction are occasionally firmly distended to the size of a thumb and feel marrowy. The subcutaneous fatty tissue is edematous and the vascular bed gelatinous. The laterally adjacent arterial bifurcation is often narrowed by spasm. For this reason Fontaine et al. (1965) recommended perivascular sympathectomy of the dissected arterial segments in addition to thrombectomy for treatment of phlegmasia cerulea dolens. Six days after the appearance of acute symptoms, the vascular sheath and adventitia become so fragile that the arterial wall easily tears. Subsequent anticoagulant therapy requires strict hemostasis with nonabsorbable sutures.

One of the chief problems of surgery of the venous system is the great risk of recurrent or early thrombosis that each venous suture entails (Mahorner et al., 1957). Attention to several technical details aids in limiting this complication.

—If venotomy is applied at the site where venous flow is strongest, the risk of suture thrombosis (Fig. 5.33*b*) is smallest. These sites are always found at the junction of large main vessels, in the case of femoroiliac thrombosis at the union of the superficial and deep femoral veins (Fig. 5.34 on Plate III and Fig. 5.37.)

Poor flow is still a valid thrombogenic factor of Virchow's triad. Hence, the femoral bifurcation

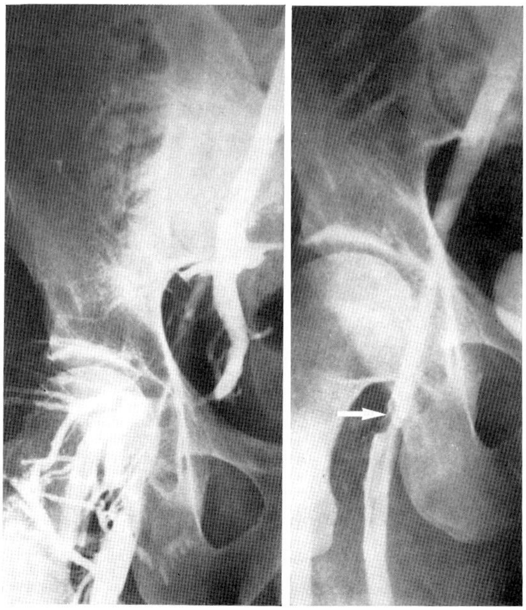

a b

Fig. 5.33. Segmental femoroiliac thrombosis on the right (man aged 30) (*a*); control phlebogram with mural suture thrombosis level with venotomy 3 months after thrombectomy (*b*).

is the site of choice for thrombectomy in the femoroiliac segment.

In the conventional procedure, only a short segment of the common femoral vein was exposed originally in order to keep the connections of the venous wall with its surroundings intact as far as possible (Fig. 5.34 on Plate III). At best, only the main trunk of the deep femoral vein, which is frequently included in thrombosis of the leg, could be cleared by this short venotomy. However, since not only the profunda femoris but up to eight branches from the thigh, that frequently are occluded by thrombi at the union, join a segment of 10 cm in length in the groin, their elective elimination by an appropriate, extensive longitudinal venotomy may produce an impressive inflow (Fig. 5.37). This intraoperative success clearly justifies more generous exposure of the inguinal venous axis, contrary to previous objections. But *all* branches must be closed by means of loops or even clamped in order to prevent much blood loss. Nevertheless, circular mobilization of the whole segment should be avoided.

In addition, a considerable advantage of the balloon catheter lies in the fact that the vein need not be approached directly over the thrombosis, as was described for other methods of extraction (Fontaine and Tuchmann, 1963; Palma, 1968), but can be opened at the site of choice, even if the thrombosis lies distally or proximally to it. Probing can be done in three directions from the femoral bifurcation. Direct approach to the thrombosed segment remains indicated only for obliteration of short distances within the limb or pelvic axis if contributory anatomic factors have to be eliminated at the same time (Gaylis, 1974).

Longitudinal venotomy is preferred to transverse venotomy since there is the risk of circular tearing of a transverse incision when the balloon is withdrawn.

Retrograde Thrombectomy from Pelvic Veins

With the vein open, the thrombus appears as a shiny, dark cherry red or, if it is older, a gelatinous or washed cast of the lumen; in femoroiliac thrombosis, it extends finger-like projections into the mouth of the profunda femoris and other collaterals (Fig. 5.28 on Plate II and Fig. 5.37).

The second 8 to 10 French balloon catheter is pushed past the thrombus (Fig. 5.26 No. 2 and 5.28 on Plate II) into the common femoral vein and into the vena cava. It is now inflated in its turn and retracted into the common iliac vein, which

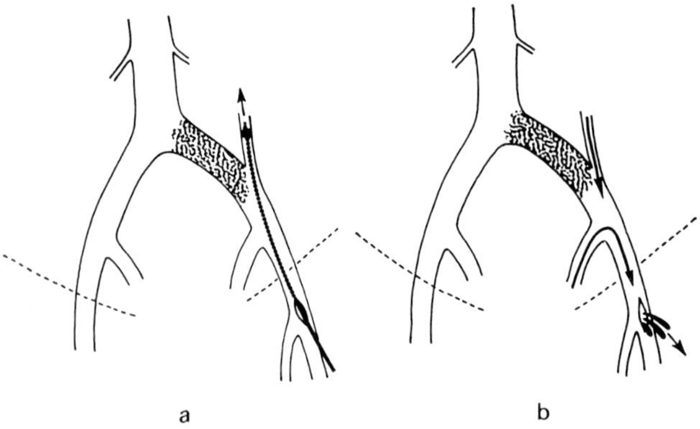

Fig. 5.35. Errors during thrombectomy. Deviation of balloon catheter (*a*); misleading good reflux in resistant obstruction in the common iliac vein (*b*). (From Mavor, G. E., J. M. D. Galloway and R. G. Mahaffy: Surg. Gynec. Obstet. 129 [1969] 57.)

is felt by a slight resistance. Here it replaces the formerly applied blockade of the balloon introduced preliminarily into the vena cava, which was emptied but left in situ for the present. Thus the system of the healthy side is free once again. Today, this second catheter in Fig. 5.26 is introduced under high-pressure respiration without preceding cava blockade.

For thrombectomy proper, the operating table is turned to give maximal elevation of the head (anti-Trendelenburg position). The third balloon catheter, 8 French, is pushed forward for extraction till it touches the second balloon. Blind cannulation of the vena cava and pelvic veins according to the original method of Fogarty does not inform the surgeon of the exact position of the catheters, however (Fig. 5.35*a*). Hence, it is recommended that the inferior vena cava be exposed by a preliminary lumbar retroperitoneal gridiron incision to permit palpation (Eriksson et al., 1967), or that the balloons be filled with contrast medium and a roentgenogram taken (Mansfield et al., 1971; Mavor et al., 1969).

Finally, clearing of clots is done with the extraction catheter assisted by active abdominal pressing in local anesthesia or high-pressure respiration in inhalation anesthesia. The common iliac vein is valveless and the external iliac and common femoral veins contain only one to three pairs of insufficient valves in 25 per cent of cases. In 37 per cent of cases, the venous column is last interrupted by a valve in the superficial femoral vein just distal to the union with the profunda (Basmajean, 1952; Eger and Casper, 1943). A strong retrograde flow of blood must be seen before radical clearance can be assumed, but it is not a reliable sign (Fig. 5.35*b*). On intraoperative phlebograms of 16 patients, Wilson and Britt (1967) observed remnants in the inferior vena cava and pelvic veins despite good reflux in 14 cases. On the other hand, inadequate reflux is a certain sign of incomplete disobstruction. Before repeated attempts at extraction are made, it is advisable to spread the common femoral vein with a curved clamp, since occasionally a pair of competent valves opposes backflow (Diethrich, 1967) (Fig. 5.36). Thrombectomy is usually complete if the clots are molded and connected. Multiple single bits of clot suggest incomplete clearance.

Clots at the unions are carefully removed with forceps, deeper seated clots are removed with 8 or 6 French catheters. Immediately afterward, all

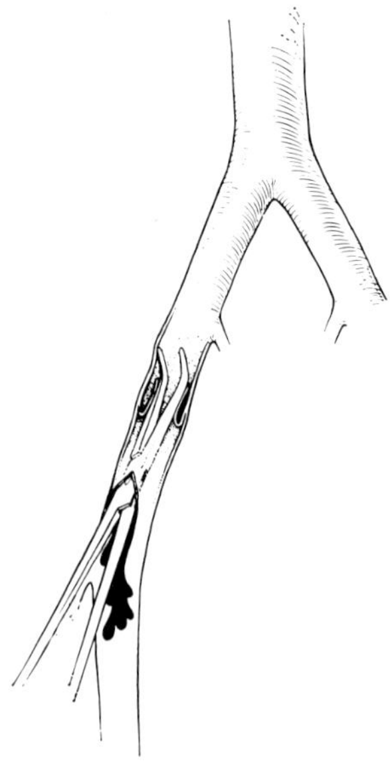

Fig. 5.36. Spreading a pair of valves in the common femoral vein. (From Diethrich, E. B.: Surg. Gynec. Obstet. 124 [1967] 1322.)

these cleared branches must be closed again by the loops or by means of fine clips in order to avoid blood loss (Fig. 5.26 No. 5 and Fig. 5.37).

Anterograde Thrombectomy from the Leg Axis

This method is more difficult than retrograde thrombectomy from the pelvic veins. Only rarely does the thrombus literally jump out of the distal vascular space when lightly touched.

Disobliteration of all Inguinal Branches

External measures. Fresh thrombi together with clots in collaterals may be expelled by centripetal bandaging of the leg with an Esmarch bandage (Fig. 5.39*b*). Supportive measures are repeated dorsiflexion of the foot and milking by foulage.

Distalward catheterization. If these external manipulations fail, the fourth catheter, 6 French, is introduced distally (see Fig. 5.26 No. 4). Difficulties may arise because of strong opposition to the catheter at the check valves. The soft catheter tip is easily caught in the valve pockets. With Fogarty's procedure, however, the valves are not injured because of the flexible tip. With twisting and slight stretching and emptying of the balloon,

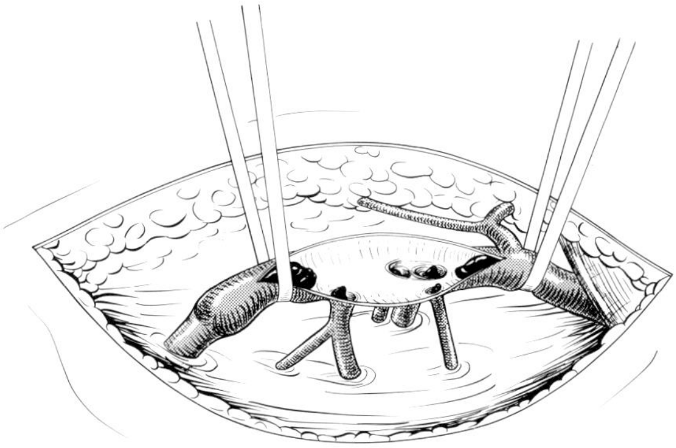

Fig. 5.37. Clots at the union of branches of different caliber in the segment including profunda femoris and superficial femoral veins with the common femoral vein. Deblocking of all these branches including long saphenous vein produces massive improvement of postoperative inflow into the pelvic axis (cf Fig. 5.34 on Plate III and Fig. 5.26 No. 5). All branches have to be closed or even clamped in order to prevent marked bleeding. Nevertheless, circular mobilization of the whole segment is to be avoided. The branches in this figure are stressed exclusively for illustration of anatomic conditions. (Drawing by G. Forster, Fachklasse für wissenschaftliches Zeichnen, Kunstgewerbeschule der Stadt Zürich.)

the tip slips through the valve (see Fig. 5.30), but frequently only after repeated trials. On withdrawal of the inflated catheter balloon, the valve pockets are also milked atraumatically. These were found by McLachlin and Paterson (1951) to be hemodynamically predisposed sites of deposit of initial thrombosis. Extended exposure of the superficial femoral vein for thrombectomy by multiple venotomy, suggested by Palma (1968), is redundant.

The catheter can thus usually be pushed into the popliteal vein; it will not pass farther distally, into the leg trunks, because of the closer position of the valves.

To overcome these difficulties, Kiely (1973) developed a new catheter technique: He introduced a guide wire into the deep veins above the ankle, pushing this into the venotomy as far as the groin and fastening the balloon to it, which is subsequently pulled down to the ankle.

External measures with or without catheterization distalward from the venotomy in the groin never completely remove thrombi from the main veins of the leg, however. But a maximal inflow from the leg into the superficial femoral vein is a very important condition for prevention of immediate recurrent thrombosis. Following the recommendation of Mercier and Tournigand (1976), the popliteal vein is exposed in principle by Szilagyi's method for removal of thrombi from the distal leg axis and is incised in order to clear visually clots in the distal venous trunks and the veins of the soleus muscle by foulage. The results achieved at the 3- to 6-armed popliteal junction are surprising in individual cases and effect perfusion of the superior femoral vein quite decisively (Fig. 5.38).

Finally, a 16 French catheter is drawn down by means of a guide wire to the level of this popliteal venotomy, and the vein is closed by interrupted sutures. The catheter is inflated just prior to the final closure of the inguinal venotomy and pulled out from the femoral axis as final clearing measure.

Temporary arteriovenous fistula. Recent experience has shown that, with intraoperative indications of threatening recurrent thrombosis, a temporary arteriovenous fistula assists in keeping the disobliterated femoral and pelvic segments patent postoperatively (Gruss and Laubach, 1971). Arterialization of the deep venous system increases pressure and flow.

Since the first communication of Bryant (1958), numerous experiments on dogs have shown that many variations of temporary arteriovenous fistulas protect free grafts in the femoral vein (Bryant et al., 1958; Levin et al., 1971) and

PLATE III

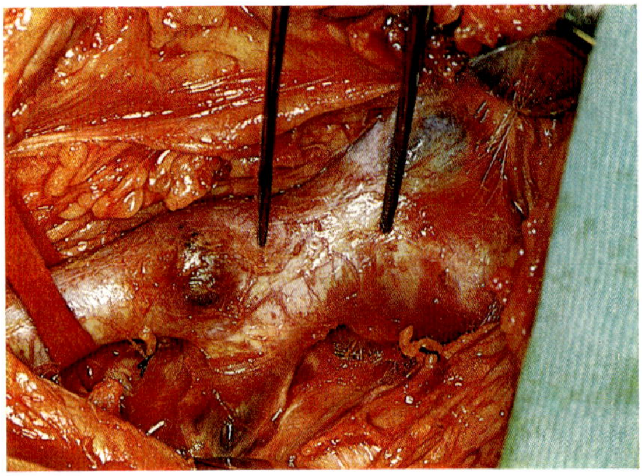

Fig. 5.34. Freeing of the junction of the superficial femoral and profunda femoris at the common femoral; tape around superficial femoral; forceps indicates zone of choice for venotomy. The venotomy is elongated according to the number and situation of the here very variable branches of smaller caliber in order to be able to remove thrombi from these as well (cf Fig. 5.37).

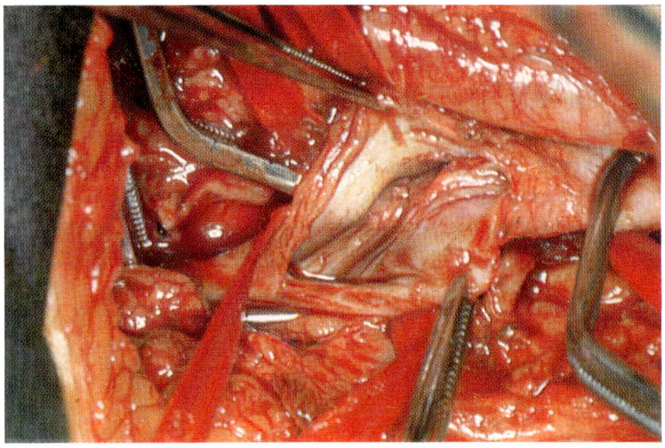

Fig. 5.43. Fourteen-day-old clots, flushed out and adherent to venous wall.

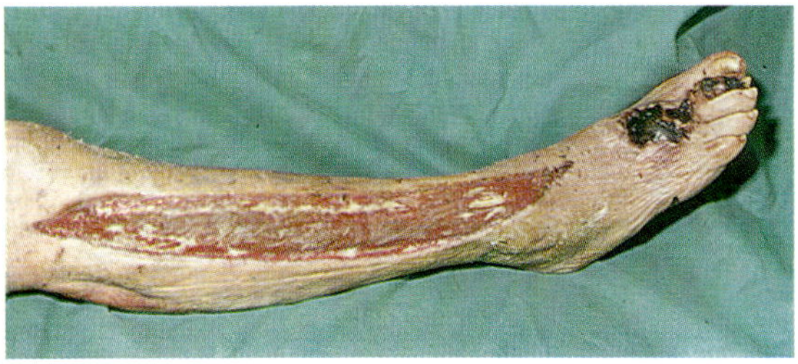

Fig. 5.44. Fasciotomy of the anterior tibial muscle compartment as palliative treatment of phlegmasia cerulea dolens (woman aged 80).

Fogarty and Hallin (1966) made their patients get up on the second postoperative day, but the stage of healing of the wound may not permit this in every case.

Active exercises. As soon as the patient has awakened from the anesthesia, he is urged to promote venous flow himself by strong muscle exercises: dorsiflexion of the foot 100 times per hour, pressure of the foot against a specially fixed board for activating soleus and gastrocnemius musculature, tension of quadriceps and, later, active movement of the whole limb—"walking in bed"—as well as forced breathing exercises. As a supplement to these measures, Völker's treadle (pedal expander) (Fig. 5.42) has proved useful. It serves mainly to empty the soleus veins, which may act as a "mud catcher," causing recurrent thrombosis during bed rest (Gibbs, 1957; Kakkar et al., 1969).

Venous segments subjected to thrombectomy will remain patent if this early mobilization is consistently enforced (Sevitt, 1960). If the thrombus was removed in one piece, the risk of dislodgment of remnants as emboli during exercises is small. Pressure bandages accelerate flow in the deep venous and deep lymphatic systems of patients confined to bed.

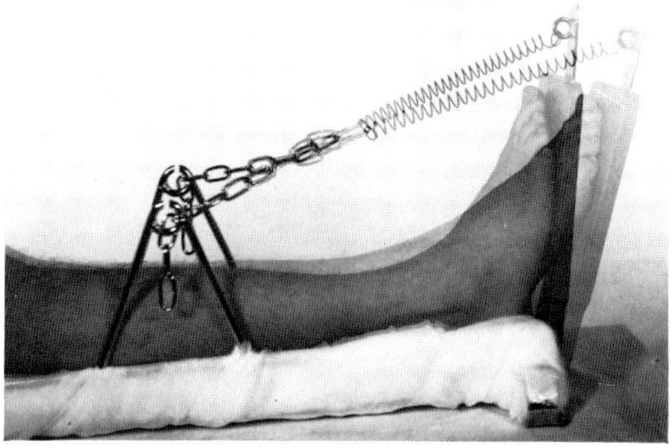

Fig. 5.42. Völker's treadle (foot expander).

Anticoagulant therapy. Systematic postoperative anticoagulant therapy must not be omitted:

—5000 I.U. intravenously, after closure of the venotomy, followed by

—10 000 I.U. heparin per liter of infusion fluid in 12 hours; the irrigation catheter is introduced into a subinguinal tributary of the long saphenous for direct flushing of disobliterated pelvic veins (see Fig. 5.31).

—oral administration of coumarin derivatives immediately after operation, and

—discontinuation of heparin when the results of the Quick test are in the therapeutic range, with continuation of oral treatment for minimal 6 months.

Phlebographic Evaluation

Certain information about the results achieved provides the basis for postoperative treatment and assessment of the outcome. As long as the irrigation catheter for flushing of the pelvic veins is still in situ, the contrast medium can be directly instilled to visualize them (Nachbur et al., 1967). Later phlebographie evaluation requires the same technique as preoperative localization of the thrombosis (Brunner and Wirth, 1971; Brunner, 1971; Wirth et al., 1971).

Conditions and Problems Relating to Thrombectomy

Local Conditions

According to our own surgical experience and examinations by other authors (Encke et al., 1966; McLachlin and Paterson, 1951), the source of a fully developed, unilateral acute thrombosis with sudden swelling of the whole limb, bursting pain, tenderness of the femoral vascular space and white or cyanotic discoloration (see Fig. 5.16 on Plate I) is, as a rule, either occlusion of the venous femoral union with the common femoral vein or a joint femoroiliac obliteration (Fig. 5.45). Isolated leg thrombosis does not cause as severe a syndrome as communis or femoroiliac thrombosis. In particular, there is no swelling of the thigh.

With this in mind, the site of the thrombosis can be roughly localized clinically; but for appraisal of results and detailed technical procedure that is carried out blindly by Fogarty's method, precise *preoperative delimitation* of the obstruction is desirable. This the more so, since according to Kakkar (1972), 15 per cent of acute swellings of the leg do not originate in the veins. For exclusion of these cases, application of the Doppler ultrasound technique is suitable as "disentangling test" (Bollinger, 1975; Cranley et al., 1975; Rickford and Negus, 1975; Hallböök and Ling, 1973; Yao et al., 1974). Genuine venous obstructions would then require preoperative phlebographic clarification. Especially important for planning the operative procedure is exact information about the inferior vena cava (Poilleux et al., 1975). The three-step combination of phlebographic methods yields a comprehensive picture (Mavor and Galloway, 1967; Wirth, 1967; Wirth and Weber, 1971; Weber et al., 1973) (Fig. 5.20):

—*Anterograde phlebography of the dorsum of the foot to determine the caudal end of the obstruction.* Although the balloon catheter advances barely as far as the popliteal vein from the venotomy of choice, assessment of the venous periphery is important for technical and prognostic reasons. In *total thrombosis* of the leg and pelvic veins, anterograde phlebography with percutaneous puncture of the veins of the dorsum of the foot does not always yield satisfactory results. Transosseous phlebography through the calcaneus, which could theoretically be employed in these cases, is to be rejected from both the surgical and radiologic viewpoints because of the risk of osteomyelitis (Maranta and Wirth, 1968; Süsse, 1956). Caudal termination of *segmental occlusions* is demonstrable by anterograde phlebography.

—*Transosseous phlebography for depiction of conditions in small pelvic veins and the common femoral vein.* The pelvic portion of the swollen limb can be visualized only transosseously, since direct puncture of the femoral is not feasible. It must be done under general anesthesia.

—*Puncture phlebography of the common femoral and pelvic veins of the healthy side for representation of the inferior vena cava and the cranial limit of thrombosis in the femoroiliac axis.*

Gillot (1974) tested occlusion phlebography via the axillary pathway for determination of conditions in the vena cava.

On the strength of this radiologic examination, which is free of complications, segmental femoroiliac venous thrombosis with a patent inferior vena cava and periphery (popliteal and leg vein trunks) proved to be the most promising condition for best results from thrombectomy (Fig. 5.33*a*). In total limb thrombosis there is a tendency to relapses, originating in the periphery, and thus to repeated subclinical pulmonary emboli if the veins in the thigh are not carefully cleared, as described above.

For pulmonary embolism arising without forewarning, the same phlebographic combination is employed.

Temporal Conditions

The reaction of the *venous wall* presents a pathologicoanatomic limit for thrombectomy by balloon catheter. In individual cases, it would be desirable to predict the stage of organization of a thrombus. This temporal limit has not been fully elucidated as yet.

Mahorner (1965) found in animal experiments that organization of a fresh thrombus had progressed greatly after 3 weeks but was not complete by 6 weeks.

Histologic examinations of Leu (1968) revealed that organization spreads over a considerable period. First fibroblasts and capillaries grow in between the fourth and twentieth days, and fibroblastic transformation of buds follows between the eighth and sixtieth days. Thus there are undoubtedly thromboses that organize early and

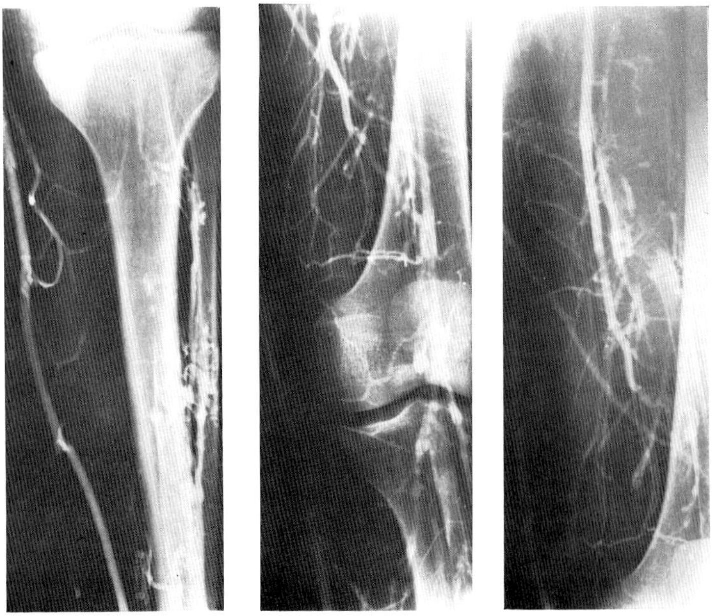

a b c

Fig. 5.45 *a–c*

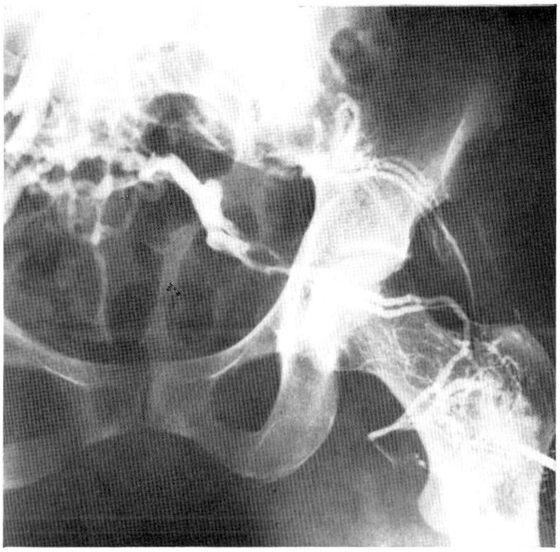

d

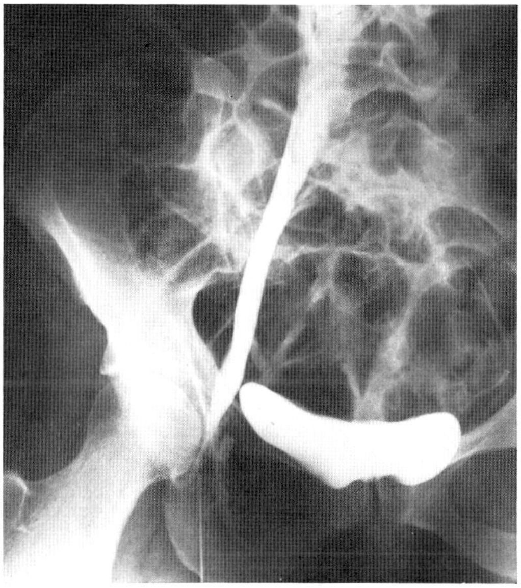

e

Fig. 5.45 *a-e*. Global thrombosis of the left lower extremity (woman aged 38). Floating thrombus in vein trunks of the leg and in the femoropopliteal segment (anterograde phlebography) (*a-c*); total occlusion of the pelvic veins (transosseous phlebography of the pelvis) (*d*); patent inferior vena cava (phlebography by femoral puncture from the healthy side) (*e*).

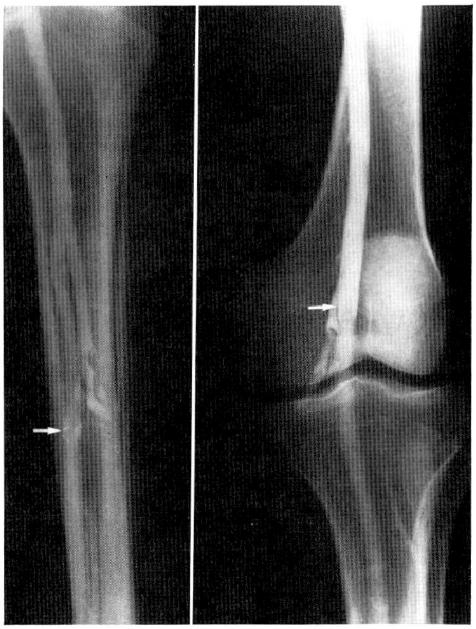

g f

Fig. 5.45 *f-l*. Six months after thrombectomy (done on the second day of acute symptoms) there is free passage in the whole deep system, and the valves are preserved (*g, f, i*).

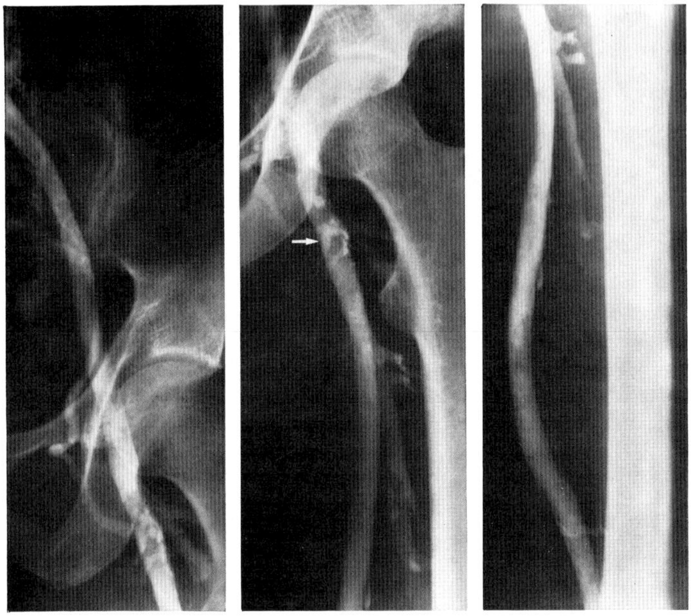

h i k

Fig. 5.45 *h-k*

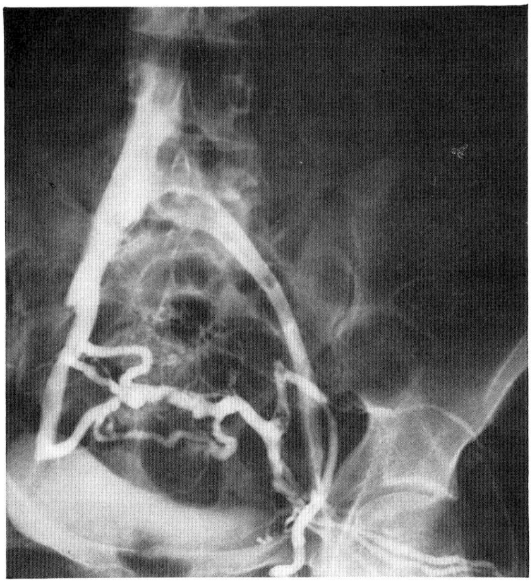

l

Fig. 5.45 *l*

others that organize late, but no clinical or laboratory methods are available to ascertain the state of organization in individual cases.

However, even if a thrombus can be extracted after 6 weeks, other factors must be considered. To avoid recurrent thrombosis, it is also essential that the thrombus can be cleanly and atraumatically lifted off the endothelium. From this point of view, the most favorable period becomes much shorter. According to Linton (1969), it is possible only within the first 18 hours. Fogarty et al. (1966), Fogarty and Hallin (1966) and Mavor and Galloway (1969) place the extreme limit at the seventh day. Haller (1962) achieved his best late results with thrombotic sequelae and recurrences after 6 months among those patients who had thrombectomy in the first 10 days after appearance of clinical symptoms. Thrombectomy done between the fourteenth and twenty-first days was incomplete, especially distally (Haller and Abrams, 1963), and consequently, late results included many relapses. Fontaine et al. (1965)

achieved their best results in phlegmasia cerulea dolens when thrombectomy was done within the first 3 days.

Our own surgical material showed that a thrombus could be extracted in one piece and without damage to the endothelium in the first 6 days. Thrombi of 1 to 2 weeks' duration were already adherent to the venous wall (Fig. 5.43 on Plate III) and disintegrated during extraction, increasing the chances of intraoperative pulmonary embolism. The thrombi were most firmly adherent to valve pockets, and remnants had to be left; this predisposes to recurrent thrombosis. This experience is in agreement with autopsy findings according to which stagnation thrombosis usually begins in valve pockets in which blood remains as in a mud barrier (McLachlin and Paterson, 1951). The margins of insertion of the valves were usually swollen and rigid in this progressive stage. The adventitia was scarred and the perivenous tissues were edematous. Partially organized thrombi could be removed with the ring stripper, similar to arterial occlusive cylinders, even after 3 months (Senn and Nachbur, 1976); but the venous wall in our own cases was grossly injured, so that rethrombosis at the end of the operation was unavoidable without temporary av fistula.

The delicate *valve cusps* can be preserved only if the adherent thrombus is removed between the second and fifth days (Eriksson et al., 1967; Mahorner, 1965). Organization of a thrombus begins at the valve cusps (Gibbs, 1957). The postoperative phlebogram showed fresh thrombosis in three of our patients who had undergone thrombectomy 3 to 6 days after symptoms appeared; no functioning valves were observed in the formerly thrombosed segments even though the vascular system was patent. One patient had functional valves after thrombectomy within 2 days (Figs. 5.39*c* and 5.45*f-l*). Lansing and Davis (1968) took phlebograms of 15 patients who, 5 years previously, had undergone thrombectomy within the first week. The lumen of the superficial femoral vein was indeed patent but valves were insufficient or absent.

The difficulty of assessing the most favorable time becomes further complicated by the fact that the onset of acute symptoms occasionally occurs after thrombosis has been developing subclinically for a few days. Hence leading questions to the patient are frequently decisive. Initial symptoms such as pain in the calf and a sensation of heaviness are often made light of by patients in the preacute stage. In addition, thrombosis often develops gradually during bed rest for disease (e.g., influenza), without the typical signs of spontaneous pain, swelling, discoloration and stagnating superficial veins. Diagnostic indications such as a discrepancy between pulse rate and temperature (Allen's sign), tender veins of the calf, calf pain on passive dorsiflexion of the foot with the knee flexed (Homans' sign), pain over the adductor canal or the calf due to subfascial edema are important signs pointing to a possible suspicion of thrombosis. (Shafer and Duboff, 1971; Cranley et al., 1976). Pelvic pain is frequently the first symptom of a descending iliac thrombosis (Kauppila, 1974). Today, diagnosis is established with radioactively labeled fibrinogen (Kakkar et al., 1969; Kakkar, 1972; Covey and Sherman, 1975; Jung et al., 1975). However, on exclusively positive findings with radioactive fibrinogen without clinical signs of thrombosis or pulmonary embolism, specific therapy will hardly be necessary (Doouss, 1976).

Rule of thumb. It is clear from the foregoing that, as regards prophylaxis of embolism and preservation of valves and wall structures, probably only thrombectomy done in the first 48 hours is of maximum value; this also applies to fibrinolysis (Kakkar et al., 1969). The vein may still be disobliterated cleanly and with little risk of intraoperative pulmonary embolism in the first 6 days. Only partial success is achieved when it is done during the second week, and none of the aims is attained after the third week. The contribution of radiology in determining the state of organization of a thrombus is visualization of a *floating thrombus* bathed in contrast medium (Fig. 5.45*a-c*) (Elliot et al., 1976; Thomas and McAlister, 1971). The appearance of this envelope on phlebography gives the impression that the venous contour has been traced with a pencil (May and Nissl, 1967). Such a floating thrombus must be evaluated as highly emboligenic and forms an urgent indication for thrombectomy (Thomas and McAlister, 1971; Poilleux et al., 1975). Senn and Nachbur (1976) enlarge this indication, possibly by application of a ring stripper, also to late thrombectomies, weeks and months after the acute manifestation.

Etiologic Conditions

Acute swelling of the limb as a sequel to a *first* spontaneous femoroiliac thrombosis occurred in only a small number of our patients. Much more frequently it meant final decompensation of hitherto subclinical chronic thrombosis or progressive malignant compression. If these cases were not recognized preoperatively, thrombectomy was at best only partially successful. This points up the importance of clinical and radiologic diagnosis in deciding on surgical intervention. In addition, patients with general diseases such as ulcerative colitis and polycythemia which occasionally cause deep vein thrombosis and those with marantic thrombosis are excluded from surgery.

Chronic femoroiliac venous thrombosis with acute exacerbation. Early experience with thrombectomy showed that, even with peracute swellings, only occasional fresh clots could be extracted from an unexpectedly chronically obliterated venous system. On direct questioning, these patients admitted to previous attacks of swelling, so that in retrospect it was realized that the occlusive process must have taken place several times. Meantime, venous reflux was provided by collaterals.

Thrombosis of the venous system frequently is evolutionary—on the one hand, because it gains a foothold in different segments of the main trunks gradually or continuously, and on the other, because of concentric lamination in the lumen, arising from mural thrombi. Thrombi of various ages are found on cross section of veins, similar to arterial aneurysms. The latest layers lie centrally. Thus a clinically peracute swelling occasionally follows many preceding subclinical events (Brunner, 1974).

On longitudinal and transverse section of the deep venous system, the surgeon is confronted with aggregates of thrombus of varying age resulting from previous clot formation (Brunner, 1974). Gradual or continuous intravascular clotting, proceeding for weeks, may spread either upward or downward, but more frequently upward (Kakkar et al., 1969; Sevitt, 1969, 1975).

On longitudinal section, one succeeds only occasionally in clearing fresh thrombi from single segments of the axis in the vicinity of the venotomy. Figure 5.21 on page 107 shows a fresh femoral event following old pelvic thrombosis. It is important for late results that the junction of the superficial femoral and profunda femoris with the common femoral vein remain free, at least for partial success. On cross section, only fresh masses of the interior of a thrombus can be eliminated by the balloon. It glides past older, adherent layers. Early phlebographic assessment reveals unevenness of the wall due to mural remnants (see Fig. 5.31). Such mural remnants are most frequently found at the level of the iliac "*vascular spur.*"

Fogarty et al. (1966) considered an established post-thrombotic syndrome with acute exacerbation a contraindication to thrombectomy. In unrecognized cases among our own patients, the acute painful episodes were stopped by the operation; but the flow achieved in the damaged system could not be counted on to keep the vessel patent. Furthermore, a patient with intraoperative pulmonary embolism, who survived after a Trendelenburg operation, showed clearly the danger of manipulation of partially organized thrombi. Since neither embolism nor the post-thrombotic syndrome is prevented, thrombectomy is only *conditionally* indicated once chronic venous thrombosis is ascertained, in our experience. However, partial success is possible (Senn and Nachbur, 1976). Transosseous pelvic phlebography can usually detect old thrombosis, revealing collaterals and recanalization, or a successive event (see Fig. 5.21).

Particularly careful investigation is required in postpartum thrombosis, which has been repeatedly observed among some of our multiparous patients occurring only as last link in a chain of insignificant swelling attacks.

An exception to this indication is phlegmasia cerulea dolens with threatening venous gangrene, for which even partial disobstruction has proved to be the best measure for decompression of the microcirculation (Mahorner, 1965; Mavor and Galloway, 1969; Senn and Nachbur, 1976). With descending femoral thrombosis and longer existing occlusions of the pelvic axis, Hilbe and Flora (1972) follow this up by a Palma anastomosis immediately after disobliteration of the leg axis.

Another exception involving urgent indication for thrombectomy is a floating thrombus occurring during an ascending chronic thrombosis with acute exacerbation.

Malignant compression. Among our patients, acute thrombosis was repeatedly the first indication of malignant processes in the pelvis and malignant lymphomas and tumors of the female generative organs. Occasionally large inguinal lymphomas escape palpation, having disappeared in the general swelling of the thigh, and are demonstrated only on lymphography. Figures 5.22 to 5.24 on page 108f show these examples of malignant compression diagnosed radiologically.

- Giant follicular lymphoblastoma (Brill-Symmers disease) in a female aged 76 with compression of the right femoroiliac trunks in several places (see Fig. 5.22). *First sign: acutely swollen right lower extremity.*
- Retroperitoneal metastasis of a squamous cell carcinoma of the right lower lobe of the lung in a 57-year-old woman 6 months after excision (see Fig. 5.23). Compression of the right external iliac vein with displacement of collateral vessels. *First sign: acutely swollen right lower extremity.*

—Compression of left common iliac vein due to carcinoma of the uterus with lymph node metastases in a patient aged 43 years (see Fig. 5.24). First transosseous phlebography was done to elucidate a discrete chronic swelling of the limb; it revealed marked constriction of the external iliac vein (see Fig. 5.24*a*). The patient returned with *peracute swelling* 14 days later. The remaining lumen was occluded by thrombosis (see Fig. 5.24*b*).

The importance of preoperative diagnosis in these cases is obvious.

Paraneoplastic syndrome. Occasionally femoroiliac thrombosis occurs along with carcinoma without direct mechanical vein compression, leaving the causal relation between tumor and thrombosis undefined. These "distant effects" of tumors are called paraneoplastic (Wichert, 1970). In addition to leg, arm and jugular vein thrombosis, changes in the blood picture and neurologic, cardiac, dermal, metabolic, endocrine, gastrointestinal and osseous paraneoplastic syndromes are known (Reisner, 1973).

Uehlinger (1966) defined paraneoplastic syndromes as follows: "They are sequels to specific and nonspecific metabolic functions of neoplastic cells. They are connected neither with spatial extent nor with histologic differentiation of the tumor. They are subordinate to the growth, regress after its resection and may return with local recurrence or metastases. *The connection between tumor and paraneoplastic syndrome is frequently realized only in retrospect.* The full significance of paraneoplastic syndromes is that they are indicators of first rather than early signs of malignant neoplasm. They contribute to increasing the number of successfully operable malignant tumors."

Paraneoplastic femoroiliac thrombosis usually manifests itself as phlegmasia cerulea dolens. Among our patients it was observed as the first sign of occult carcinomas of the stomach, pancreas and lungs. Since the principal disease continually causes thrombosis in more vein segments, thrombectomy does not treat the causal factors. In addition, massive anticoagulant therapy in the presence of occult gastrointestinal carcinoma promotes unexpected hemorrhages.

In the acute stage, the history and general state occasionally suggest occult carcinoma. However, an unremarkable history easily obscures the real cause of thrombosis. The value of history (phlebitis migrans) and clinical (Virchow's gland) and radiologic examination is evident. In any case, it is advisable to consider malignancy in patients beyond the age of 40, when the cause of phlegmasia cerulea dolens appearing out of the blue is not obvious. The indication for thrombectomy then depends on the general situation and is even then only conditional, despite threatening venous gangrene. Of course, radiologic examination of the gastrointestinal tract is frequently precluded by the acute state of the limb. But it is not advisable to disregard contraindications knowingly.

Intraoperative Complications

Left-sided Obstruction in the Common Iliac Vein

In three of our patients with left-sided femoroiliac vein thrombosis, the catheter did not reach the inferior vena cava on probing because it hit the "vascular spur" where the right common iliac artery rides on the left common iliac vein, described by Schilling (1926) and precisely defined by May and Thurner (1956) (p. 23ff) (Dale and Allen, 1975).

—In the first case, thrombectomy proved incomplete and was discontinued. Result: early recurrent thrombosis.
—In the second case, the segment was repaired by laparotomy and venotomy. The "vascular spur" was enucleated. Result: early recurrent thrombosis.
—In the third case, the obstruction was broken by repeated inflation of the balloon and the pelvic veins were completely cleared. Result: clinical success; the pelvic veins remained radiologically patent.

Conclusions. Eliminating the left-sided "vascular spur" is essential for full success of thrombectomy. Occasionally the obstruction can be removed with the balloon. If this does not work, only partial success and recurrent thrombosis can be expected. However, this can possibly be avoided when applying the above described flow-preventing details of surgical technique, especially temporary av fistulas (Fig. 5.26 Nos. 5 and 6, Fig. 5.40, Fig. 5.41).

Intraoperative Pulmonary Embolism—Trendelenburg Embolectomy (H. Schwarz)

In order to prevent thromboembolic complications, ligatures of the venous trunks after thrombectomy have been recommended in recent years by American authors (Brunner and Lanz, 1964; DeWeese, 1964; Fontaine et al., 1969). Taking into account all the technical details of the balloon method, such ligatures are not necessary. They are unphysiological measures that forcibly interrupt venous drainage. Even the caval ligature is always followed by some signs of venous stasis in spite of extensive compensating collaterals (Nabseth and Moran, 1965). Therefore it would seem that these ligatures are indicated only as embolism prophylaxis in the case of aged patients with manifest thrombosis and as a screen against septic thrombosis.

Theoretically, we have to take into account the possibility of an embolism after every venous thrombectomy. But intraoperative and postoperative mortality is significantly lower than embolism mortality under conservative treatment. Fontaine and Tuchmann (1964) reported one death (1.2 per cent) out of 86 thrombectomies in the region of femoral, common and external iliac veins and the vena cava. As opposed to this, 12.3 per cent of their conservatively treated cases died of massive embolism.

The therapeutic approach is decided by the extent of pulmonary embolism. All stages of transition are possible, from massive bilateral embolism with instant death to small repeated emboli with barely recordable tachycardia. A rule of thumb derived from large numbers of deaths due to pulmonary embolism is that one fourth of the patients survive 1 hour, one fifth 4 hours and one sixth at least 6 hours (Carcia, 1969). There is therefore sufficient time for exact diagnosis in a great number of patients. The extent of the embolization must be determined, either by the noninvasive method of lung scintigraphy or by angiography. There is no doubt, especially in bilateral pulmonary embolism, that best results with embolectomy are achieved when the heart-lung machine is used. Various diagnostic examinations are inestimable preoperative aids, the resulting loss of time, however, may mean death for a patient with massive pulmonary embolization. Cardiac arrest soon follows if the embolism causes acute cor pulmonale with high central venous pressure, tachypnea, tachycardia and cyanosis, or the small minute volume causes drop in blood pressure and coronary failure. Only prompt intervention can save the patient. Ideally, partial bypass (femorofemoral) with the oxygenator will circumvent the pulmonary block and much improve circulatory conditions. Up to 1 hour can be gained for induction of anesthesia, thoracotomy and continuation by total bypass (heart-lung machine) (Beall, 1965).

For the actual embolectomy there is more time at our disposal if a heart-lung machine is connected. In this way the arterial blood supply of the periphery, in particular of the brain, is ensured, so that the embolic masses can be removed more quietly and carefully. Therefore the heart-lung machine is to be recommended in principle.

However, a heart-lung machine is not available to every surgeon who performs venous surgery. In emergency, in cases of cardiac arrest there is no time to connect it and the classic Trendelenburg operation (Trendelenburg, 1908) is indicated, since the alternative means death. One of our cases proved that even in a hospital with complete cardiopulmonary and vascular facilities prompt decision to perform the traditional Trendelenburg operation may be the correct solution: massive pulmonary embolism occurred on withdrawal of the last balloon during an operation for chronic venous femoroiliac thrombosis in subacute exacerbation:

The anesthetist reported cardiac arrest while the skin was being sutured. The diagnosis of pulmonary embolism in this 45-year-old patient with healthy lungs was beyond doubt. Immediate extrathoracic cardiac massage was accompanied by speedy preparation for thoracotomy and heart-lung machine. When the anterior mediastinum was opened and the pericardium split, a tense right atrium, a tightly filled right ventricle and empty flaccid left ventricle were found. With cardiac action practically absent, connection to the heart-lung machine had to be abandoned, since any further loss of time would have proved fatal (see technical procedure below). The patient recovered fully from both the thrombectomy and the pulmonary embolectomy, and asked to have the cardiac surgeon again at hand for his hip joint operation 4 years later.

Technique

Precautionary measures serve as preparation for the Trendelenburg operation with every thrombectomy for femoroiliac venous thrombosis: favorable scheduling, disinfection and draping of the thorax (cf Fig. 5.25 on Plate II), connection of the electrocardiograph, working respirator and, if possible, a heart-lung machine in readiness.

Procedure by the following steps:
- Longitudinal and slightly paramedian incision from the jugular notch to the xiphoid process with division of the skin and soft tissues down to the bone.
- Longitudinal sternotomy in the very middle by means of the circular saw; the bone is severed full length.
- Insertion of a sternal retractor or spreading of the sternal halves with sharp hooks.
- Displacement of loose mediastinal connective tissues plus thymus remnants down to the pericardium; sharp severing of the fibrous ligaments in the jugular region.
- Longitudinal opening of the pericardium from the exit of the ascending aorta down to the diaphragm.
- Hemostasis is dispensed with until the embolectomy is over.

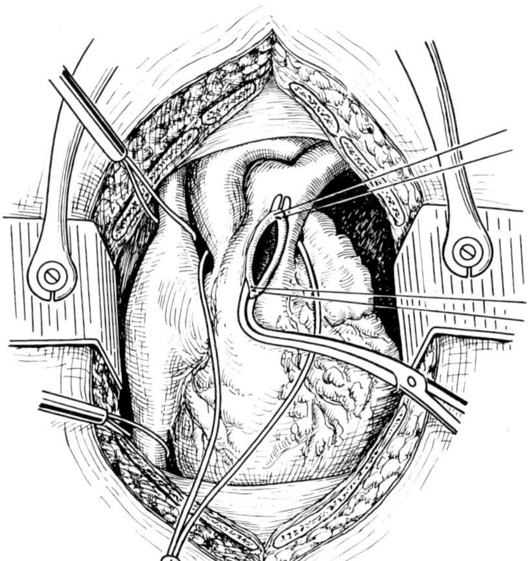

Fig. 5.46. Trendelenburg operation. Thorax opened by longitudinal sternotomy. Superior and inferior vena cava tied with single sutures; aorta and pulmonary vein tied with a common suture. The trunk of the pulmonary artery is longitudinally opened over a tangentially applied hemostat. (After Encke et al.)

Embolectomy can now be performed:
- Brief cardiac massage in case of cardiac arrest; it will be seen that effort is required to press blood into the pulmonary arteries.
- Placing a tape around both the aorta and the pulmonary artery by drawing it through the transverse sinus of the percardium.
- Intrapericardial clamping of both the superior and the inferior vena cava with a vascular clamp (Fig. 5.46).
- After the clamping of both caval veins the trunk of the pulmonary artery is opened longitudinally for approximately 3 cm between 2 stay sutures.
- After the emptying of the overfilled right ventricle, the proximal pulmonary stump is clamped by pulling the tape.
- The actual embolectomy is now performed by means of a sucker which is introduced first into one, then into the other pulmonary artery; it clings to the clots; by careful withdrawal, the embolic masses are evacuated.
- Repeated strong inflation of the lungs by the anesthesiologist pushes distal emboli back toward the sucker. The pulmonary vessels are free when bright red blood appears in the sucker; in case of doubt, the pleural duplication is opened to "milk" the lung.
- In order to close the pulmonary incision, the vascular clamp is placed tangentially.
- Opening of the venous inflow by releasing first the superior, then the inferior vena cava. Volume replacement and cardiac massage if necessary.
- The pulmonary artery is sutured with continuous atraumatic 4/0 silk.
- Fenestration of the pericardium to the left thorax or insertion of a through drainage into the pericardium.
- Loose knotted sutures in the pericardium: catgut 3/0; meticulous hemostasis.

The *closing of the thorax* terminates the operation:
- Wiring of the sternum (approximately 6 wires).
- Periosteal suture with single catgut button sutures.
- Subcutaneous suction drainage if necessary.
- Skin sutures.

Perspectives

(U. Brunner)

Newer perspectives are based on a combination of thrombectomy with fibrinolysis of clots in the trunk veins of the lower legs. The following case provides an illustration:
The patient was a 22-year-old man with acute spontaneous thrombosis of his left leg; the anterograde phlebography on the first day of treatment shows a femoropopliteal thrombosis

with partial blocking of the leg veins (Fig. 5.47a, b). On the second day of treatment the initial dose of 242,000 U streptokinase was administered, followed up on the third day by a maintenance dose which constituted 2/3 of the initial dose per hour. On the fourth day a control phlebography reveals lysis of the thrombus at the level of the poplitea (Fig. 5.47c). The femoropopliteal block persisted. The determination of the prothrombin time suggested that no further result was to be expected from a continuation of fibrinolysis. In this situation the patient was treated with epsilon-aminocaproic acid and later with heparin. On the fifth day retrograde thrombectomy was successfully performed. The phlebography taken six weeks after the operation revealed a completely patent venous system (Fig. 5.47d, e).

Other experience has taught us that in the combined treatment fibrinolysis must always be undertaken before the surgical intervention and not after.

Combined Surgical Thrombectomy and Fibrinolysis

Nachbur (1976, 1977) recently developed a combination therapy, whereby the vascular system of the extremity is perfused by itself immediately subsequent to the thrombectomy with about 20 000 to 25 000 U. streptokinase for 1 to $1\frac{1}{2}$ hours by means of extracorporal circulation. Residues in the main venous trunks of the leg may be removed due to this regional fibrinolysis and the venous in-

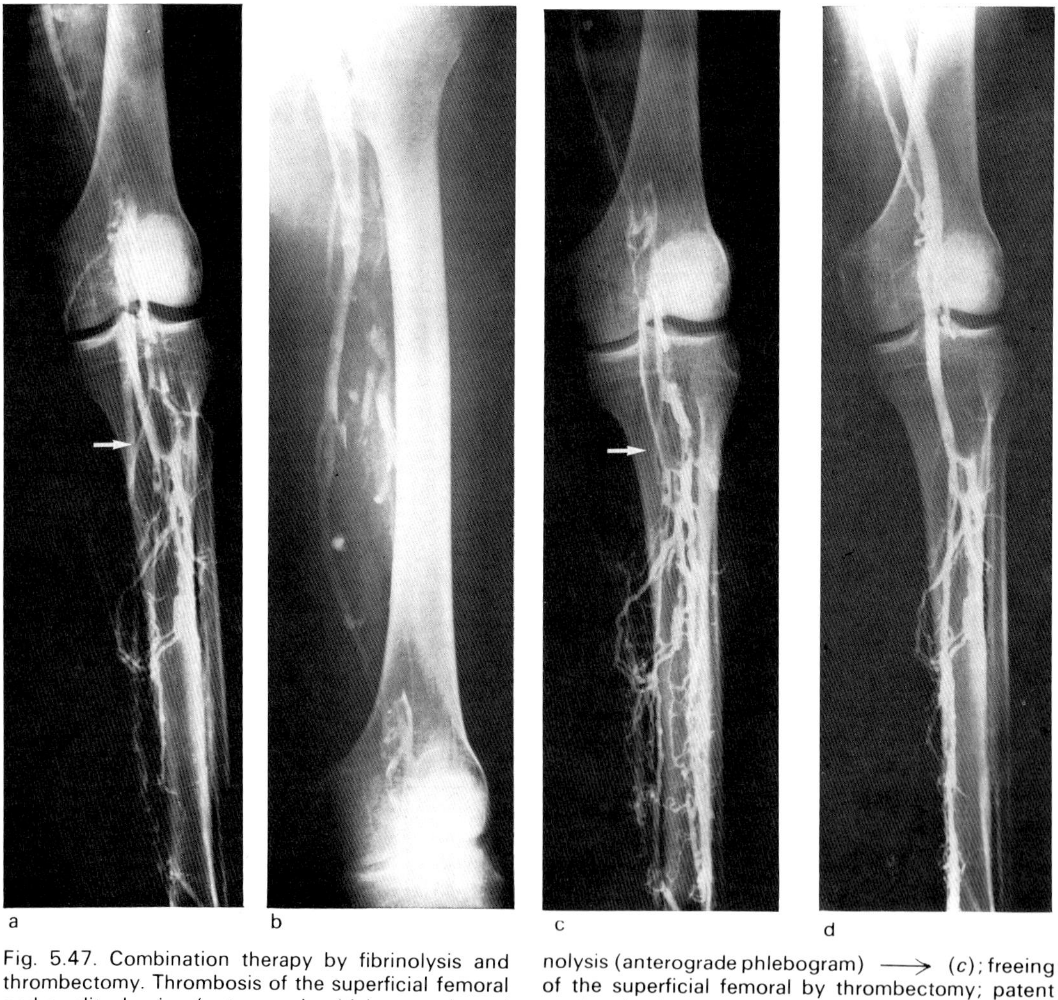

a b c d

Fig. 5.47. Combination therapy by fibrinolysis and thrombectomy. Thrombosis of the superficial femoral and popliteal veins (anterograde phlebograms), and floating thrombus in the popliteal bifurcation ⟶ (*a,b*); freeing of the popliteal vein by fibrinolysis (anterograde phlebogram) ⟶ (*c*); freeing of the superficial femoral by thrombectomy; patent trunk veins in phlebogram 6 weeks after fibrinolysis and thrombectomy (*d,e*).

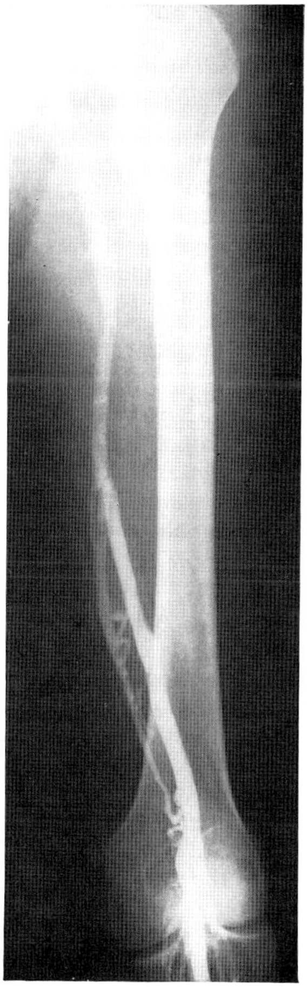

Fig. 5.47*e*

flow into the axis of the thigh thus be enhanced. Results compared with conventional thrombectomy were decisively improved in this manner. Nevertheless, the technical expenditure is considerable.

Late Results

With the technique described above, pure thrombectomy without additional resection of venous segments and ligatures of the inferior cava is the method of choice for the surgical treatment of femoroiliac venous thrombosis. Based upon clinical and radiologic controls of our own medical material, complete and partial success was seen to have been achieved 2 years after the operation in 64 per cent of the cases (Brunner and Wirth 1971). Mavor et al. (1969), using similar methods to check their material radiologically, achieved complete and partial success in 69 per cent of the cases. Phlebographic checks are important for the evaluation of results since clinically satisfactory early results are often misleading with regard to an incompletely patent venous system (Fig. 5.48). Admittedly, the clinical and radiological results of thrombectomy are variously assessed in literature. Enthusiastic reports (Edwards et al., 1970; Harris, 1968; Senn, 1969) are opposed to others expressing total resignation (Karp and Wylie, 1966; Lansing and Davis, 1968).

The radiological checking of early and late results showed above all that not only full success, but also anatomical partial success is of great functional significance. If we manage to disobliterate the femoral bifurcation, the profunda femoris provides an adequate collateral circulation even if the superficial femoral remains interrupted as far as the popliteal vein. The result is usually acceptable clinically (Fig. 5.48).

Indication

Due to the natural course of thrombosis as a

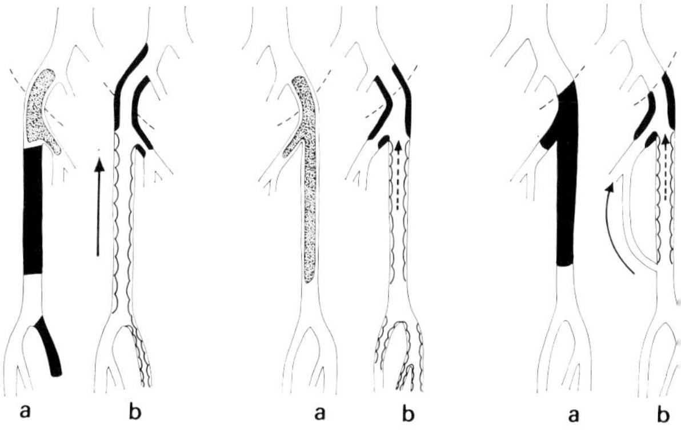

Fig. 5.48. Drawing of radiologic findings in three partial successes. The hemodynamically most important success of the operation is disobliteration of the femoral bifurcation. Floating thrombi (dotted), old occlusion (black), recanalization (wavy), partial success (heavy line). Preoperatively (*a*); postoperatively (*b*). (From Brunner, U., W. Wirth.: Schweiz. med. Wschr. 101 [1971] 1327–1334).

system is well recanalized. The course and arrangement of the deep venous system correspond with normal anatomic conditions. The venous walls are slightly irregular. The valves are destroyed. In the differential diagnosis, congenital absence of the valves and primary

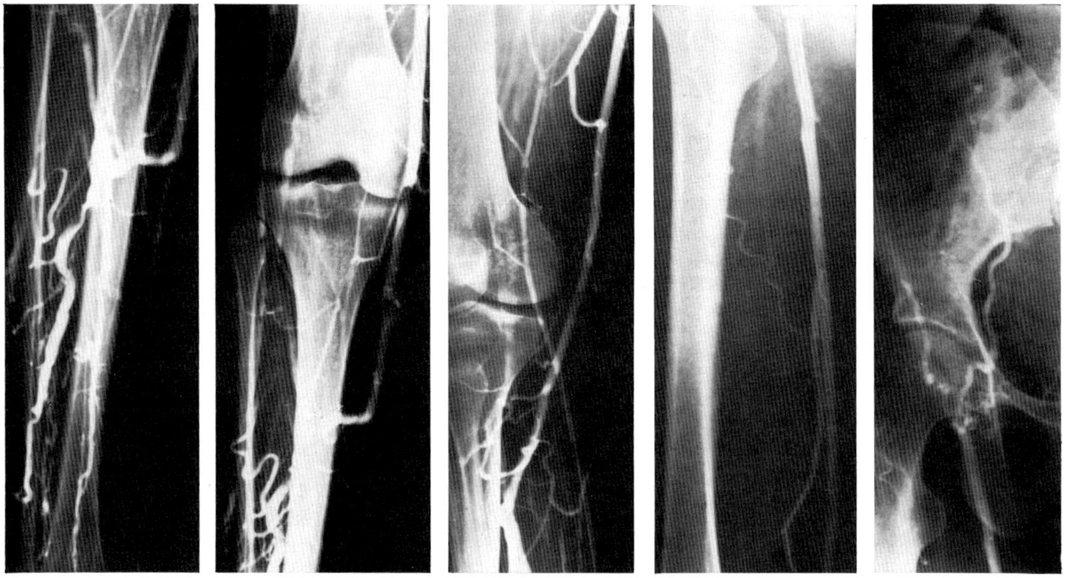

Fig. 6.9. Post-thrombotic damage, Stage IV. Failure of recanalization, with marked pelvic vein damage. First order collateral circulation still mainly insufficient.

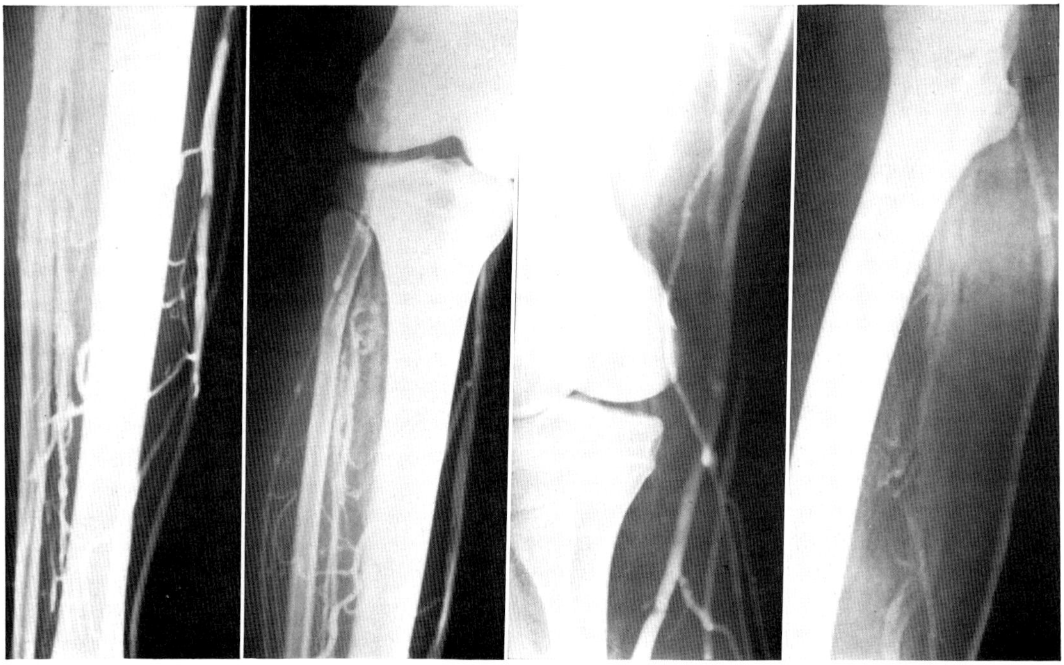

Fig. 6.10. Beginning recanalization of the deep venous system. First and second order collateral circulation sufficient.

varices of the deep venous system must be considered.
- Stage II (Figs. 6.4 to 6.6). Considerable changes of the venous wall, but drainage in the deep venous system corresponds to normal topographic conditions. The contour is markedly irregular. The valves are destroyed.
- Stage III (Figs. 6.7 and 6.8). Severe destruction of the deep veins, which are replaced by a maze of collaterals.
- Stage IV (Fig. 6.9). Recanalization has not occurred. In addition, the state of the superficial collateral circulation must be assessed in each stage; i.e., it must be ascertained whether it is sufficient or already insufficient, and varicose.

Evaluation of the extent of recanalization is always important (Fig. 6.10).

Phlebography provides information about the function of the damaged venous system. In practice, only phleboscopy permits assessment of drainage. The following points must be observed: whether drainage is approximately normal, delayed, or much retarded; and whether the contrast medium remains in the distal parts of the leg or flows off. Phleboscopy also shows whether drainage of venous blood occurs via the superficial or the deep venous system.

Finally, the communicating and perforating veins are assessed. Their valves are frequently insufficient, because of either occlusion during thrombosis and later recanalization or pressure overload (Figs. 6.11 and 6.12).

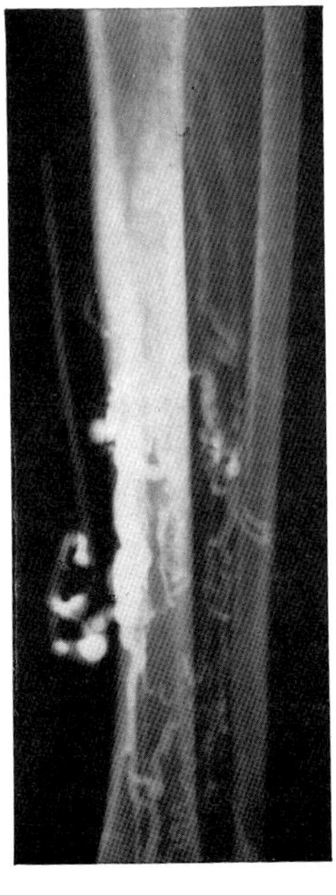

Fig. 6.11. Post-thrombotic damage, Stage III. Insufficient Cockett vein with "ulcer bolster." First order collateral circulation is otherwise still sufficient.

Thus, phlebography permits an objective appraisal of the damage to the deep venous system in the post-thrombotic syndrome and makes possible evaluation of the superficial venous system; on this basis, appropriate therapeutic measures can be undertaken and a prognosis given.

Surgical Measures

The damage following thrombosis of the deep leg veins is so extensive that venous backflow can only be improved by conservative or surgical measures, present or future. There is no hope of creating normal circulatory conditions, as with plastic surgery of arteries.

Conditions

Conservative treatment, both before and after operation, is the *foundation* on which surgical management must be based. Luke (1953) established rules that the patient must follow all his life. Our patients are given a similar, more detailed *thrombosis memorandum*.

Basically, it contains precise instructions regarding
- correct pressure bandages of whatever type, elastic stockings or dressings;

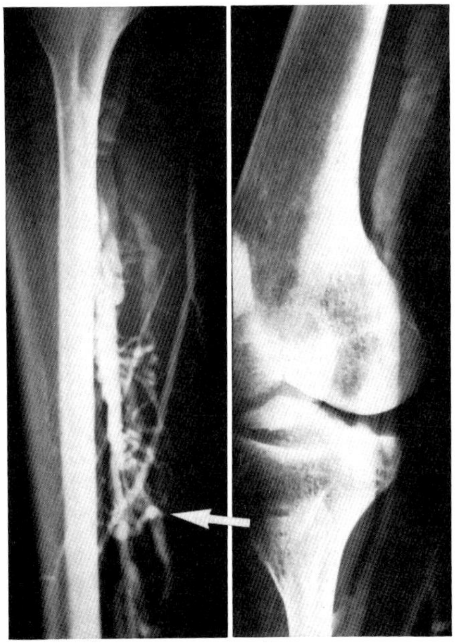

Fig. 6.12. Post-thrombotic damage, Stage I. Insufficient Cockett vein.

— correct elevation at night and possibly in the afternoon;
— regular systematic exercises, brisk walking for 2 hours daily, light athletics, especially swimming, and so forth;
— avoidance of exposure of the extremity to strong sunlight;
— weight control;
— regular defecation; and
— avoidance of any constriction (rubber bands, tight bodices, and elastic tops on socks.

Determination of normal arterial circulation is *self-evident* for any surgical treatment of the veins. It should be confirmed by oscillography, if doubt remains after angiography. If mixed arterial and venous circulatory disease is present, restoration of the arterial element takes precedence. With certain exceptions, when leg ulcers on a post-thrombotic leg and arterial obstruction occur simultaneously, the patient should be treated as if the arterial obstruction alone were the cause.

For *surgery*, precise *roentgen diagnosis* of the veins of the lower extremity *and* pelvis is essential in each case. *Roentgen demonstration* of *pelvic veins*, in addition to that of the leg veins, is always necessary, even when the pelvic vessels are clinically normal (negative history, absence of collaterals in the inguinal and lower abdominal regions).

In addition, *venous pressure measurements* are proving increasingly valuable.

Pressure measurements in the *peripheral veins during exercise* alone are adequate for the construction of curves showing an exact picture of the *extent of functional damage*. The superficial and deep venous systems are closely linked during walking. Hence, pressure measurements of the superficial venous system on exercise also provide information about the state, or strictly speaking, about the function, of the deep veins.

We introduce a catheter into a branch of the long saphenous vein at the ankle or the dorsum of the foot. The catheter is coupled with a Statham element, to which a curve plotter is attached. The patient bends his knees ten times. Characteristic curves are obtained for healthy and diseased veins (Fig. 6.13).

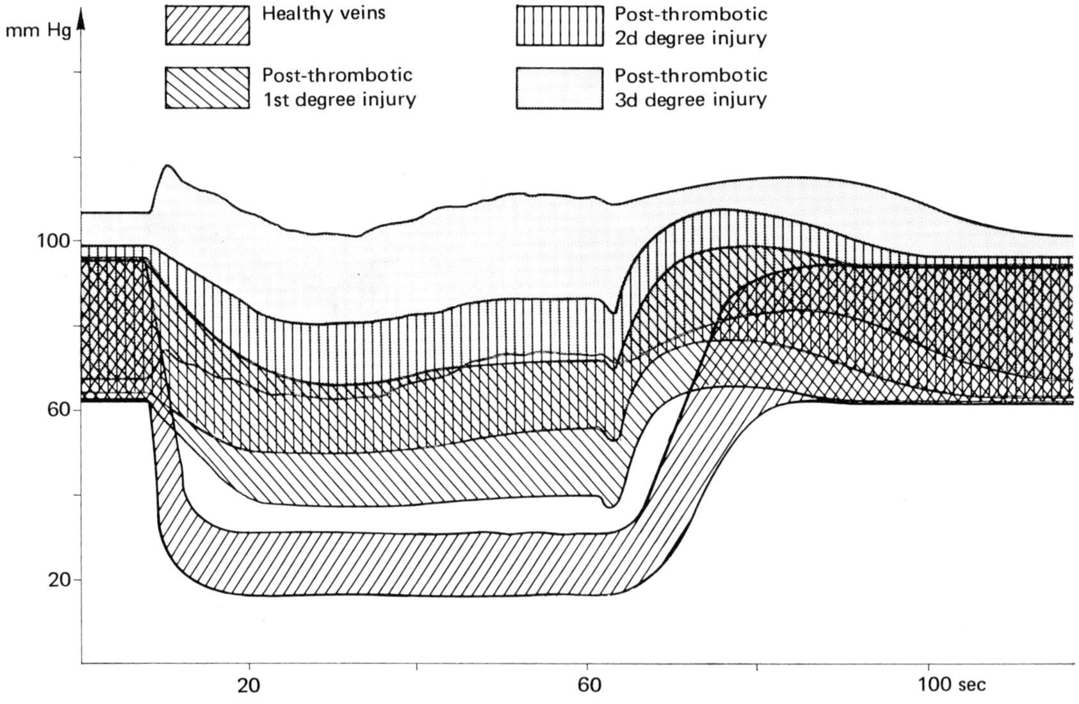

Fig. 6.13. Peripheral vein pressure measurements during exercise from healthy persons and patients with the post-thrombotic syndrome of the first to third degree. The relatively wide range of the individual areas of a large population is caused by the inclusion of the factor of height (peripheral venous pressure also depends on the level of the blood column above the puncture cannula).

The injuries are divided into three groups.
- Slight post-thrombotic damage: first degree injury.
- Moderate post-thrombotic damage: second degree injury.
- Severe post-thrombotic damage: third degree injury.

Technical details are given in *Messmethoden in der Venenchirurgie* (May, 1971a).

Surgical Measures for Improving Venous Backflow

Sympathectomy

Operations on the sympathetic trunk, especially blockades, for acute thrombosis were abandoned many years ago. The importance of vasospasm, postulated by Ochsner (1940), was considerably overestimated. Mandl (1953) recommended elimination of the lumbar chain for the post-thrombotic syndrome. May et al. (1970) reported their extensive studies on histologic findings in lumbar ganglia in this condition. Apparently irreversible damage of the ganglia, parallelling the degree of injury due to thrombosis, was consistently demonstrated (Figs. 6.14 and 6.15). It is responsible for several symptoms, including the cold clammy skin that follows thrombosis in some cases. Thus, resection of lumbar ganglia would also be justified pathophysiologically.

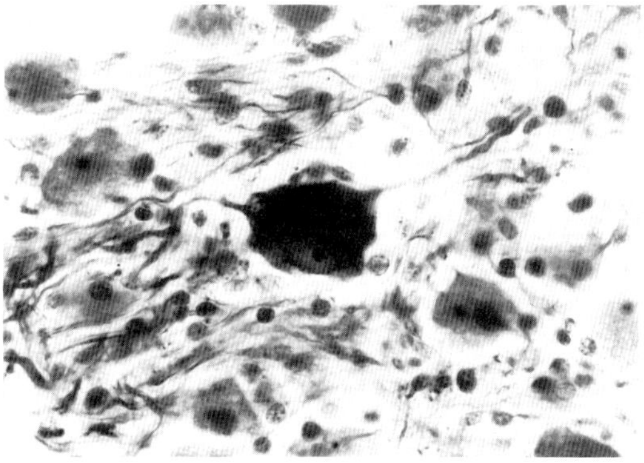

Fig. 6.14. Normal ganglion cell.

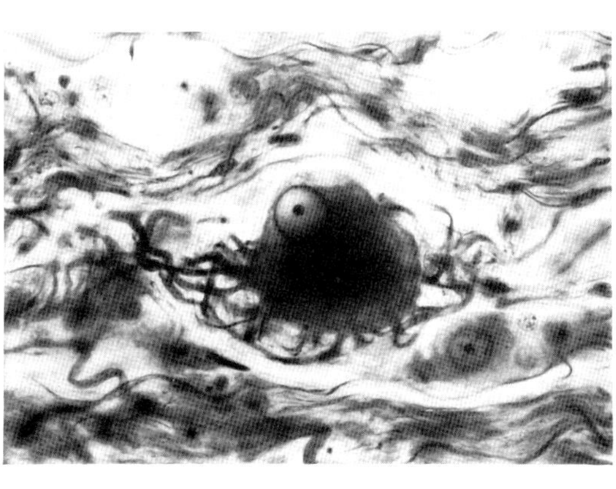

Fig. 6.15. Post-thrombotic, damaged ganglion cell.

May reexamined 22 patients in 1969 on whom he had operated 10 to 15 years previously. Objective improvement of the natural course of the syndrome was not recorded in a single case, but two-thirds of the reexamined patients were subjectively improved, the leg being warm and dry. The procedure should be reserved for those rare cases in which complaints of a cold sweaty extremity are marked. Pratt (1964) shares this opinion. Linton (1953) described the rare complication of chronic painful ulcers on dorsum of the foot or toes appearing after sympathectomy. He called it "post-thrombotic postsympathectomy syndrome." We have never seen it, but it should be noted that Schönbach and Thorban (1959) demonstrated organic injury to the arterial wall after sympathectomy. Venous tone after sympathectomy has been studied by Beaconsfield (1954) and circulatory changes by Gilbertsen (1960) and Messent and Beaconsfield (1954).

Ligation of the Popliteal Vein

Buxton et al. (1944) proposed ligation of the superficial femoral vein for the post-thrombotic syndrome. This method became known only after Linton and Hardy (1947) and Piulachs (1956) in the United States, Vidal-Barraquer (1950) in Spain, and Halse (1959) in Germany advocated it.

According to Halse, the *principle* is as follows:

The deep femoral vein is only rarely changed after thrombosis. There are numerous cross connections between the superficial and deep femoral veins above the popliteal space. After partial resection of the superficial femoral below the junction with the deep femoral, the venous blood is drained from the popliteal into the femoral and, via communicating veins, into the deep femoral. The *functional result of the operation* lies in the fact that the barrier to drainage is repaired, and functional collaterals provide reflux by the path described.

Technique

Under local anesthesia, a 10 to 15 cm long incision is made on the ventral aspect of the upper third of the thigh, and a 3 to 4 cm segment of the femoral is resected below the union with the deep femoral (Halse, 1959). Piulachs (1956) and Vidal-Barraquer (1950) go further, resecting a segment of the superficial femoral and popliteal, and later performing resection of varices of the long saphenous if necessary (Fig. 6.16)

Ligation of the Popliteal Vein

Bauer, in a large series of publications since 1948, has recommended ligation of the insufficient popliteal.

Indication. Marked swelling of leg in the evening, with "bursting" pain—the patient feels as if the leg were bursting (Bauer). *Leg ulcer* is not an indication for popliteal ligation. Bauer advises ligation of insufficient perforating veins for its elimination. The indication is confirmed by phlebography if it shows that a great deal of contrast medium adheres in the insufficient deep veins.

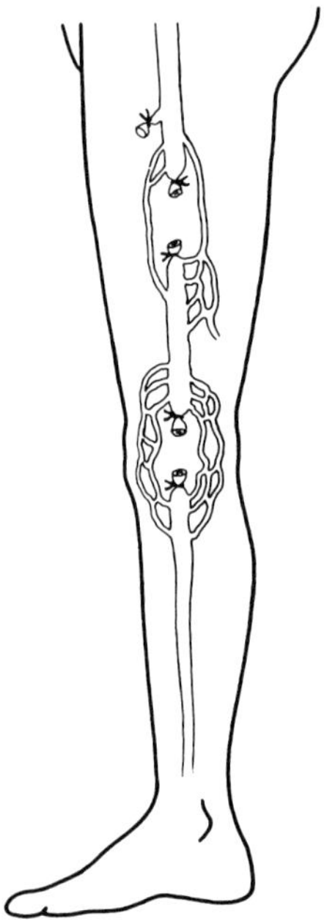

Fig. 6.16. Ligation of the popliteal and femoral veins.

Technique

The patient lies prone on the operating table. The distal portion of the leg is supported by a pillow large enough to prevent the toes from touching the table. The muscles are thus relaxed. The level of the skin incision is important. Phlebographic studies showed that the popliteal has received all its tributaries at the level of the upper margin of the patella and has become a uniform vessel. Therefore, the vein should be exposed and ligated at this level, which should also be the center of the transverse section through the skin. Transverse section is preferred to longitudinal section. Muscle and fatty tissues are carefully displaced and the popliteal is isolated. It is dissected from its common vascular sheath and from the artery for about 5 cm. Two ligatures are applied and a segment of vein of 1 to 2 cm is resected. It must be ascertained with great care that a second popliteal is not present; if it is, it must be ligated also. Ligation of the popliteal must be as radical as practical.

Bauer (1965) reported disappearance of edema and pain in 69.4 per cent of 136 patients operated on. The result was unsatisfactory in 20.6 per cent.

Criticism

Most vascular surgeons carried out ligation of the femoral and popliteal veins for many years, but skeptical arguments were expressed early. De Camp (1951) and Boyd (1953) demonstrated that the peripheral venous pressure curve, recorded during exercise, always deteriorated after ligation of both the femoral and popliteal veins (Figs. 6.17 and 6.18).

We published the same venous pressure curves 2 years ago. We know of no case in which the venous pressure curve improved after ligation of the femoral or popliteal vein. Even if the bursting sensation disappears, the tendency to edema does not, and cannot, improve in the long run if the curve does not do so. The tendency to edema is mainly due to failure of the calf muscle pump. The suction action on relaxation of the calf muscles is decisively reduced. This is the chief significance of the venous pressure curve, which is an unerring indicator for the advisability of operation. Operation on the popliteal vein, or on a post-thrombotic leg in general, cannot be successful if the suction effect on diastole is not improved and venous pressure thus lowered. Hence, surgery is generally not worth the effort.

If improvement of post-thrombotic sequelae is seen, it is frequently due to simultaneous ligation of insufficient perforating veins or simply better supervision of elevation and compression applications. Thus, improvement is usually the result of supportive treatment and not of surgery. Actually, all vascular surgeons known to me

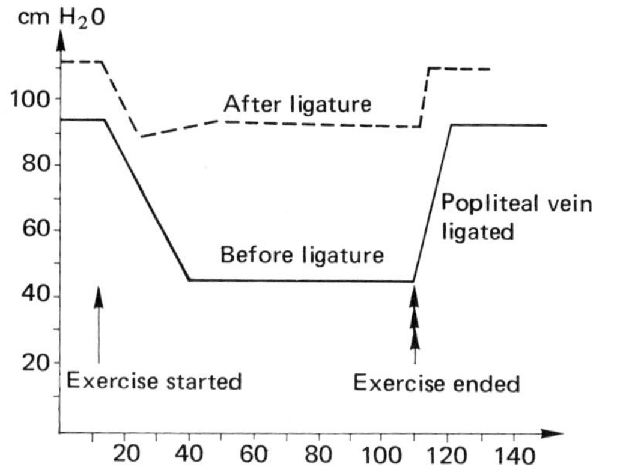

Fig. 6.17. Venous pressure before and after ligature of the popliteal vein.

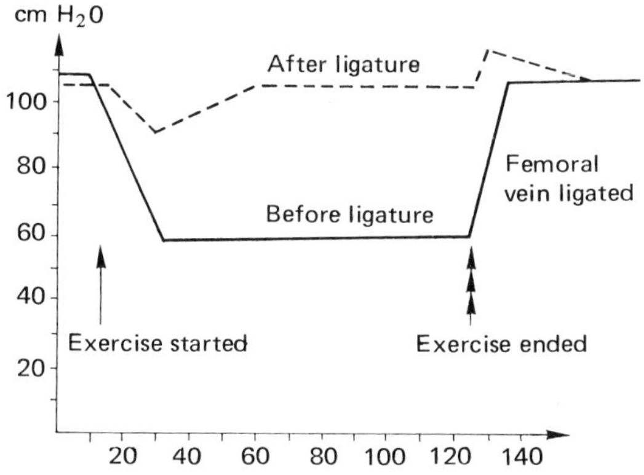

Fig. 6.18. Venous pressure before and after ligature of the femoral vein.

have become reticent and skeptical vis-à-vis femoral and popliteal ligation. Blood flow measurements of post-thrombotic veins with thermistors performed by Netzer (1968) also made these operations appear questionable. We agree with Haeger and Sandber (1966): The only indication is severe orthostatic cruralgia, the sensation of bursting, if pressure bandages, elastic stockings and other supportive measures are inadequate, and this is rarely the case.

Gracilis Transfer of Psathakis

In 1964 Psathakis proposed pulling the gracilis tendon under the popliteal vein in deep vein insufficiency (Fig. 6.19). A kink is produced in the vein that is supposed to act as a replacement valve. *Indications* are, again, all variants of the insufficiency syndrome, mostly post-thrombotic

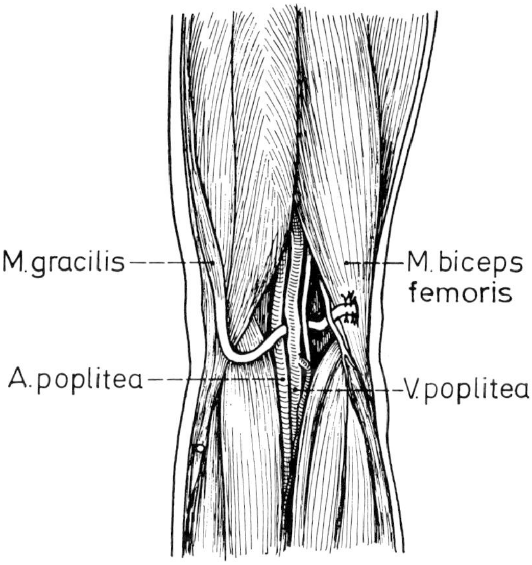

Fig. 6.19. Gracilis transfer of Psathakis.

insufficiency, if the femoral and popliteal veins are recanalized.

Technique

The popliteal fossa is opened posteriorly by a lateral longitudinal incision. The gracilis tendon is located from a medial skin incision over the pes anserinus, divided and moved subcutaneously from medial to lateral to the biceps femoris across the tendons of the semitendinous and semimembranous muscles. The tibial and common peroneal nerves remain dorsal to this tendinous loop. The gracilis tendon is sutured to the tendinous portion of biceps femoris to form a kind of sling. The tendon should not be taut when relaxed, since this may lead to thrombosis by compression of the vein. If the gracilis tendon is too tense, the tendinous portion of the biceps muscle can be elongated by longitudinal incision. Psathakis chiefly stresses the importance of sufficient length of the gracilis tendon. It should be not tight like a "string" but loose like a slack "washing line" in the popliteal fossa after suture to the biceps tendon. Here, the reduced muscle tone during anesthesia should be taken into account. During relaxation of the gracilis muscle, the gracilis tendon lies in the popliteal fossa like a washing line, but it is stretched on contraction of the gracilis. The popliteal vein is pulled dorsally and kinked by leverage, the semitendinous and semimembranous tendons serving as pivot. If the gracilis tendon is too short to guarantee regular function as a "substitute valve," which almost always is the case, it must be extended. If the length of the gracilis tendon has been underestimated, the situation can be rectified by a second operation two weeks later.

Postoperative Care

The patient starts leg exercises on the day of operation in order to prevent thrombosis and to preserve the gliding ability of the gracilis tendon.
Prophylaxis of thrombosis with anticoagulants is contraindicated, since hematomas in the popliteal fossa could endanger gliding of the tendon. The patient gets out of bed on the ninth postoperative day. Only natural weight bearing produces the desired results, because it is the only way of activating the muscle pump (calf musculature). Prolonged standing and sitting should be avoided. Occasionally, brief periods of walking in place suffice to relieve venous stagnation.
If superficial venous insufficiency is present at the same time, it should be removed by stripping.
If leg ulcers or preulcerous skin changes are present, the insufficient communicating veins should be eliminated. For large ulcers, skin grafting is required.
All operations can be carried out in one session.

Results

Psathakis lists as results:
— disappearance of edema and pain,
— healing of eczemas and ulcers,
— "lighter" feeling of the legs, and
— softening of infiltrated tissues.

Haeger (1968) performed such operations 46 times. The state was improved in four cases, remained stationary in 41 and deteriorated in one. Loose, in whose clinic Psathakis carried out a number of these operations, also has reservations about the procedure (personal communication, 1969).
In contrast, Berger and Brücke (1970) reported disappearance of edema and pain in eight of ten patients after operation, healing of ulcers in two and death in one.
Unfortunately, systematic preoperative and postoperative venous pressure measurements, the only decisive method of evaluation, are not available.
Netzer (1968) recommends preoperative popliteal pressure measurement. The operation would then be performed only if increased pressure was observed during breaks in walking—diastole (May, 1969, 1971).

Surgery of Secondary Varicosities

Varices of injured deep veins are called *secondary*, or better, according to Santler (1968), *complicated* varices. This terminology is not intended to distinguish between originally primary idiopathic varicosities of a leg, on which thrombosis of the deep veins is superimposed, and varix formation due to overloading of the superficial circulation because of obstruction in the deep veins.

Diagnosis

If damage of deep veins is suspected, radiologic study is imperative for confirmation. Suspicion is aroused by a positive history, that is, if the patient reports previous phlebitis or postoperative swelling of the leg. Past fractures are also suggestive, as are unilateral edema and prolonged swelling of the legs and induration and discoloration of the distal portion. Since history and clinical impression are wholly unreliable, the only means for clarification remains phlebography.

Indications

Varicosities may be removed without hesitation if the deep veins are only slightly involved. We have even gained the impression that surgical removal causes less reaction and is gentler than sclerotherapy. A problem arises, however, when damage of the deep veins is marked. In these cases, the varices may become the main carriers of venous backflow if recanalization has not taken place (this occurs in only about 10 per cent of cases), or if recanalization was inadequate. Resection of varicosities results in impressive increase of edema and, in grave cases, therapy-resistant leg ulcers around the ankle, the "gaiter area" (Fischer, 1969), that are due to a failing escape mechanism, rather than incompetent perforator veins. Naturally, the patient is soon aware of the casual connection with the operation, and claims for compensation have increased recently with omission of phlebography being an issue raised.
These aggravating sequels of varicectomy occur in only a very small percentage of cases. In practice, the more or less well recanalized deep veins are usually sufficient to cope with reflux.

Roughly 20 years ago, most textbooks contended that secondary varices should not be operated on. Around 10 years ago, this taboo was completely negated by well known vascular surgeons, who supported varicectomy if thrombosis dated back at least one year. After a year the deep venous system is more or less well recanalized in about 90 per cent of cases. Although they operated without phlebography, notable deterioration due to surgery was expected in only 20 per cent of cases. This figure includes 10 per cent in which the deep veins are occluded, and 10 per cent in which the deep veins are poorly recanalized. These cases are frequently concealed by postoperative bandaging, as is increasing edema in milder cases, which is certainly more common.

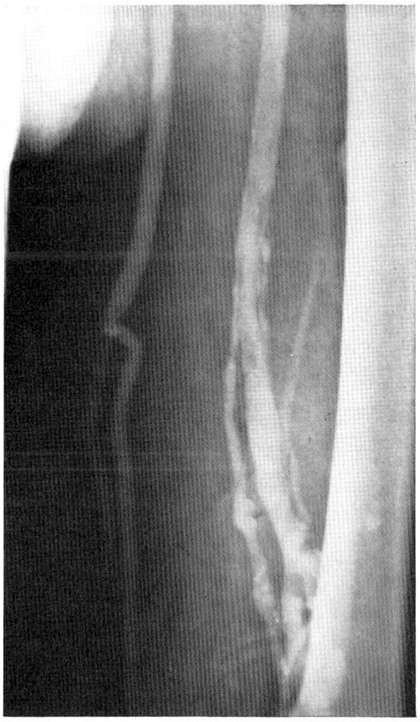

Fig. 6.20. Phlebography. Deep vein well filled with contrast medium. The great saphenous can be eliminated.

One cannot simply say that secondary varicosities may or may not be operated on; the problem is more complex. We agree with Santler (1968), who states that superficial veins are essential only in the phase of acute obstruction of deep veins. Although some superficial veins do fail, circulatory collapse does not follow, because the superficial venous system is arranged in several layers. The result is only increased edema. But the superficial veins are never an ideal substitute for failing deep veins, since they are not directly connected with the calf muscle pump, the most important mechanism aiding drainage. The basically insufficient auxiliary pathways of drainage may prove to be additional barriers if they become varicose. Santler writes: "If deep drainage difficulties arise because of narrowed lumens, it ought not be assumed that the great reservoir of subcutaneous veins will be a substitute. Rather, the contrary applies. For with the insufficient communicating veins releasing passage to the surface,

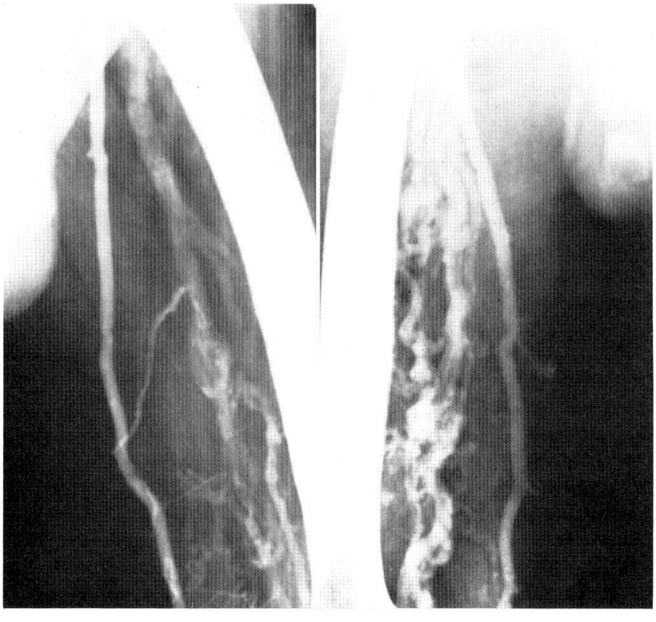

Fig. 6.21. Femoral vein incompletely or poorly recanalized. The long saphenous is therefore necessary for reflux and must not be eliminated.

the blood is forced into paths that are not constructed for rapid and ample transport and that lack corresponding driving power. The sequelae—varicosities, phlebectasia, corona phlebectatica, congestive discoloration and eczema—are impressive witness to this.

It should rather be considered that the capacity of the venous system of the lower extremity is approximately four times as great as that of the corresponding arterial system, and that it may be greatly augmented by establishment of new channels, by their enlargement and, most important, by varix formation. The blood volume of the leg is alleged to be 400 ml, and this amount may be doubled in extreme cases of varicosity.

For therapy this means that the capacity in post-thrombotic varices is superfluous, even injurious, and must be reduced. The resulting acceleration of flow is important not only for drainage but also for prevention of thrombosis.

It may be that elimination of secondary varices has no definite effect on venous backflow. This occurs in the majority of cases. Removal of varices may be either injurious or desirable; only objective tests can elucidate this.

We can only caution against reliance on clinical impression and clinical experience, and advise use of objective, verifiable principles in making the decision. These are:

— *phlebography* and
— *peripheral vein pressure measurement during exercise.*

Until two years ago, our radiologist was exclusively responsible for the decision regarding operation. In phlebography, 30 ml of 60 per cent contrast medium is injected into a vein on the dorsum of the foot after application of a tourniquet above the ankle, with the patient obliquely upright (tilting table, inclination 60 degrees). Drainage of the contrast medium is checked by screening, and the most important phases are photographed. This usually shows clearly whether drainage is mainly by way of deep or superficial veins (Figs. 6.20 and 6.21). If the contrast medium flows mainly through the superficial varices, they must not be removed. Insufficient perforating veins are also visualized. In borderline cases, though, the radiologist may not be willing to commit himself.

We are fortunate, therefore, in having a complementary method of investigation—*venous pressure measurement*. It is true that Perthes designed a test long ago meant to predict patency of the deep veins. A tourniquet is applied to the thigh and the patient is asked to walk. Supposedly, the superficial veins empty if the deep veins are patent. This test is subject to many subjective impressions, however, and recording venous reflux by curves is a considerable advance.

Venous pressure measurement. A catheter is introduced into a vein on the dorsum of the foot and is connected with an Atlas apparatus type EM 50. Pressure is transmitted by Statham element. A Multicord 250 recorder, which contains an intensifier, is attached to the pressure apparatus. Measuring pressure at rest is of little value. What is important is registration of curves following pressure changes on exercise, and therefore the patient is asked to bend his knees a few times. The pressure changes—normally there is a considerable drop on moving—are recorded by the apparatus in a characteristic curve. We call this the electrocardiogram of the peripheral heart. Normal curves are never to be expected after deep vein thrombosis, because the deep veins are always damaged (for details, see May, 1971).

The function of the calf muscle pump, the most important adjuvant of venous reflux, is destroyed by failure of valves and insufficient recanalization of the deep veins. When muscles are relaxed, which we call diastole, a considerable drop in pressure is supposed to occur normally because of an aspiration effect. This pressure decline is absent in deep vein insufficiency.

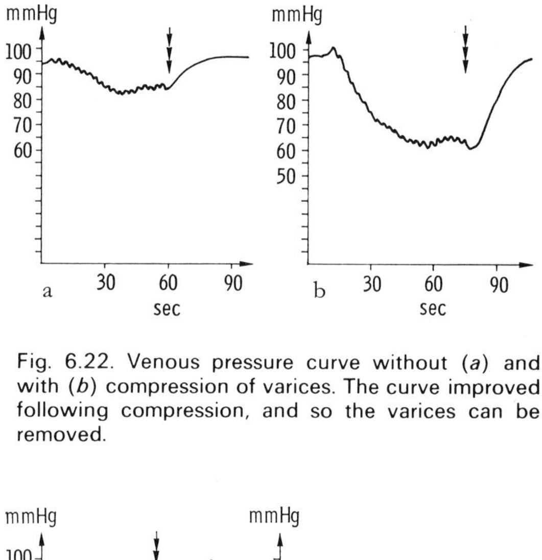

Fig. 6.22. Venous pressure curve without (*a*) and with (*b*) compression of varices. The curve improved following compression, and so the varices can be removed.

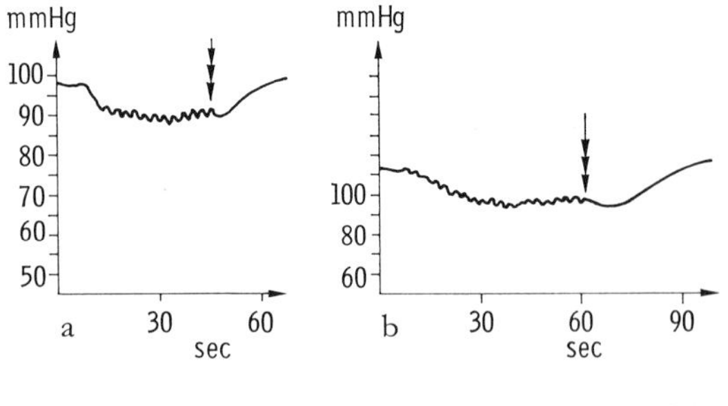

Fig. 6.23. Venous pressure curve without (*a*) and with (*b*) compression of varices. Because the curve deteriorated, the varices must not be eliminated.

Impaired diastole is the most important measure of the degree of deep venous insufficiency. Each degree of severity has its corresponding curve. After the exercise curve has been obtained, the thigh is bandaged, for compression of the insufficient great saphenous vein. The patient is again asked to bend his knees. Varices are removed only if there is great improvement in the curve after bandaging (Figs. 6.22 and 6.23).

To conclude, we should like to add two points:

— In severe damage to the deep veins, we are generally very reticent about removal of varices. We operate only on varices that are cosmetically really troublesome, contain large aneurysmal dilatations in the groin or in their course or maintain eczemas, and when the venous pressure curve clearly permits expectation of improvement.
— We consider it necessary to explain to the patients in writing that the deep venous injury remains irreparable despite varix operation, that edema will persist and that they will have to continue to wear elastic stockings. We have found time and again that, in spite of verbal explanation, patients erroneously believe that operation is synonymous with cure and cannot understand why bandaging must be continued.

Insufficient perforating veins are operated on in any case.

Ligation of Insufficient Perforating Veins

An important accompaniment to the post-thrombotic syndrome is the occurrence of insufficient perforating veins, mainly in the distal portion of the leg. They also occur in normal deep veins, with or without varicosities. Phlebographic examination reveals whether the deep veins are normal or not. This is significant for prognosis and therapy. If insufficient perforating veins, and perhaps varices, are eliminated in the presence of normal deep veins, the patient is healthy. If the deep veins are damaged, only a symptom has been removed, and the patient must continue using compression bandages.

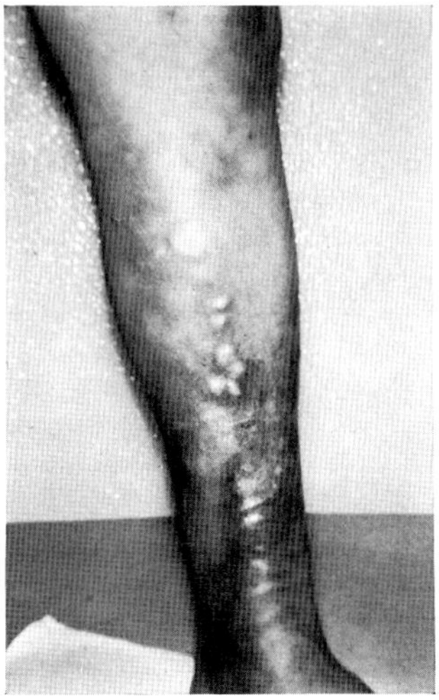

Fig. 6.24. Post-thrombotic induration.

Indications

Elimination of all insufficient perforator veins during surgery for primary varices is recommended (p. 89ff). In the post-thrombotic syndrome, elimination of insufficient perforators, but only of the leg, is still more important. We remove them in all these cases on principle.

Sequelae to Insufficiency of Perforators

Pressure waves are transmitted from the deep venous system to the surface by loss of valves in the perforating veins. The arteriovenous pressure difference in the capillary bed decreases, and relative hypoxia, *induration* typical of the post-thrombotic syndrome (Fig. 6.24) and post-thrombotic leg ulcers following minor trauma ensue. The leg affected by thrombosis reveals two syndromes that should be kept separate:

—*edema* subsequent to failure of the calf muscle pump; and
—*induration* of the distal portion of the leg with alternating inflammation and eczema, and finally leg ulcers.

The latter are almost never direct sequels to injuries of deep veins but rather result from insufficient perforators. Formerly it was assumed that induration stemmed basically from insufficient perforator veins, but Fischer (1969) pointed out that induration, particularly around the ankle, also arises from failure of the drainage mechanism. This affects only a small percentage, however. On principle, insufficient perforating veins must be looked for in all legs damaged by thrombosis. Particularly thick insufficient perforators frequently appear as "varicose spheres" at the upper margin of indurations touching the mouths of the perforators, the fascial gaps.

Clinical examination is fraught with so many errors that phlebography of perforating veins is preferred in all cases. If the leg is swollen, pressure bandages are applied and the leg is elevated at night until the swelling recedes. The patient lies on a slightly tilted table. A superficial vein of the inner or outer aspect of the ankle or the dorsum of the foot is punctured. The table is further tilted and the flow of the contrast medium is observed under the screen. As soon as a perforator is visualized, an exposure is made. More contrast medium is then injected into another superficial vein above this perforator, perhaps with mild stasis applied below the knee, and this process is repeated until the whole leg has been examined roentgenologically medially and laterally.

Bernink (1971) stated that occasionally insufficient perforating veins are not demonstrable on x-ray examination. With increasing experience and care, these cases become rare. At times, it may be difficult to distinguish on a film whether a perforator is sufficient or not. We treat every large perforator vein as if it were insufficient.

Patil (1970) showed that insufficient perforating veins may be demonstrated *thermographically*. We do not believe that this method is suitable to replace phlebography.

Anatomy

Cockett showed in fundamental publications (1955; Dodd and Cockett, 1956) that certain insufficient perforating veins at the inner aspect of the leg and outer aspect of the ankle are of main importance. He further pointed out that these are usually not connected directly with the main trunk of the great saphenous; this means they remain unaffected by stripping. Instead, they are attached to a posterior branch of the great saphenous.

The three most important perforators are called *Cockett perforators*. All three roughly occupy *Linton's line*, which runs along the long axis of the leg, one fingerbreadth behind the internal malleolus. They flow into the posterior tibial veins.

The *lowest perforator, Cockett I*, lies close behind and below the medial malleolus. It is the smallest and is thus frequently overlooked.

The *intermediate perforator, Cockett II*, lies about four fingerbreadths above the tip of the medial malleolus, roughly one or two fingerbreadths posterior to the tibial crest.

The *uppermost perforator, Cockett III*, is the most constant. It lies at the transition of the lower and middle thirds of the leg, near the margin of the tibia. It is joined to the long saphenous by a short branch. It flows directly into the long saphenous only occasionally. In this case, it has a small branch to the venous arch which connects the other two perforators. If the uppermost perforator is very large, the intermediate is smaller, and vice versa.

A thrombus may extend from deep veins into perforating veins. During recanalization, the valves of these perforators are destroyed.

Exact measurements were made by Sherman (1949), and by Gundersen (1966). Sherman found the most important perforating veins 13.5, 18.5, and 24 cm above the sole of the foot (Fig. 6.25).

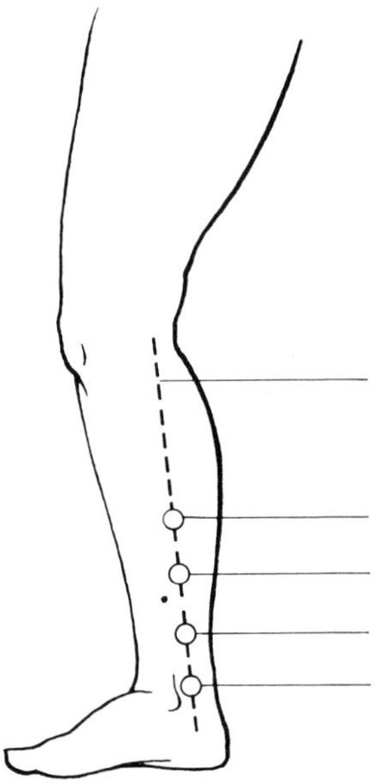

Fig. 6.25. Drawing of the most important perforating veins on the inner aspect of the leg. (After Sherman and after Gundersen.)

The first corresponds with the Cockett II perforator, and the second with Cockett III (p. 17).

Gundersen examined 104 legs in detail and found insufficient perforating veins at 13.5 cm in 27.2 per cent, at 16 cm in 8.2 per cent, at 18.5 cm in 37.8 per cent and at 24 cm in 10.4 per cent of cases.

All other reports on insufficient perforating veins are single observations. These figures are important indicators of where to look for perforator veins, but are not a substitute for systematic phlebographic examinations.

Nylander and Hager (1970) described a surgically important variant. They noted in 22 of 92 cases of chronic insufficiency that the three perforating veins leave the superficial veins for the depths of the leg at the common sites, crossing the superficial fascia of the leg at the typical location and passing the deep fascia under the belly of soleus. They join to a short trunk and flow into the posterior tibial veins (Fig. 6.26). In these cases, a small incision suffices for elimination of all three perforators.

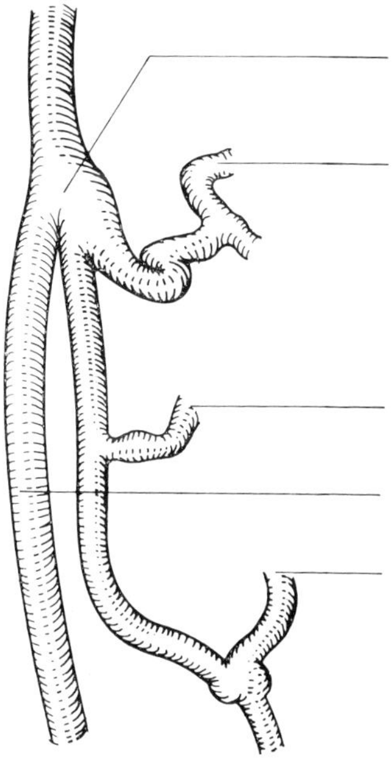

Fig. 6.26. Variant. All three Cockett perforators join in a common trunk before flowing into the posterior tibial. (After Nylander and Haeger.)

The perforating veins at the *external malleolus* are far more inconstant. The range is so wide that we will not name them individually. Each patient must be carefully examined under the screen.

Technique

We mark the site of the perforating veins under the screen (Fig. 6.27). The perforators are exposed by small transverse sections, and the fascial gap is closed. Before ligation we pull at the clamped perforator (Fig. 6.28) so that the ligature is placed close to the deep vein without stump formation, just as we do for ligature of the great saphenous. For indurations, we prefer longitudinal section directly above the perforating veins if feasible. We deviate dorsally only when there are severe skin changes so that the skin incision goes partially through healthy skin. Undermining skin is a poor principle, but unavoidable in this case. It should be as sparing as practical.

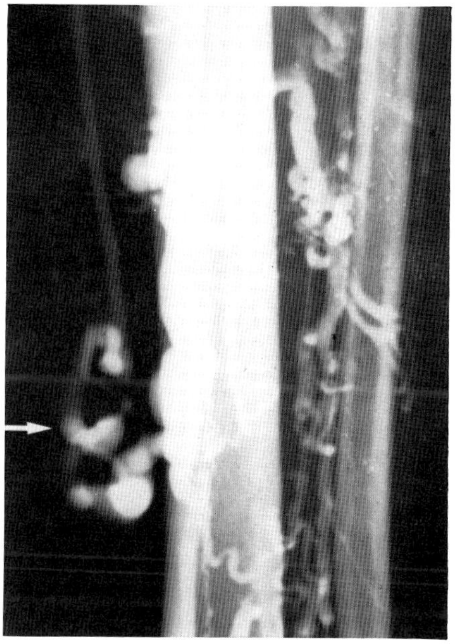

Fig. 6.27. Insufficient perforating vein with severely injured deep veins.

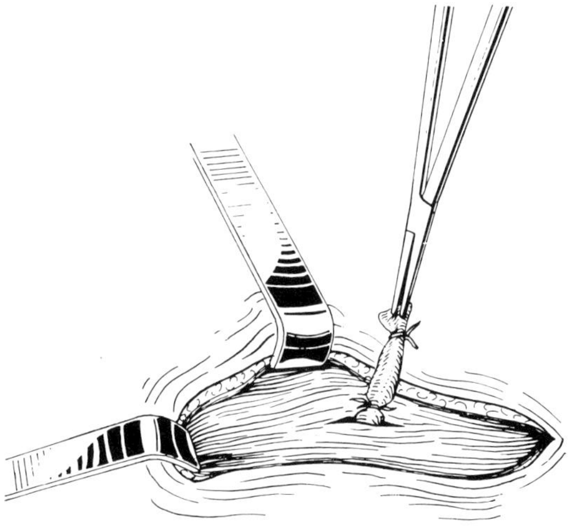

Fig. 6.28. The insufficient perforating vein is pulled forward and ligated at the level of the fascial gap.

We believe it is most important not only to avoid injury to the fascia, but also to close fascial gaps carefully, since a firm fascia is necessary for a properly functioning calf muscle pump. If the skin is damaged, skin sutures should be avoided and dermal deficiencies should be closed with adhesive strips. We insist that the patient get up immediately after operation. Bandages are applied until the hematomas are absorbed and the main wound is properly healed.

Bassi (1962) described a method for destroying insufficient perforators semisurgically in outpatients. A hooklet is introduced through a minute skin incision and the perforating vein is torn away. Hemostasis is brought about by pressure. This method does not provide precise surgical exposure and is rather inexact in indurations, where the perforators are barely palpable.

A very difficult question is how long this operation "lasts," that is, when new insufficient perforating veins will have formed. The literature provides no answer; all reports suggest that an insufficient perforator vein was overlooked at the first intervention. Our experience shows that the older the patient, the better the prognosis; continued activity is the main cause of new formation. Even in the most unfavorable case, the patient will be free of symptoms for an interval of 5 to 10 years.

Finally, we consider it necessary to draw attention once again to the need for preoperative explanation to the patient, always in writing. Despite surgical measures, the fate of the leg will depend largely on the care with which the patient adheres to the life style prescribed for the post-thrombotic syndrome.

Femoral Bypass

Approximately 10 per cent of patients are left with occluded deep veins after acute thrombosis has subsided; in 35 per cent (this figure is perhaps too high), recanalization of the deep veins is practically total. Only the valves of the deep veins remain nonfunctional. There are few late sequelae in these cases. But in at least 55 per cent of patients the deep veins are incompletely recanalized. In addition to the 10 per cent in whom the deep veins remain occluded, these are patients with marked clinical aftereffects. It is impossible to give more exact figures on the incidence of deficient or failing recanalization. The latter is largely dependent on therapy. If treatment with anticoagulants is started early and continued long enough, cases of deficient recanalization are correspondingly fewer, as we showed years ago. If the patients are promptly treated with streptokinase, it is possible in most cases to reduce aftereffects to local valvular damage, as Widmer showed (1971). But thrombosis is so rarely treated with streptokinase. In any case, most patients retain incompletely recanalized deep veins. The seriousness of destruction of valves was formerly overestimated. The essential valvular action is prevention of retrograde pressure waves during walking, pressing, laughing and so forth. That inadequacy of valves is not serious, apart from producing slight swelling of the leg, is proved by the state of persons with congenital aplasia of valves.

But if the deep veins are poorly recanalized, late sequelae of thrombosis are considerably more grave. Severe stagnation appears, which is treated hopefully with lifelong pressure bandages, stasis relief and other supportive measures. Normally, 90 per cent of the venous blood flows through the deep veins. It is now forced to deviate via superficial veins, which are not an adequate substitute because they are not directly connected with the calf vein pump, which, as the "secondary heart," presents an essential aid for venous backflow.

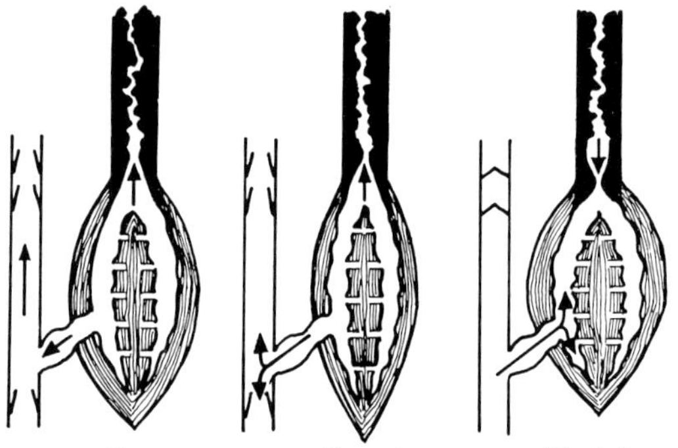

Fig. 6.29. Venous circulation in a poorly recanalized femoral vein. The blood flows proximally at rest, but there is slight flow from deep to superficial; in systole, there is deficient emptying owing to partial obstruction of outflow; in diastole, there is deficient aspiration as a result of inadequate emptying.

We made a special study of patients in whom the femoral vein was poorly recanalized (Fig. 6.29). The calf muscle pump works against a partially obstructed outflow. This factor promotes deterioration of the venous pressure curve during exercise. The great saphenous vein has to overcome the main reflux, but is not connected with the muscle pump. An attempt is made to establish such a connection surgically, as shown in Figures 6.30 to 6.32. We anastomose the great saphenous with the most distal portion of the popliteal. So far, we have performed this operation only when the long saphenous has competent valves, but if our suppositions are correct, the operation should also be of value when the great saphenous has insufficient valves. The *emphasis* is not on *venous valves* but on *free drainage*.

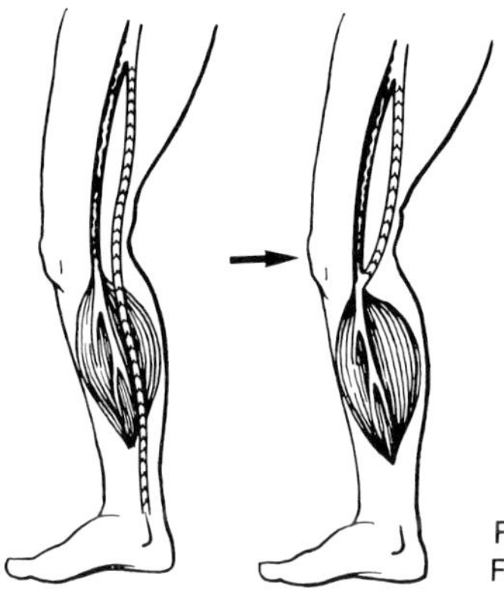

Fig. 6.30. Femoral bypass.

Conditions for the operation are:

—The valves in the great saphenous may be competent or incompetent, but the vein should be of good caliber and fairly free of varicosis.

—The post-thrombotic damage should chiefly be in the long saphenous. If the pelvic veins are much injured, the method is as useless as it is when there is severe damage to the leg veins.

—The most distal portion of the popliteal must be at least half patent; otherwise the anastomosis does not receive sufficient inflow.

It is self-evident that the operation is carried out only after x-ray examination of the leg and pelvic veins. The caliber of the long saphenous frequently cannot be correctly judged on general films, but direct injection of a contrast medium into the distal portion of the long saphenous must be warned against. We paid for exact demonstration of the vein by partial thrombosis due to the contrast medium several times, and had to end the operation.

Similarly, we have been surprised during operation a few times to find that the x-ray demonstration of the popliteal vein did not reveal actual conditions. Although it appeared sufficiently recanalized on the film, we found, after exposing and freeing it, that it was much occluded, with only a crescentic slit left open. The erroneous picture resulted from obtaining radiographs in only one plane. Two planes are essential in all cases.

Technique

The patient lies supine. The leg is slightly externally rotated and the knee moderately flexed. An 8 cm incision is made dorsally and parallel with the tibia, just below its medial condyle. After the skin is split, the very superficial long saphenous should be looked for. It should have been marked before operation with the patient standing so that it can be protected. The vein is exposed for only a short distance in order to see whether it is large enough and patent. It must never be gripped by forceps or pinched by a hook. The deep fascia is then divided and the medial head of the gastrocnemius displaced. The soleus is thus exposed. The pulsating artery is

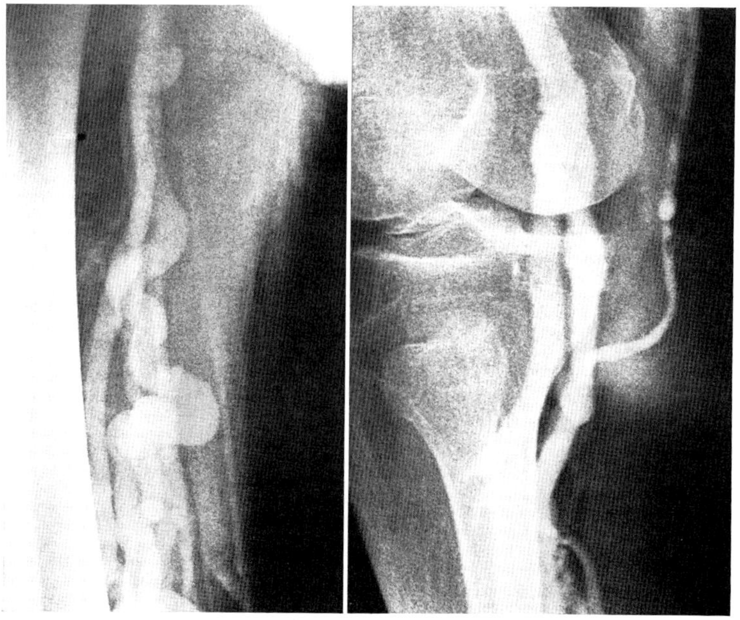

Fig. 6.31. Femoral bypass. Ideal indication: femoral severely damaged, popliteal normal; incompetent valves in the great saphenous.

palpated in the loose fatty tissue between the margin of the soleus and the tibia. With the artery as a guide, the vein is easily found, lying *in front* of the artery. It may become necessary to divide the semitendinous tendon, which narrows the upper angle of the wound. It must be sutured when the wound is closed.

In the post-thrombotic syndrome, the vein is usually tightly adherent to the artery underneath as a result of previous perivenous inflammation. Cautious freeing of the vein from the artery presents the only technical difficulty of the operation.

The popliteal is dissected for 3 to 4 cm. Exposure of its most distal portion is important, for the lumen is best preserved here, even in unfavorable cases. The vein is looped with two thin rubber catheters and pulled forward. Maximal opening is secured by self-retaining retractors. The long saphenous is dissected. Again, care should be taken not to grip it with forceps or irritate it mechanically in any way. Two milliliters of heparin is injected in order to prevent blood clotting. The long saphenous is now sharply divided into the distal angle of the wound and the distal stump is ligated. The proximal end is flushed with heparin-saline, which dilates the vessel slightly. However, veins can be stretched much less than arteries. The vein has markedly contracted since it has been freed. The popliteal is throttled proximally and distally by two rubber catheters and opened. Hemostats should be avoided. The long saphenous is slit for 2 cm and joined by a 2 cm end-to-side anastomosis to the popliteal. Bleeding at the suture line after release of the throttle is stopped by saline compresses, never by puncture. The long saphenous must be left in a loose loop—remember that the knee is bent. The knee is now extended. There must be no tension in the saphenous and it must not be coiled. The wound is closed in layers. A large enough window must be left in the deep fascia to avoid restricting the saphenous. Suction drainage is very important.

Postoperatively the patient receives heparin intermittently for 5 days so that the clotting time is prolonged two or three times normal. This is followed by administration of a coumarin preparation, which is continued for 6 months with monitoring of prothrombin time. Bed rest and elevation, with vigorous exercising, are necessary for 7 days. Radiologic studies should be performed only under additional heparin protection.

There is one decisive test for the success of the operation. Roentgenologic studies show whether the anastomosis is still patent (Fig. 6.32), but the operation is successful only if function has improved. Venous pressure curves on exercise provide this information. Complete return to normal of the curve cannot be expected, but the

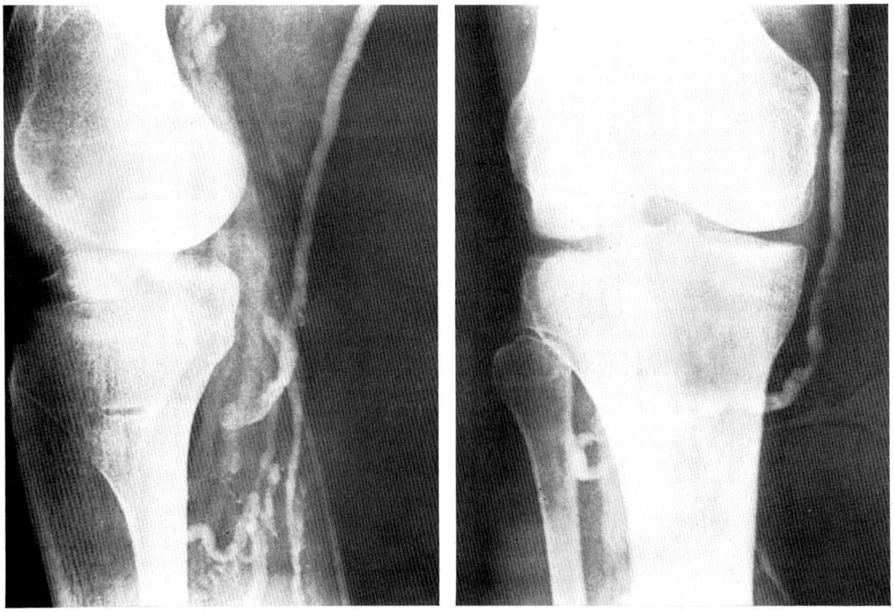

Fig. 6.32. Femoral bypass in two planes. The popliteal is poorly recanalized, but there is good drainage. Great saphenous contains incompetent valves.

surgical aim is to promote the patient to the next best group (Fig. 6.33).

Late results cannot be yet predicted. It is quite possible that functioning valves in the great saphenous degenerate as a result of altered pressure conditions. This may be of no functional importance. Possibly the great saphenous dilates in its new function, and drainage improves further in the course of years. Nonetheless, some skepticism is in order for any venous anastomosis. All venous anastomoses are threatened by shrinkage, as described by Kunlin and May (1965). Fibrin threads form, and eventually strands of scar tissue, that slowly close the anastomosis. We call this *progressive* stenosis. The cause is slow flow in the venous system. Future observations will show whether it may be necessary to apply a temporary distal arteriovenous fistula in order to keep the anastomosis open.

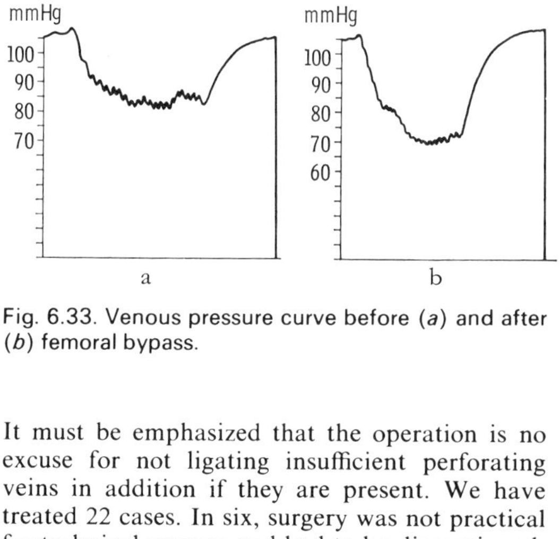

Fig. 6.33. Venous pressure curve before (*a*) and after (*b*) femoral bypass.

It must be emphasized that the operation is no excuse for not ligating insufficient perforating veins in addition if they are present. We have treated 22 cases. In six, surgery was not practical for technical reasons and had to be discontinued. Of the remaining 16 cases, the anastomosis closed in three, the venous pressure curve naturally remaining unchanged; in one case it deteriorated slightly. The expected improvement in the curve was seen in the other 13 cases. We are informed that Husin (1970) conceived the same idea almost simultaneously.

Frileux et al. (1972) published a report of 20 bypass operations on the post-thrombotically damaged femoral vein. Unfortunately, only six cases were evaluated roentgenologically; the anastomosis was patent in four. The technique described by Frileux in 1970 differs considerably from our own for most cases: All branches of the great saphenous are ligated, and the long saphenous is filled with heparin solution, clamped distally and proximally, extracted and pulled through under the sartorius muscle; it is then anastomosed at the level of the adductor canal with the distal femoral or popliteal vein. Frileux remarked that Warren and Thayer reported the idea of a venous bypass in 1954, and so they deserve priority.

Leg Ulcers

We recommend as the basis for the treatment of leg ulcers:

—verification of intact arterial circulation by oscillometry or oscillography, and if suspicion remains, angiography;
—x-ray demonstration of the deep veins; and
—x-ray demonstration of the superficial and perforating veins.

We are well aware that this systematic basic recommendation is not necessary in many cases. But a considerable part of the success of Böhler (1938), the founder of modern trauma surgery, is due to this uncompromising fundamental demand, that x-ray pictures be obtained in two planes for every fracture without exception: before treatment, after application of plaster of Paris and at the end of treatment. Böhler surely must have realized that fractures of the radius and many others could be set without x-ray evaluation, but who would guarantee this 100 per cent? Thus we are convinced that decisive progress in angiology, and in as socially important a disease as leg ulcers, can be achieved only by uncompromising systematic application of all objective means of examination available.

Classification

Following extensive comparative roentgen examinations, we divide leg ulcers as follows (May, 1962):

—venous leg ulcers, and
—post-thrombotic leg ulcers.

Discussion of leg ulcers not due to venous disease—for example, subsequent to arteriovenous fistulas, arterial disease, hypertension, nerve damage, trauma, carcinoma, tuberculosis—would be beyond the scope of this book.

In venous ulcers the deep veins are normal or approximately so. According to investigations of Fischer (1969), the deep veins are frequently measurably broader in the presence of varices. Piulachs (1956) noted that valves of the deep veins were likewise insufficient. At times, it is difficult or impossible to decide whether these valves are incompetent because of progressive degeneration, constitutionally inherent in aging, or because of nondiagnosed intramural thrombosis (Degni et al., 1965). Hence, the term *chronic venous insufficiency* is certainly good, because it is noncommittal about etiology. Slight deviations from normal may be disregarded during surgery.

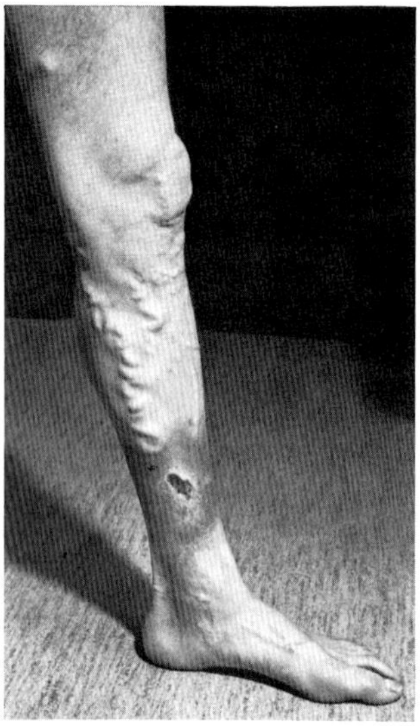

Fig. 6.34. Leg ulcer in primary varicosity and insufficient Cockett III perforator vein. The insufficient perforating vein at the level of the adductor canal (Dodd's perforator) is also visible.

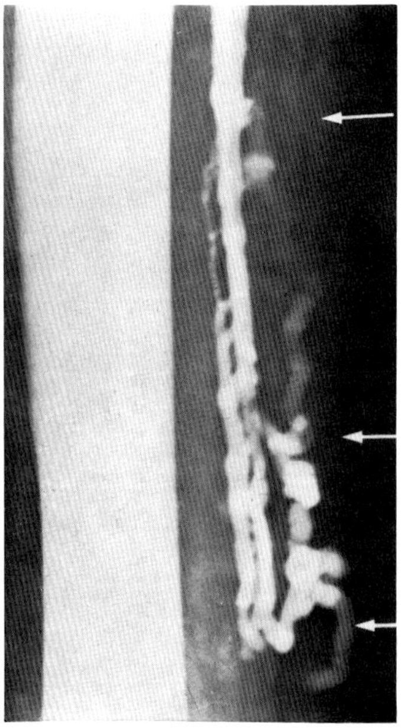

Fig. 6.35. Ulcer blowout; incompetent perforating veins with normal deep veins.

The predominant cause of venous ulcers is insufficient perforating veins (Figs. 6.34 and 6.35). Occasionally, burst, incorrectly treated varicosities may cause ulcers. Insufficient perforating veins *may* but need not be associated with primary varices. These may be present but do not cause the ulcers, unless a varix has burst, as mentioned above. Less than a third of all leg ulcers are venous ulcers.

Most ulcers are post-thrombotic leg ulcers. Our own investigations (May, 1962) agree with the findings of Arnoldi (1964), Cockett (1955) and Haeger (1965) that lesions of the deep veins cause leg ulcers only very rarely. They are responsible for edema of the leg and induration in the distal part. Varicose eczema is not infrequently caused by secondary varices.

The cause of post-thrombotic leg ulcers is almost always the additional development of incompetent perforating veins. An exception are the relatively infrequent *ulcers in the gaiter area* (*Fischer*). They form around the ankle, accompanied by severe stasis edema, and are due to stagnation of the cutaneous venous plexus in the opposite direction to drainage.

Mechanism of Development

The fundamental explanation for the development of leg ulcers due to insufficiency of perforator veins was given by Cockett (1955); later publications complemented but did not correct his

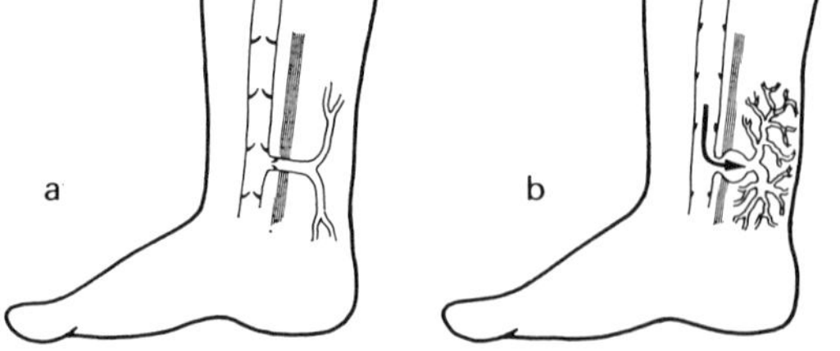

Fig. 6.36. Development of an ulcer. Normal conditions (*a*); ramming effect due to incompetent perforator vein (*b*). (After Cockett.)

interpretation. Valvular incompetence of the perforators permits transmission of deep venous pressure, which is increased during calf muscle contraction, to the venules of the skin. Cockett calls this a ramming effect. An ulcer precursor state arises in the form of a mesh of finely dilated venules around the ankle, called an "ankle flare" by Cockett (Fig. 6.36). Finally, the poorly nourished skin breaks down, usually after minor trauma. The leg ulcer is fully established. Fischer (1969) confirms that these blowout ulcers usually lie at the emergence of a Cockett perforator. Arnoldi (1964) performed very detailed venous pressure measurements, and we carried out similar studies. We share the opinion that these are thrusts of pressure waves, which occur during each muscular contraction and continue up to the skin. They decrease the arteriovenous difference in the capillary bed, causing relative hypoxia and, finally, ulcer. The development of the ulcers was imitated on a frog model by van Limborgh et al. (1966).

Treatment

The few cases in which the ulcer is a sequel to a burst varix are easy to treat. The ulcers soon heal under pressure bandages and a subsequent varix operation removes the cause. Apart from these exceptions, the cause of all other ulcers is one or several insufficient perforating veins. The only practical therapy, therefore, is elimination of the incompetent perforators. We prefer surgical dissection and ligature of the perforator veins to all other procedures, such as sclerotherapy and percutaneous destruction with special instruments.

The ulcer must be healed before surgery. The guidelines established by Sigg (1968) for healing

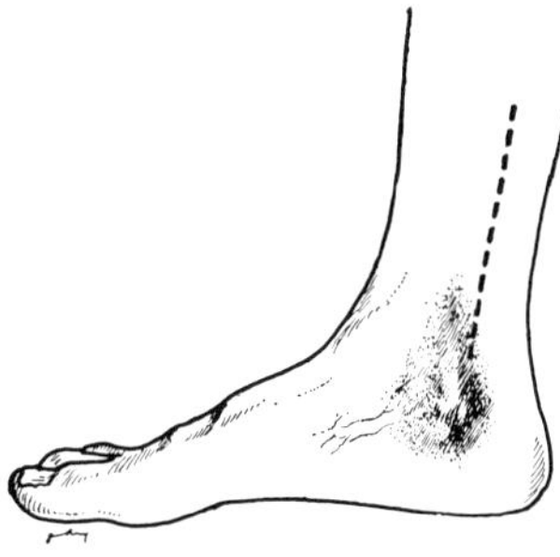

Fig. 6.37. Line of incision for ligation of perforators responsible for the ulcer.

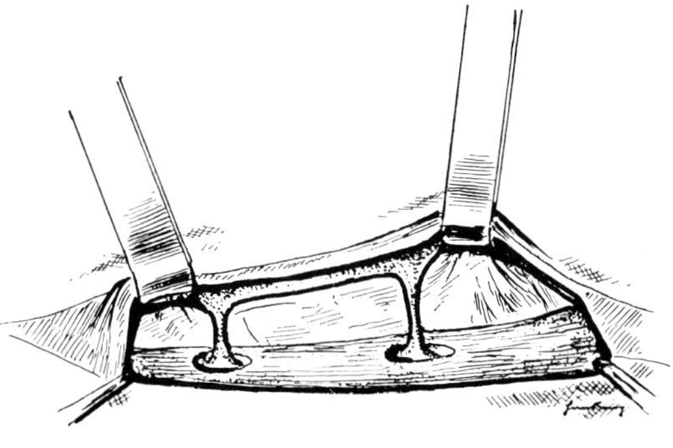

Fig. 6.38. The perforators are exposed and can be ligated.

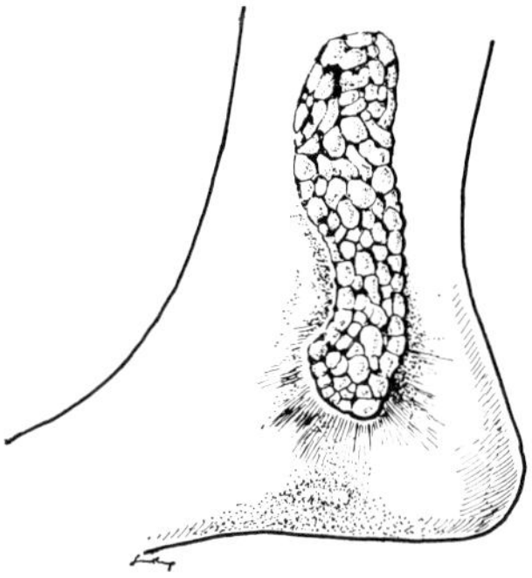

Fig. 6.39. Ulcer covered with pinch grafts.

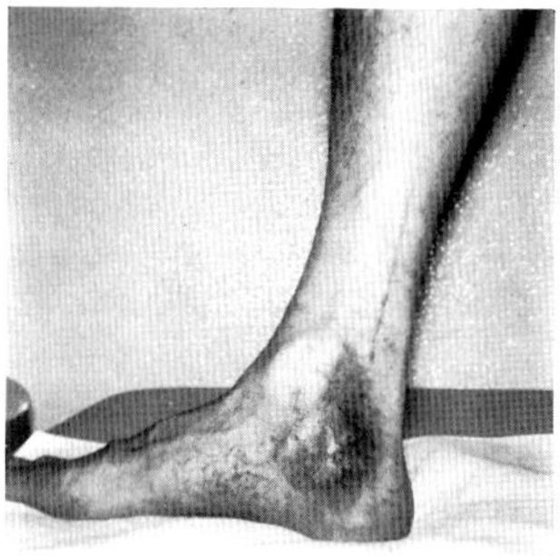

a

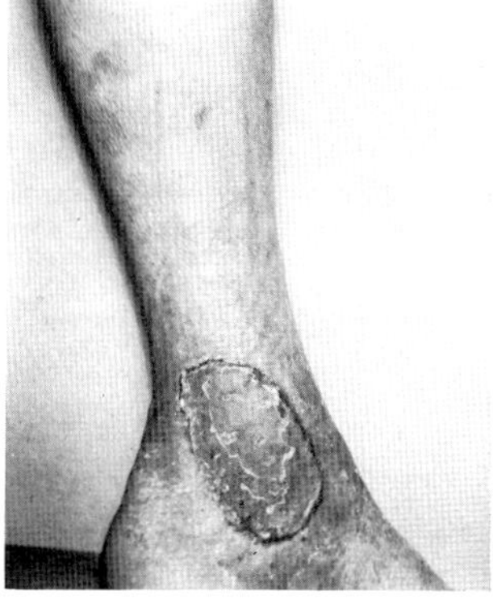

b

Fig. 6.40. Leg ulcer covered with split-thickness skin graft. The healed incision for ligation of the insufficient perforating veins is still visible.

leg ulcers are undoubtedly the treatment of choice.

The *principles of treatment* according to Sigg are:

—no need for bed rest,
—proper pressure bandaging of the whole leg, from the toes to below the knee, with two elastic bandages, and
—local wound treatment.

Any type of ointment is contraindicated. The popular antibiotic-containing ointments are not suitable; at best, they promote sensitization against the antibiotic. Superinfection of the ulcer is almost natural but it is never the cause of nonhealing. Sigg is entirely correct in his view that each ulcer would heal with application of normal saline by itself, provided the pressure bandages are properly applied. We prefer boric acid solution, or with severe infected ulceration, ethacridine (1:1000). This always suffices. It is important to apply a large piece of foam rubber that covers well the gauze pad drenched in boric solution over the ulcer. Elastic bandages are applied on top of this. Eczema in the surrounding area is treated with corticoid-containing ointments or other appropriate dermatologic preparations.

Proper bandaging must be explained to the patient. He should also be instructed how to raise his legs at night. If a patient is simply told to elevate the legs, he is likely just to carelessly push a wedge bolster under his heels. This is entirely inadequate. The foot of the bed should be raised by 30 cm, or a 22 cm wedge bolster that tapers in the popliteal fossa should be pushed under the whole leg. Only in this way is a venous pressure of zero guaranteed at the level of the ulcer when the patient is lying down. Any venous ulcer heals with this treatment.

Subsequently, the incompetent perforating veins are examined roentgenologically and removed surgically, as described in the previous chapter (Figs. 6.37 and 6.38).

After removal of the perforator veins, the ulcer usually heals with a firm scar.

If the scar is rather large, it should be excised and covered with healthy skin. We advise excision not only of the scar but also of the indurated surrounding tissues, that is, all the diseased tissue. We also remove the underlying fascia, for only then is the base of the wound well vascularized, to ensure lasting healing of the skin transplant. The base of the wound may be covered with *patch grafts* (Fig. 6.39). This yields the worst results cosmetically but we use this method occasionally when the base is avascular.

Cosmetically better results are achieved by grafting with *split-thickness skin* removed by a dermatome (Fig. 6.40). This in turn may be improved with *retiform split-thickness skin*, obtained by a *meshgraft dermatome*.

In rare cases, even this skin does not hold. We are then compelled to achieve solid coverage by means of a *sliding graft*.

References

Arnoldi, C. C.: The venous return from the lower leg in health and in chronic venous insufficiency. Acta orthop. scand. Suppl. 64 (1964)

Arnoldi, C. C.: On the pathogenesis of the venous leg ulcer. Acta chir. scand. 134 (1968) 427

Bassi, G.: Le Varici degli Arti inferiori. Minerva Medica, Torino 1962

Bauer, G.: Rationale and results of popliteal vein division. Angiology 6 (1955) 169

Bauer, G.: Indications for popliteal vein ligation. J. cardiovasc. Surgery 4 (1963) 18

Bauer, G.: The long term effect of popliteal ligation in 136 cases of severe bursting lower leg pain and oedemae. J. cardiovasc. Surg. 6 (1965) 366

Beaconsfield, P.: Veins after sympathectomy. Surgery 36 (1954) 771

Berger, A., P. Brücke: Zur chirurgischen Behandlung der Insuffizienz tiefer Beinvenen. Acta chir. aust. 2 (1970) 97

Bernink, B. P.: Sind die phlebographisch als inkompetent gedeuteten Venae communicantes auch physiologisch insuffizient? Zbl. Phleb. 10 (1971) 41

Böhler, L.: Die Technik der Knochenbruchbehandlung, 6. ed. Maudrich, Vienna 1938

Boyd, A. M.: Major venous ligation in the treatment of post-phlebitic sequelae. Lancet 1953, 113

Buxton, R. W., F. A. Coller: Surgical treatment of long standing deep phlebitis. Surgery, Suppl. 11 (1945) 749

Buxton, R. W., J. M. Farris, C. A. Moyer, F. A. Coller: Surgical treatment of long standing deep phlebitis of leg. Surgery 15 (1944) 749

Cockett, F. B.: The pathology and treatment of venous ulcers of the leg. Brit. J. plast. Surg. 43 (1955) 260

Cotton, L. T., V. C. Roberts: The value of blood flow measurement in reconstructive arterial surgery. Proc. roy. Soc. 67 (1974) 445

DeCamp, P. T.: Ambulatory venous pressure studies in post-phlebitic and other disease states. Surgery 29 (1951), 365

DeCamp, P. T.: Funktionelle Pathologie der Venen. Langenbecks Arch. klin. Chir. 325 (1969) 839

Degni, M., V. Toth, W. Lanfranchi, Maja A. Chaim: Chronic mural phlebitis. Rev. bras. Cardiovasc. 1 (1965) 65

Dodd, H., F. B. Cockett: Varicose Veins and the Pathology and Surgery of the Veins of the Lower Limb. Livingstone, Edinburgh 1956

Dormandy, J. A., E. Hoare, J. Postlethwaite: Importance of blood viscosity. Rheological claudication. Proc. roy. Soc. 67 (1974) 446

Fischer, H.: Phlebologie heute. Fortschr. Med. 87 (1969) 1001

Frileux, C.: Transposition ou greffe veineuse. In: Nouveau traité de technique chirurgicale, Vol. V, J. Patzl, L. Leger (eds.), Masson, Paris 1970 (p. 552)

Frileux, C., P. Pillot-Bienayme, C. Gillot: Bypass of segmental obliterations of ilio-femoral venous axis by transposition of saphenous vein J. cardiovasc. Surg. 13 (1972) 409

Gilbertsen, V. A.: Blood flow in postsympathectomy patients. Angiology 11 (1960) 139

Gracey, L.: Simultaneous calf and thigh blood flow measurements by selective femoral vein occlusion plethysmography. Proc. roy. Soc. 67 (1974) 444

Gundersen, J.: Incompetent perforating veins of the leg. Vasc. Dis. 3 (1966) 273

Haeger, K.: Ischaemic ulcers of the lower limb. Acta chir. scand. 130 (1965) 584–592

Haeger, K.: The treatment of the severe post-thrombotic state. Angiology 19 (1968) 439
Haeger, K.: Indications for surgery in ankle perforator insufficiency, Zbl. Phleb. 8 (1969) 158
Haeger, K.: The treatment of venous hypostatic edema and its complications. Zbl. Phleb. 9 (1970) 23
Haeger, K., J. Sandber: Zur operativen Behandlung der tiefen Veneninsuffizienz. Zbl. Phleb. 5 (1966) 93
Halse, Th.: Das postthrombotische Syndrom. Z. Kreisl.-Forsch. 48 (1959) 782
Husin, E. A.: In situ saphenopopliteal bypass graft for incompetence of the femoral and popliteal veins. Surg. Gynec. Obstet. 130 (1970) 279
Kuiper, I. P.: Perifere venenze druk meting. Diss., Nijmwegen 1966
Lewis, J. D.: Pressure measurements in the long-term follow up of peripheral vascular disease. Proc. roy. Soc. 67 (1974) 443
van Limborgh, W., W. Boersma, L. van der Lugt: Experimental production of ulcus cruris venosum conditions in frogs. Zbl. Phleb. 5 (1966) 66–75
Linton, R.: The post-thrombotic postsympathectomy syndrome. Arch. Surg. 67 (1953) 2
Linton, R. R., J. B. Hardy: Post-thrombotic sequelae of the lower extremity treatment by superficial femoral vein interruption and stripping of saphenous veins. Surg. Clin. N. Amer. 27 (1947) 1171
Linton, R. R., J. B. Hardy: Postthrombotic syndrome of the lower extremity. Surgery 24 (1948) 452
Lofferer, O.: Arteriovenöse Kurzschlüsse der Extremitäten. Zbl. Phleb. 8 (1969) 2
Luke, J. C.: Venous disorders of the lower extremity. Ciba Symp. 5 (1953) 116
Mandl, F.: Blockade und Chirurgie des Sympathicus. Springer, Vienna, 1953
May, R.: Das röntgenologische Venenbild des Ulcus cruris. Zbl. Phleb. 1 (1962) 201–203
May, R.: Die Problematik der Venenplastik Zbl. Phleb. 4 (1965) 43
May, R.: Die Wiederherstellung der postthrombotisch geschädigten venösen Strombahn. Zbl. Phleb. 7 (1968a) 24
May, R.: Grundprinzipien der Venenplastik. In: Das postthrombotische Zustandsbild der Extremitäten. A. Kappert, R. May (eds.). Huber, Bern 1968b
May, R.: Funktionelle Pathologie der Venen. Langenbecks Arch. klin. Chir. 325 (1969) 839
May, R.: Die chirurgische Behandlung des postthrombotischen Syndroms. Hefte Unfallheilk. 107 (1971) 129
May, R.: Meßmethoden in der Venenchirurgie. Huber, Bern 1971a
May, R.: Physiologie und Pathologie der Wadenmuskelpumpe. In: Meßmethoden in der Venenchirurgie. R. May (ed.). Huber, Bern 1971b (p. 22)
May, R.: Venentransplantation beim postthrombotischen Zustandsbild des Beines. Act. Chir. 7 (1972) 1
May, R., R. Nissl: Die Phlebographie der unteren Extremität. Thieme, Stuttgart 1959
May, R., H. Brinkmann, D. Peters: Lichtmikroskopische Betrachtungen an operativ entfernten Lumbalganglien des menschlichen Grenzstranges beim postthrombotischen Zustandsbild. Zbl. Phleb. 9 (1970) 2
Messent, D., P. Beaconsfield: Circulatory changes in the lower limb following lumbar sympathectomy. Surgery 35 (1954) 382
Netzer, C. O.: Die Strömungsverhältnisse beim postthrombotischen Zustandsbild. In: Das postthrombotische Zustandsbild der Extremitäten. A. Kappert, R. May (eds.). Huber Bern 1968
Netzer, C. O.: Zur Physiologie und Pathophysiologie der Wadenmuskelpumpe. In: Meßmethoden in der Venenchirurgie, hrsg. von R. May. Huber, Bern 1971
Nylander, G., K. Haeger: A variety of perforator veins of the lower leg. Zbl. Phleb. 9 (1970) 160
Patil, K. D.: Thermographic localisation of incompetent perforating veins in the leg. Brit. med. J. 1970/I, 195
Pinlachs, P.: Ulcers of the Legs. Thomas, Springfield/Ill. 1956
Pratt, G. H.: Classification and surgical treatment of the post-thrombotic syndrome. Surg. Gynec. Obstet. 118 (1964) 284
Psathakis, N.: Ein neues operatives Verfahren zur rationellen Behandlung des Insuffizienzsyndroms der unteren Extremität. Chirurg 35 (1964a) 79
Psathakis, N.: Das diagnostische und operative Problems des Insuffizienzyndroms der tiefen Beinvenen. Zbl. Chir. 89 (1964b) 177
Santler, R.: Die konservative Behandlung der postthrombotischen Varicen. Zbl. Phleb. 7 (1968) 278
Schönbach, G., W. Thorban: Funktionelle und organische Gefäßwandschäden nach Sympathectomie und partieller Nervenschädigung. Langenbecks Arch. klin. Chir. 291 (1959) 217
Sherman, R. S.: Varicose veins. Further findings based on anatomic and surgical dissections. Ann. Surg. 130 (1949) 218
Sigg, K.: Varicen, Ulcus cruris und Thrombose. Springer, Berlin 1968
Vidal-Barraqer, F.: Resultados de los distintos métodos de ligaduras venosas en el tratamiento de la insuficiencia profunda de la extremidad inferior. Angiologia 2 (1950) 1
Warren, R., Th. Thayer: Transplantations of the internal saphenous. Surgery 35 (1954) 867–876
Widmer, L.: Zum Verlauf der akuten tiefen Thrombophlebitis. In: Meßmethoden in der Venenchirurgie. R. May (ed.). Huber, Bern 1971

7 Surgery of the Pelvic Veins

R. May and J. A. DeWeese

Compression Phenomenon of the Femoral Vein

Although this syndrome affects a part of the common femoral, it will be discussed with surgery of pelvic veins, since the affected segment forms a functional unit with the pelvic veins.

Gullmo (1957) observed that application of pressure to the femoral vein produced a dent in the lacuna vasorum medially on x-ray films in roughly 60 per cent of patients with venous disease of the lower extremity (Fig. 7.1). The vein can also be displaced laterally. In 27 per cent of cases it is completely compressed.

He called this phenomenon the *strain obstruction syndrome of the femoral vein.*

May (1964) called it the *compression occlusion phenomenon of the femoral vein.* Today, the term *femoral obstruction syndrome* or *femoral compression phenomenon* is preferred.

The syndrome is observed only when the erect patient exerts abdominal pressure during phlebography.

Gullmo believes that the ligamentous attachment around the lacuna vasorum is weakened—that is, there is a *latent femoral hernia,* which compresses the vein on abdominal pressure (Fig. 7.2).

The femoral vein is compressed with each increase in intra-abdominal pressure in these cases, whereas the calf muscle pump tries to propel the

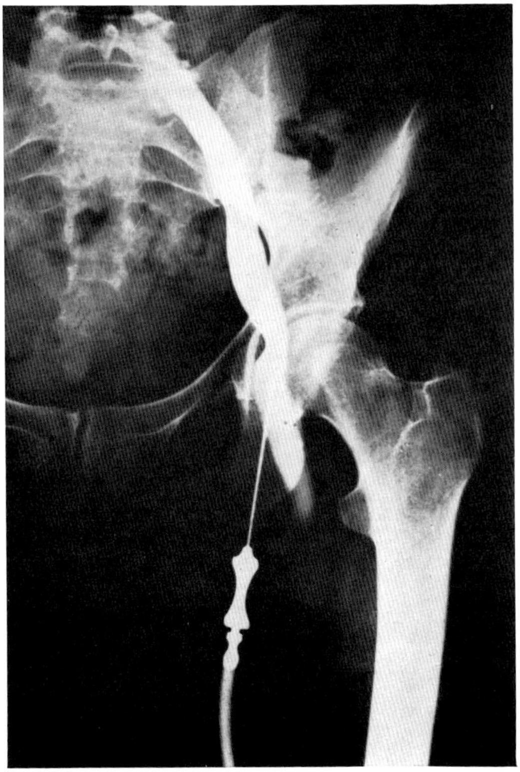

Fig. 7.1. Femoral vein compression syndrome.

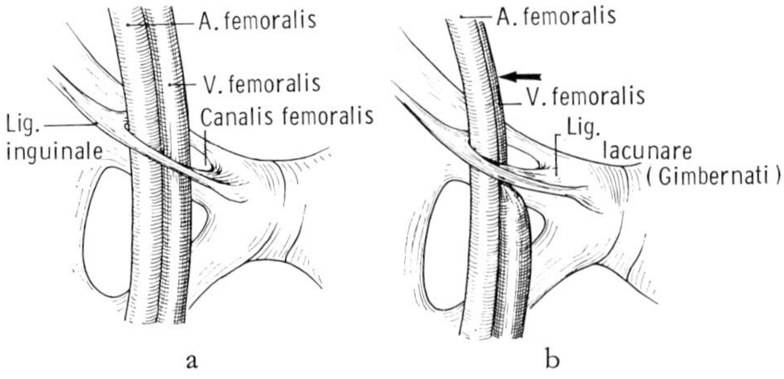

Fig. 7.2. In latent femoral hernia (*a*), the femoral vein is compressed by abdominal pressure (*b*).

blood proximally. Therefore, it is quite possible, according to Gullmo, that this syndrome promotes formation of varicosities and favors recurrence following varix operation.

Gullmo proposed operating on the latent femoral hernia. He performs hernioplasty of the superior pubic ligament (Cooper). It is important to eliminate the weak transverse fascia at the posterior inguinal wall. Occasionally, a lipoma that presses on the vein is found in the hernial opening. Gullmo considers this operation to be indicated in all severe cases.

We have performed the operation only in patients in whom a femoral hernia was present. We are still wary about it, although Gullmo demonstrated on phlebograms that the syndrome disappeared after operation.

Nylander (1961) explained the phenomenon differently. If a patient with normal deep veins presses, (raises intra-abdominal pressure), the uppermost valves of the femoral and long saphenous veins oppose this pressure, and the vein fills to capacity proximal to these valves.

However, if these valves are incompetent, there is no counterpressure, and the external iliac vein is squashed. If latent femoral hernia were the cause, only local compression would occur in the lacuna vasorum, even in severe cases. Indeed the syndrome can be prevented if the incompetent valves are equalized by a tourniquet placed at the proximal part of the thigh.

Furthermore, Nylander is of opinion that the vein, tensely filled by the raised intra-abdominal pressure, shuts off the weak portion of the lacuna vasorum by supporting the frequently poor femoral septum of Cloquet. If this protective action fails, owing to valvular incompetence, the femoral canal is wide open and a femoral hernia has a clear passage.

According to Nylander, *incompetent valves are primary, and latent femoral hernia is the result.*

Gullmo (1968) published the results of studies on 1500 patients with clinically normal conditions in the groin. The compression test was employed during phlebography, followed by urography. Accordingly, the venous indentation was found only in *incipient or manifest femoral hernias*. In the last analysis, a distinctly dilated femoral canal was observed even in the few apparently normal probands. Hence it may be said that patients with the *compression phenomenon* (practically all of them women in our series) have a femoral hernia or at least a tendency to it.

According to Gullmo, the compression phenomenon can be used to determine whether an unexplained bulge is a femoral hernia or not. Femoral hernia is accompanied by the compression phenomenon, since the hernial sac is closely apposed to the vein, but inguinal hernia is not. With inguinal hernias, only a marked deviation of the vein is found. The femoral vein remains normal in acute medial hernias, a fact that is important in evaluation.

The compression syndrome is not for us as yet an indication for surgery, but manifest femoral hernia is.

Venous Spur of May and Thurner

As described in detail on page 23ff, May and Thurner (1956) found that a *venous spur* is present in the left common iliac vein in approximately 22 per cent of adults. It is a result of intimal irritation, the vein being squeezed between the right common iliac artery ventrally and the fifth lumbar vertebra dorsally (Fig. 7.3 and Figs. 1.49*b*; 1.50*b* and 1.51*b*).

This spur produces turbulence that almost certainly promotes thrombosis with reduced venous flow, e.g., after operations and labor. We are of opinion that the predominance of left-sided pelvic vein thromboses can thus be explained. Pelvic vein thrombosis occurs on the left side in 65 per cent of cases and on the right in 15 per cent.

Diagnosis

After the existence of spur formation was established, we confronted the problem of its *diagnosis in living persons*.

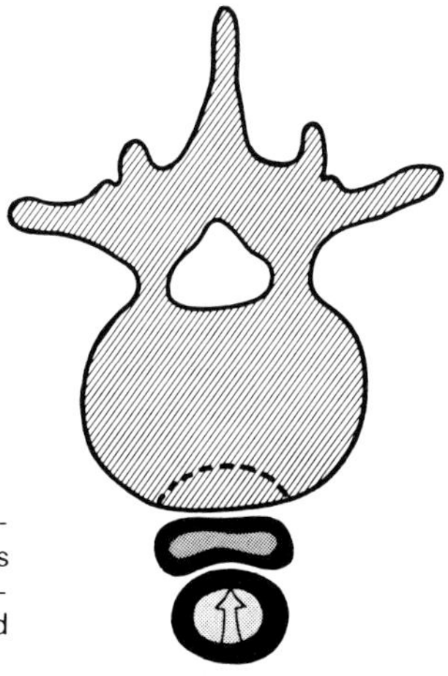

Fig. 7.3. The common iliac vein is compressed between artery and vertebra.

Roentgenologic Findings

Direct roentgenologic demonstration of the spur occurs only rarely (Fig. 7.4).

More important is recognition of *spur formation with hemodynamic consequences*. This can be achieved, and the film answers both whether a spur is present and whether it impedes the flow.

Arterial compression produces a contrast medium defect in the left common iliac vein, the "*normally invisible zone*" (Guilhem and Baux, 1954) (Figs. 7.5 and 7.6).

Collaterals normally are not shown or are only insignificantly visualized roentgenologically. Slight back pressure in the internal iliac vein is not abnormal (Fig. 7.6).

Spurs that do not interfere hemodynamically do not show on x-ray films. Possibly these spur formations might be visualized after local injection with the Seldinger catheter, but as long as they do not cause stagnation they are of no surgical interest.

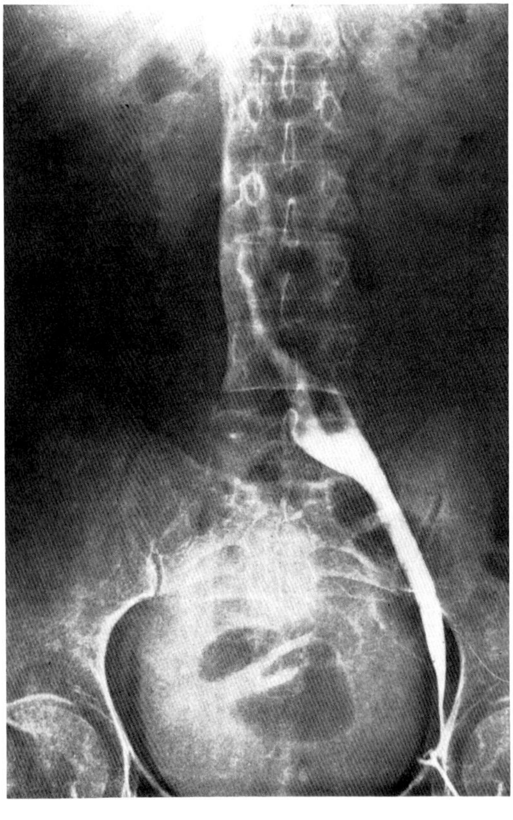

Fig. 7.4. Direct demonstration of a central venous spur.

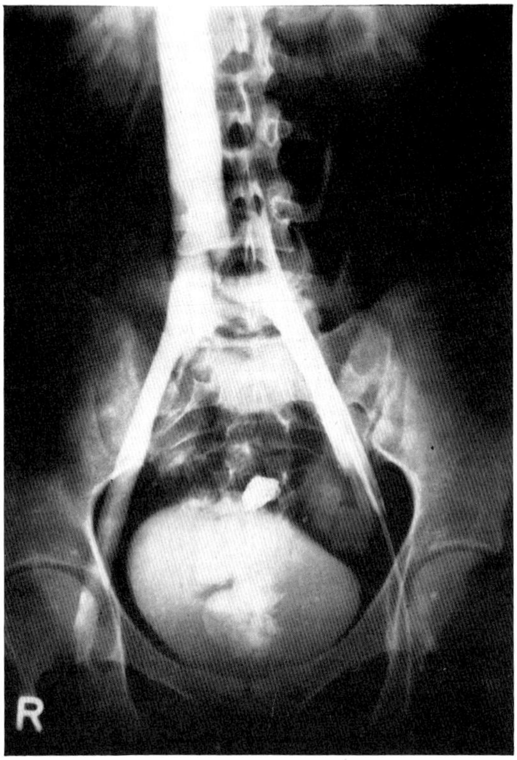

Fig. 7.5. Normally invisible zone. Contrast medium defect in the left common iliac vein due to compression by the artery. Spur formation not excluded with certainty. Transitional form.

More marked formation of collaterals (Fig. 7.7), as well as demonstration of the ascending lumbar vein, indicates that a block is present: most probably it is due to a spur. Although 100 per cent proof of the correctness of roentgen films would require a large number of operations, surgical findings so far have confirmed our views. It is currently impossible to ascertain by radiologic studies *which type of spur* is present. One can only say with certainty that there is flow impairment, no tumor and no acute or old thrombosis, and predict that the cause is probably a spur. This suffices for our procedure.

Venous Pressure Measurement

Recently venous pressure measurement has become a valuable aid, but it too cannot by itself reveal the presence of a spur. It does confirm functional impediment to flow, which is more important. In conjunction with the x-ray film, it permits diagnosis of a spur that acts as drainage barrier. We recommend this examination as a supplement.

Technique

The measurements are performed by the technique of Negus (1969). We use an Atlas pressure apparatus, type EM 50. If need be, a simple disposable manometer may be employed. The right and left femoral veins are punctured in the groin. Pressure in each is measured at rest and again after the patient has flexed the forefoot ten times. Normally, in man and the dog, the values of the two sides are identical (Neistadt and Schwartz, 1966). A pressure difference at rest is significant, as is a rise in pressure with exercise, which is impressive if drainage is impaired (Table 7.1).

Table 7.1 Average Values of Venous Pressure Measurement

	Normal	Pathologic	Pressure/Gradient (limits)
Rest	5.6 mm Hg	8.6 mm Hg	2.0 mm Hg
Exercise	7.0 mm Hg	18.5 mm Hg	3.0 mm Hg
Difference	1.4 mm Hg	9.9 mm Hg	

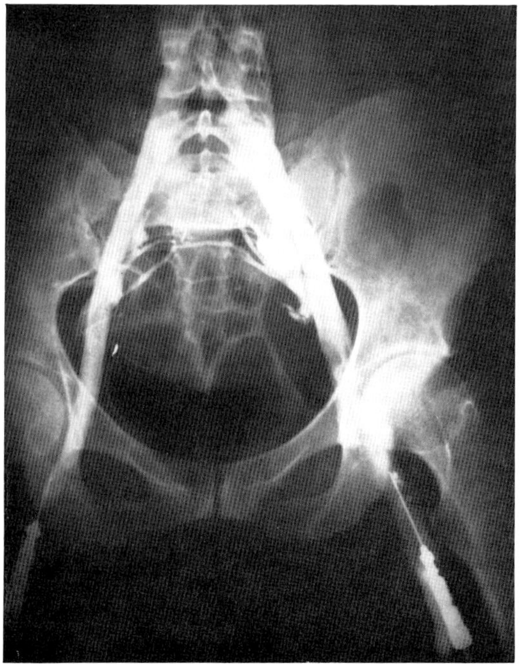

Fig. 7.6. Normal collaterals, normally invisible zone.

With unimpeded drainage, the pressure rises only slightly with exercise. The extent of the pressure rise is therefore an exact measure of the scale of the block. The degree of normalization is an objective test of surgical success.
Also of practical importance are investigations by Negus in which adequate pressure values were obtained from the recumbent patient. This should not be underestimated, for it is difficult to puncture the femoral vein in the groin of both sides and take measurements on an erect and frequently apprehensive patient.
In the presence of a venous spur that obstructs drainage, values of measurement are indeed above normal, but never to the extent typical of post-thrombotically occluded veins. Besides, it is not the absolute figures that are decisive but the difference between right and left.

Differential Diagnosis

The differential diagnosis from post-thrombotic occlusion of the common iliac vein is always

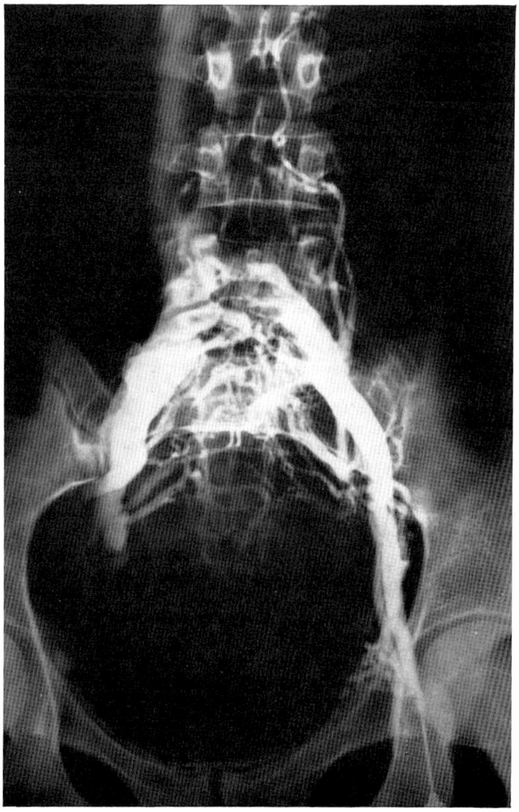

Fig. 7.7. Spur collaterals

simple. In post-thrombotic occlusion, formation of collaterals is incomparably more massive, and mural changes are always found in the external iliac vein (Fig. 7.8).

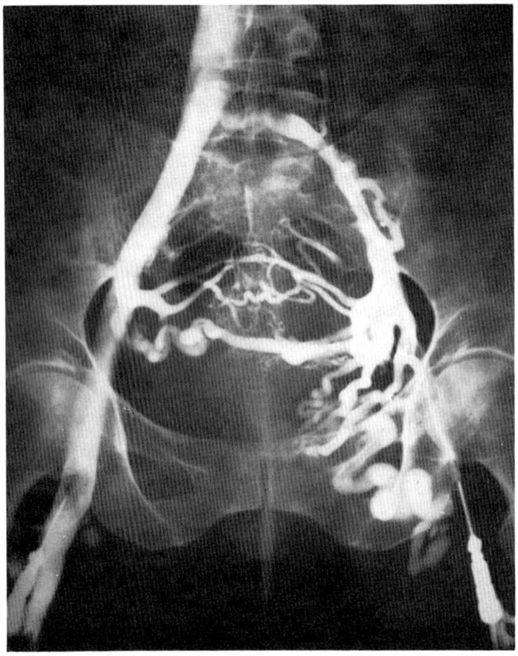

Fig. 7.8. Post-thrombotic collaterals.

Surgical Procedure

Dick (1962) proposed two methods for elimination of the compression.

Dick himself does not favor the first, resecting the right common iliac artery and replacing it with a slightly curved prosthesis (Fig. 7.9).

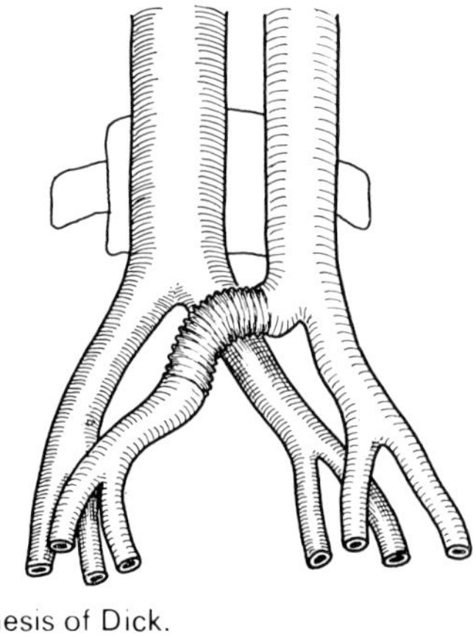

Fig. 7.9. Resection of proximal right common iliac artery and vascular prosthesis of Dick.

His second method, which has been used in several patients, consists of hollowing out the underlying vertebra (Fig. 7.10). If necessary, the groove is enlarged by removal of parts of the intervertebral disk.

Initial results appeared satisfactory. No callus formed. The disadvantage is that this serious intraperitoneal procedure can bring about only modest success, since it does not remove the intravascular block. It is too late for prophylaxis, since the spur has already formed. Nevertheless, there is no doubt of the hemodynamic success of Dick's operation. Even if decompression does not remove the spur, the spur becomes hemodynamically silent, at least at first. Only long-term follow up will show whether the improvement is lasting.

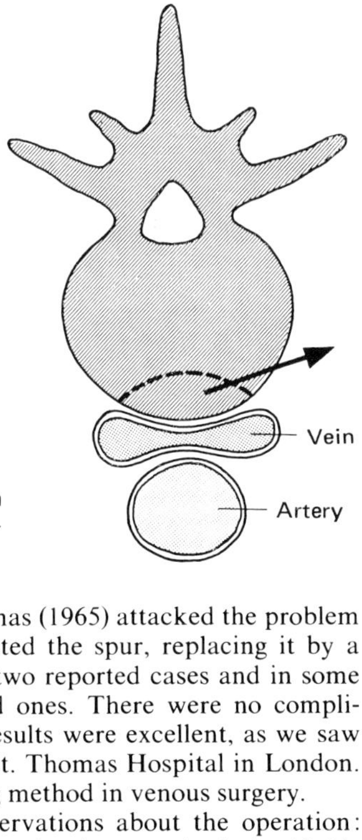

Fig. 7.10. Groove in vertebra recommended by Dick.

Cockett and Thomas (1965) attacked the problem directly and resected the spur, replacing it by a venous patch, in two reported cases and in some other unpublished ones. There were no complications and the results were excellent, as we saw during a visit to St. Thomas Hospital in London. It is an interesting method in venous surgery.

We have two reservations about the operation: First, the procedure is of a magnitude justifiable only exceptionally in so common a defect that produces minor complaints. Second, the compression persists, and this raises the question whether spur formation will recur. Hence, the hollowing-out procedure of Dick should be combined with this operation, and this makes it an even more serious intervention.

Niedner (1966) pointed to the interesting feasibility of reducing the pressure of the artery on the vein. The artery, or the whole aortic bifurcation, is fixed to the vertebral column by parietal branches, especially the superior gluteal artery. Phylogenetically, man has been erect only for a short time. In the upright position, the axis of the human sacrum forms an angle of 120 degrees, and its tip, the promontory, juts far anteriorly. The vessels overlying it are thus under tension. Compression and resulting spur formation are a tribute we pay for walking erect, a position to which we are not yet adapted. Our experience has shown that when the gluteal artery is divided, the internal iliac artery does deviate ventrally, as if it had been released from fixation (Fig. 7.11), giving the impression of a wall tree severed from its fixtures.

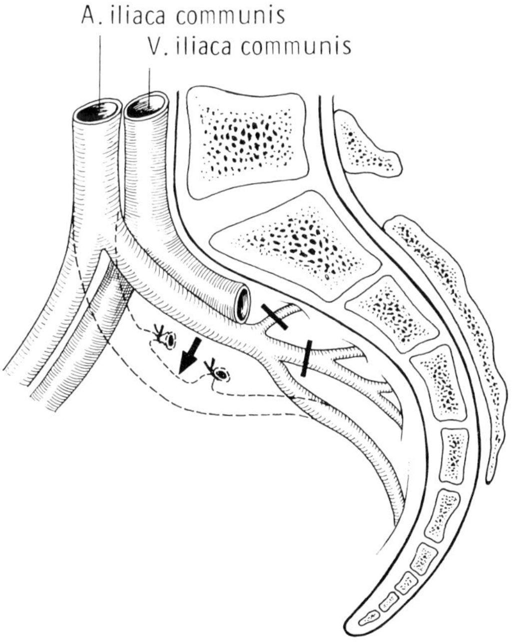

Fig. 7.11. Resection of the superior gluteal artery as proposed by Niedner.

If the whole bifurcation of the aorta is to be lifted anteriorly, it must be done bilaterally.
Gumrich (1969) has for some years used a technique of enucleation of the right common iliac artery and aortic fork and loosening of the compressed venous segment of the left common iliac vein, with lateral retraction of the right pelvic artery. The split peritoneum is drawn under the artery so that it loops around the artery like a muff. The margin is fixed to the retroperitoneum far to the right. Gumrich stresses particularly that the artery must be displaced from its bed so that it can no longer compress the vein against the promontory. This operation has been performed 62 times so far.
Follow-up studies are in progress.

Niedner's Technique of Gluteal Resection

The method does not present any difficulty. After a deep gridiron incision between the umbilicus and the superior anterior iliac spine, the peritoneum in the medial area is ablated with moist swabs. Deep spatulas are placed along the psoas muscle, on which the finger moves medially to palpate the artery. The artery is followed proximally to the bifurcation of the common iliac artery. The upper portion of the external iliac artery is dissected; care is taken to spare the vein, lying medially. With a fine rubber catheter a loop is placed around the artery. If pull is exerted on this loop, the internal iliac artery is easily exposed; proceeding along the artery, the superior gluteal artery is found. It is doubly ligated and divided. Niedner originally divided all branches of the internal iliac artery; this can be done from a unilateral approach only because of the blood supply to the uterus. A bilateral approach is necessary if the aortic bifurcation is to be lifted off. Furthermore, it has been shown that the tension actually derives from the gluteal arteries that branch off from the apex of the posteriorly convex arch formed by the internal iliac arteries.
Accordingly, we continually follow all the patients we have operated on. It will be seen in the next few years whether collaterals form—proof of blockade—or not.
Unlike Dick's method, this operation is harmless because it is extraperitoneal, and major complications are not anticipated if it is skilfully performed. We observe the principle of primum non nocere.
In summary, since even severe spur formation does not cause symptoms as long as it has not produced thrombosis, cases are found only accidentally; there is no indication of the need for phlebography and venous pressure measurement. Unfortunately, no other method reveals spur formation.
Likewise, surgical treatment has not progressed beyond early attempts. All the possible techniques proposed have been performed only a few times, and no normal controls are available.
Of little importance is *compression of the external iliac vein* by the internal iliac artery riding on it. On exposure, the adventitia of the artery is found to be tough and thickened. If the artery is freed, and the superior gluteal artery is divided in addition, the compression is removed.

Chronic Pelvic Vein Obstruction

So far, we have paid attention only to intraluminal changes following thrombosis—the extent of recanalization. This is understandable, for it is what the x-ray film conveys. Wanke and Gumrich (1950) noted during surgery of roentgenologically occluded pelvic veins that these vessels were firmly walled in their surroundings and indurated. This process involved not only the vein but also the artery. The walling-in was due to the presence of sclerosed scar tissue in the vascular sheath that contains both vein and artery. The authors called this condition *pelvic vessel obstruction*, not just pelvic vein obstruction.

The predominant cause of this pelvic vessel obstruction was past thrombosis, but at times old lymphadenitis, e.g., after osteomyelitis or carcinomatous lymphadenitis, tumors or radiation damage of tissues—in brief, chronic inflammation of all kinds and malignant and benign tumors of varied origin—were responsible.

Pelvic Vein Obstruction Due to Scarring of the Vascular Sheath

Originally, serous inflammation of perivascular sheaths produces sclerosis of the connective tissue of the sheath.

Roentgenologic Findings

The phlebographic picture of this pelvic vein obstruction was described by Gumrich and Kübler (1955). The radiologic aspect is in no way typical. More or less poorly recanalized pelvic veins are found with corresponding collateral circulation. May (1964) described slowly increasing narrowing of the vessel, resembling an elongated paper bag, that was suggestive of marked perivenous thickening. But involvement of the perivascular sheath must be assumed with *any* poorly defined pelvic vein.

Surgical Measures

Wanke (1950, 1956) described the consequences of surgery. He dissected the vein and artery from their common thickened perivascular sheath (Fig. 7.12). The indurated, often whitish, discolored vein does not regain its former circumference but dilates noticeably. Unfortunately, firm ridges can be palpated in its interior that represent old organized thrombi.

Wanke (1956) recommended transperitoneal entry and resection of the external iliac artery in all cases in which it appeared to compress the external iliac vein (Fig. 7.13).

Technique of Venous Exposure of May

We considered this operation soon after Wanke's report and have had many years of experience with it.

The transperitoneal approach is no longer defensible. We make a slightly oblique incision through the skin of the lower abdomen and split the aponeurosis of the external oblique muscle along its fibers in thin patients, or else in the direction of the skin incision. But just lateral to the rectus sheath and parallel with it, we divide the fascias of the internal oblique and, proximally, of the transverse abdominis muscles. There is no bleeding except from two or three vessels. The peritoneum-covered bladder is displaced with a damp swab and protected with wet cloths. Retractors are applied and the psoas is looked for. If it is closely followed upward, the artery is found on its medial side. The artery is freed along its wall, and lifted, with two catheters used as reins. Access to the vein is now easy. It is first exposed above the inguinal ligament, which may occasionally have to be notched. Frequently the walls show slight changes. The vein is dissected from them. It is always surprising how well the freed vein dilates. Shelling out may be difficult and mural injury barely avoidable. Any defects that result are sutured with the finest material.

Occasionally, artery and vein are tightly adherent in a tough ridge at the crossing of internal iliac artery and external iliac vein. As mentioned, Wanke suggested resection of the internal iliac artery. *This is by no means justifiable any longer.* To be sure, unilateral resection produces no immediate aftereffect, but sparing this important vessel can ensure preservation of the limb in later years, should arterial occlusion occur. The internal iliac artery is easily lifted by resection of the superior gluteal artery, as recommended by Niedner.

Results

It is always impressive to see how the vein dilates on operation. Later results are often disappointing. Figure 7.14 illustrates such a case. The

operation appeared to us to be a paradigm of satisfactory shelling out. But radiologic evaluation showed no improvement.
Oddly enough, the patient feels subjectively improved, an observation also made by Kunlin (1950). It is difficult to say whether this is simply a psychologic effect or a result of also freeing the artery. Numerous sympathetic fibers are divided at the same time. In our experience as well, the objective findings were in stark contrast to statements by the patient. Objectively, only modest improvement was registered. The lumen remained practically the same, but the collateral was no longer visualized. It had *not* been ligated during operation. A single x-ray film proves nothing. *In evaluating control films, we always have at our disposal a series of four exposures, of which only one is reproduced here because of space limitations.*
The most favorable cases are those in which local

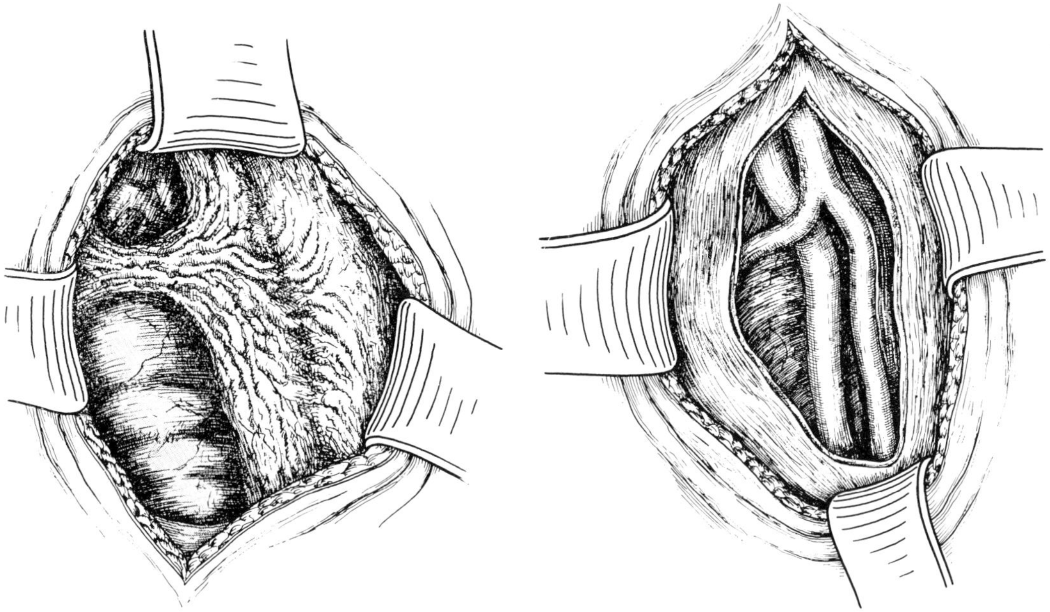

a b

Fig. 7.12. Pelvic vein obstruction due to scarring (*a*). Appearance after dissection by Wanke's method (*b*).

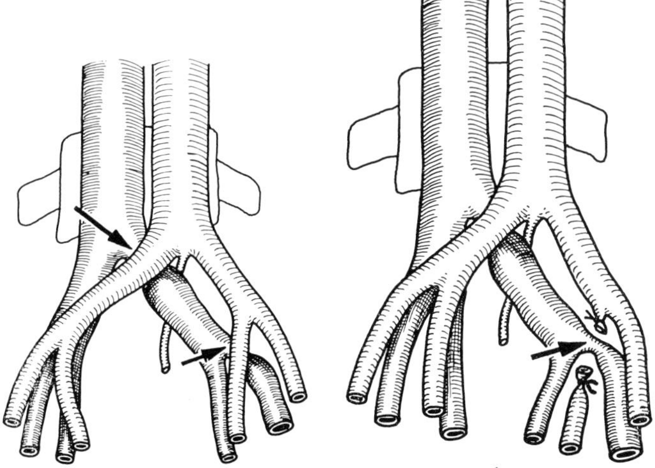

a b

Fig. 7.13. Relief of compressed external iliac vein (*a*) following resection of the internal iliac artery (*b*).

constrictions of the vein are due to scars of other pathogenesis than thrombosis. Bales and DeWeese (1966) reported such a case and reviewed the American literature, which also described best results in cases in which stenosis was due to scars from retroperitoneal abscesses, for example, psoas abscess.

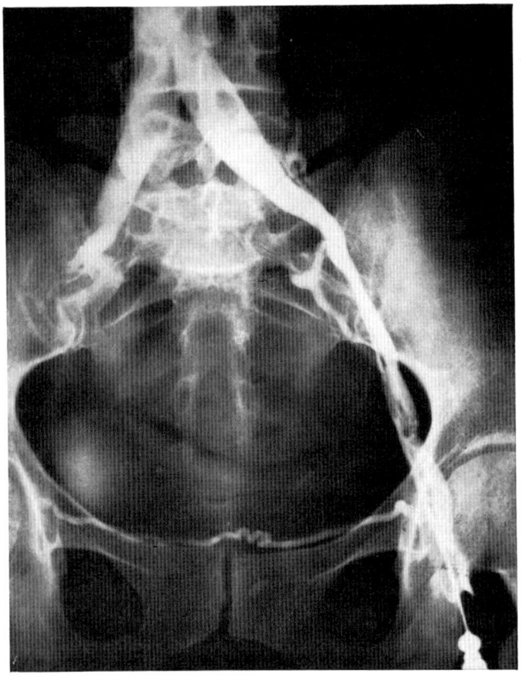

a

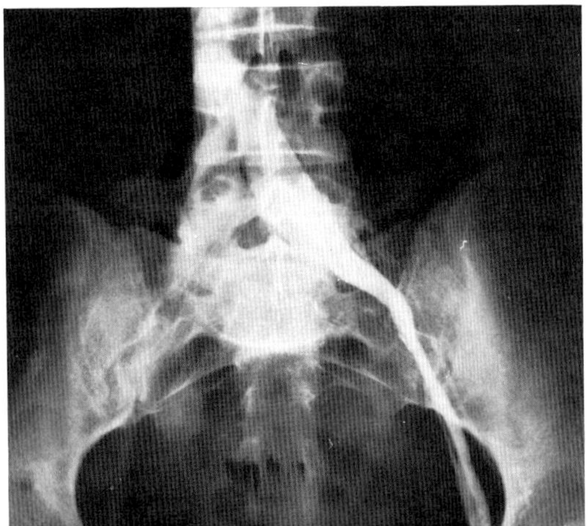

b

Fig. 7.14. Pelvic vein obstruction. Phlebography before (*a*) and after (*b*) dissection.

In the *post-thrombotic syndrome*, we now advise *shelling out* only for very *limited localized constrictions*. Even then, the results are often disappointing, as seen in Figure 7.14. A further reason for these disappointing results may be that we rely too much on x-ray appearances. We see marked constriction of a vein, the shelled out vein dilates satisfactorily at operation, and the postoperative x-ray film confirms it, but the leg remains swollen as before.

Cockett and Thomas (1965) deserve the credit for having demonstrated that lymphatic channels coursing along pelvic veins are easily implicated in pelvic thrombosis, which means that the edema in these cases is predominantly lymphogenic. This would explain the discrepancy between successful shelling out of veins and unchanged, poor clinical findings on the leg.

For *extended obstructions*, the difficult, time-consuming operation, in which the vein is frequently torn, is not justified by the meager results. Cockett and Thomas (1965) have investigated this problem in detail over the last few years. They call chronic pelvic vein obstruction the *iliac compression syndrome*, but include spur formation in it. A visit to his clinic showed that Cockett shares our views of the limited chances and results of surgery by shelling out.

However, it is possible that the operation will regain importance, once it becomes practicable to improve the technique of *removal of old thrombi* (p. 62).

In any case, preoperative and postoperative venous pressure measurements should be made, as described on page 161, because only in this way can objective evaluation of success be expected.

Compression of Veins by Tumors

In each case of venous compression, pressure due to (usually malignant) tumors, conglomerations of lymphatic glands in blood diseases, and so forth, has to be excluded before a diagnosis of thickening or post-thrombotic syndrome can be made. Even if there is no way of treating most of these cases, the patient should be spared a useless intervention, which is what venous shelling out would constitute (Fig. 7.15).

Roentgenologic Findings

For *x-ray diagnosis of compression of the inferior vena cava*, the reader is referred to the basic

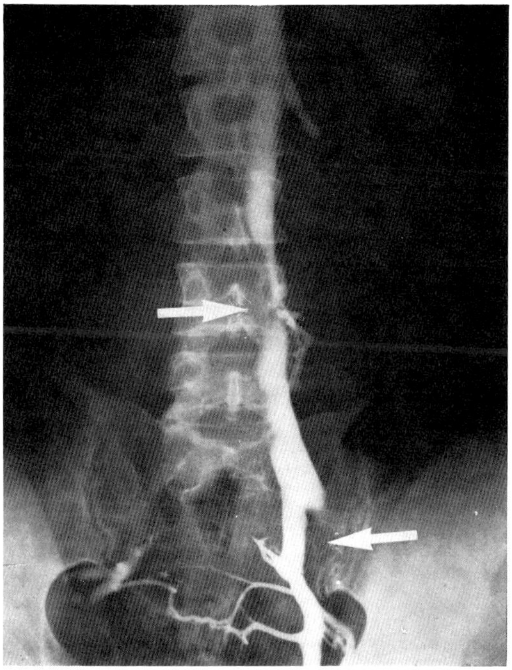

Fig. 7.15. Compression by tumor.

publications of Helander and Lindbom (1956), of Holtz and Powers (1962), and especially of Doppmann (1967), who emphasized presentation in two planes. The diagnosis of caval compression of tumors in children was elaborated by Bennek (1966).

Increasing numbers of cases of *retroperitoneal fibrosis* (*Ormond's disease*) have been reported in Europe in the last few years. Inflammatory retroperitoneal thickening constricts the inferior vena cava and ureters (May, 1968). We attempt at least to free the ureters from the constriction, but there seems little that can be done with the vena cava.

Diagnosis in the region of the *pelvic veins* is particularly difficult but is imperative. Patients with chronically swollen legs are frequently seen, but it must be determined whether the condition is due to post-thrombotic states, in which case it can be alleviated surgically, or to recurrent carcinoma, in which surgery is useless. Gynecologic and laboratory examinations are frequently ambiguous. Several radiologists, particularly Antonopoulos (1955), have dealt with the problem of differential diagnosis. May (1964) described differential diagnostic indicators, as did Kainberger (1967). We were not much impressed by these studies. Diagnosis is easy in clear-cut cases, when there is an abrupt break in the large vessels and corresponding collateral circulation. In difficult cases, requiring decision, these signs are vague. It is misleading to try to construct clear radiologic signs where there are none, and too much is asked of phlebography in these cases. We urge clarification by additional aortography, ureterography and lymphangiography. Even if each of these investigations is of little value on its own, a combination of them usually gives a reliable answer.

Marked constrictions of arteries and ureters make the presence of a malignant process highly probable.

Obstruction of Pelvic Veins by Vascular Prostheses

In the last few years, a peculiar form of pelvic vein barrier, in fact a blockade, has been observed—obstruction of the left external iliac vein by an arterial prosthesis. Jackson reported such a case in 1967.

Reconstructive Surgery of the Pelvic Veins

Chronic post-thrombotic injuries to pelvic veins and their sequelae present a grave problem affecting many thousands of patients all over the world. Unlike those in post-thrombotic venous damage in the lower extremity, symptoms in post-thrombotic damage to the pelvic veins are insufficiently relieved by conservative measures such as compression bandages. Many investigations have detailed the social consequences of early retirement, change of occupation, and so forth.

In severe cases, patients complain of venous claudication, that is, pain on prolonged walking. Surgical intervention directly to damaged veins was, as we have shown, hardly more than tentative, with occasional successes, but could not be established as a routine method.

The idea of applying to veins measures that had been successful in arterial surgery was proposed. However, before operation we demand:

- a chance of success, making surgery worthwhile;
- little surgical risk, since these are relatively harmless complaints which, unlike arterial occlusion, do not threaten survival of the limb; and
- a prospect of lasting success, at least for many years.

Kunlin (1950) established a bypass from the great saphenous to the contralateral external iliac vein

(Fig. 7.16). Thrombotic obstruction followed after 3 weeks of patency.

Today, we should propose addition of a temporary arteriovenous fistula. This would almost certainly ensure patency of the graft.

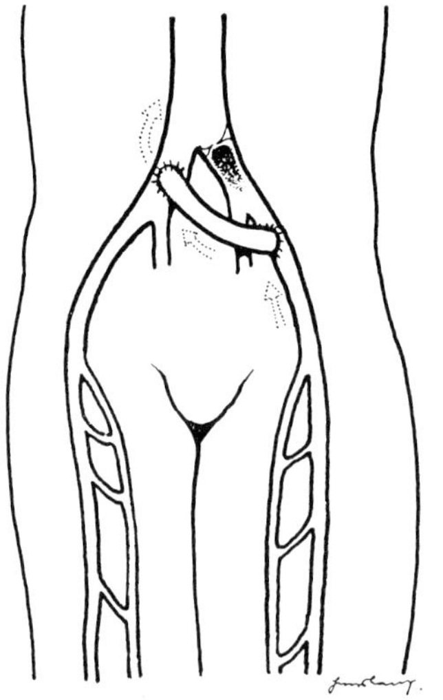

Fig. 7.16. Bypass by the method Kunlin.

Hardin (1962) described five patients in whom obstruction of pelvic veins was bridged by a venous bypass using the ipsilateral great saphenous vein, which had been turned up (Fig. 7.17). He added a venous patch at the lower end. A patent vein was seen on subsequent phlebography. Dale and Scott (1963) and Harris (1965) were similarly successful.

The decisive breakthrough from experimental surgery to a method meeting the demands listed above was made by Palma et al. (1958).

Palma Operation

The principle of the operation is to sever the great saphenous vein on the healthy side at the level of the knee, to free it from all collaterals up to its junction and to transpose it in a subcutaneous tunnel across mons pubis to the diseased side, where it is anastomosed with the femoral vein (Figs. 7.18 and 7.19).

Technique

The operation is carried out after heparinization under general anesthesia. The femoral vein on the diseased side is first exposed, and the most suitable segment for anastomosis is prepared. If the vein is obliterated in the groin, a more distal portion is used. The long saphenous vein on the healthy side is then exposed and all tributaries are carefully ligated. A subcutaneous tunnel is bored through the mons pubis with the finger or with dressing forceps close to the deep abdominal fascia. The saphenous of the healthy side is now separated above the knee and pulled through the tunnel; care is taken to avoid torsion. After clamping of the femoral vein, the saphenous is anastomosed end to side with the femoral vein. The patient soon begins active exercises in bed. Anticoagulant therapy is maintained for 3 weeks.

Our Own Experience

Unlike Palma, we have for some time now exposed the *healthy side* first, not the diseased side. If the vein is found to be too small or to branch immediately, it is useless for anastomosis and the operation must be discontinued. Pre-

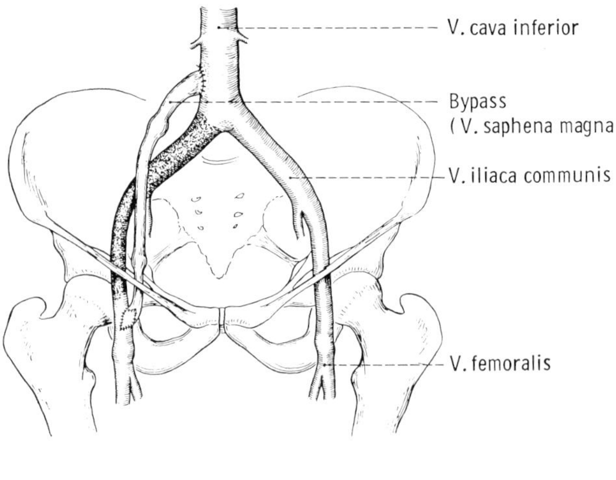

Fig. 7.17. Bypass operation of Hardin.

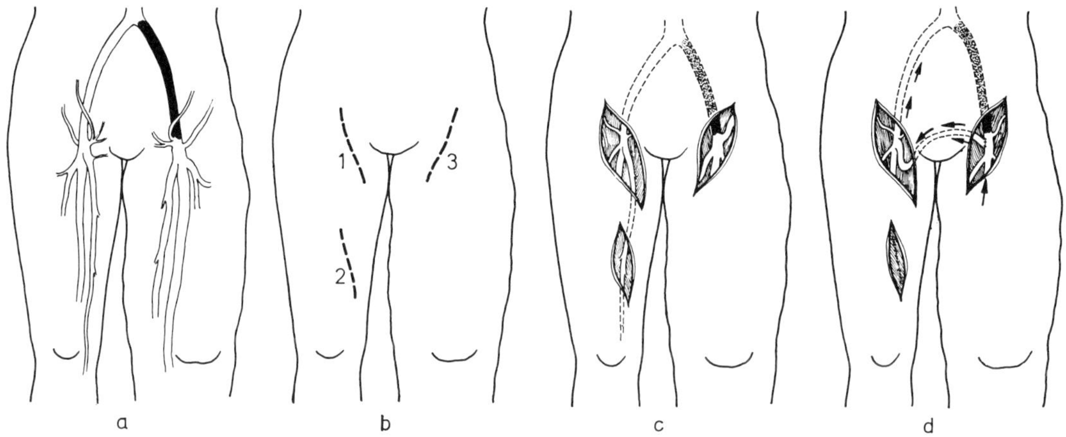

Fig. 7.18. Palma operation. Common and left external iliac veins occluded (*a*); skin incisions for exposure of veins (*b*). Left: common and superficial femoral veins exposed; right: long saphenous exposed (*c*). The distally clamped long saphenous of the right is pulled through a subcutaneous tunnel to the left where it is anastomosed with the common femoral vein (*d*).

operative roentgen demonstration of the long saphenous might easily reveal its size, but it risks thrombosis of the vein. We inject 10,000 IU heparin before separating the vein, so that the blood becomes completely incoagulable. We do not give protamine sulfate postoperatively to neutralize the heparin effect; instead, sufficient heparin is administered in the first 5 days after operation to keep the clotting time prolonged, at approximately 15 minutes. We then employ

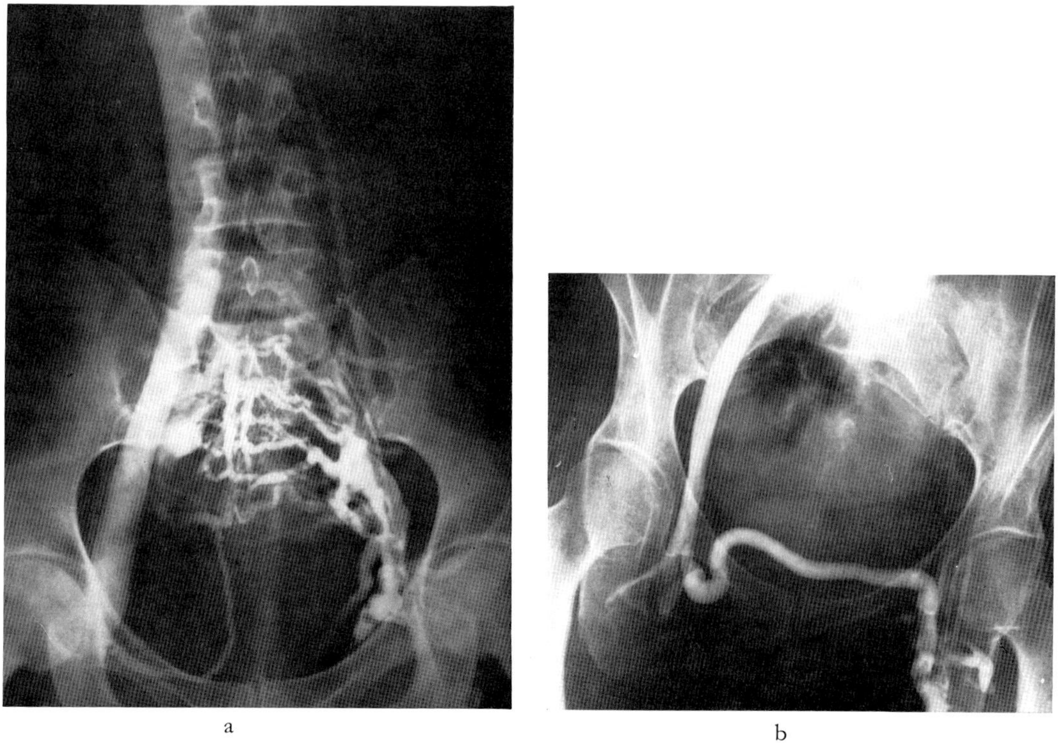

Fig. 7.19. Palma operation. Preoperative (*a*) and postoperative (*b*) films.

nicoumalone, keeping the prothrombin level low for at least 3 months. Healing should be complete by this time.

For cosmetic reasons we expose the long saphenous by short longitudinal incisions and avoid a long incision.

It is very important to expand the long saphenous properly with saline-heparin solution, as Palma et al. (1958) emphasized. It is just as important to see that the long saphenous forms a flexible loop on the healthy side. Compared with an artery, a vein can be expanded but not distended, since there is hardly any muscle in its wall.

Marked tension provokes a fatal kink.

In order to prevent torsion, we first push a rigid plastic tube through the tunnel and pull it through the vein.

We avoid any clamping of the vein. Thin rubber tubes, tightened by assistants, suffice. In suturing the anastomosis, magnifying spectacles are used.

Intermittent suction drainage of both groin wounds is considered necessary. The anastomosis is applied as obliquely as practicable.

Sites of Anastomosis

Basically there are five sites for anastomosis:
—at the common femoral vein,
—at the superficial femoral,
—at the long saphenous,
—at the junction with the long saphenous, and
—end to end with the other long saphenous vein.

Anastomosis to the common femoral would appear to be preferable (Fig. 7.20*a*), since the flow is considerably increased by union with the deep femoral. But this anastomosis should not be forced. The femoral is frequently severely damaged up to four fingerbreadths below the inguinal ligament, even in so-called pure pelvic vein thrombosis. It is senseless to construct an anastomosis in a poorly recanalized region. The incision should be elongated distally, where mural conditions are usually quite satisfactory. Palma et al. extend this to the distal portion of the thigh, a practice we would not advise.

However, if the femoral does not appear to become normal up to two fingerbreadths below the groin, we prefer to apply the anastomosis with the long saphenous as obliquely as practical (Fig. 7.20*b*). In these cases, the anastomosis is particularly strong as compensation for the obliterated deep vein. In a few cases, we have separated the long saphenous at its junction and anastomosed it there, expecting that the ring at the junction, as a natural opening, would produce less scarring. This may be correct; but we are awaiting late results before repeating this procedure. From the point of view of primum non nocere, it has to be considered that an important drain has been injured if the anastomosis closes.

Indications

The pelvic veins must be greatly obstructed.

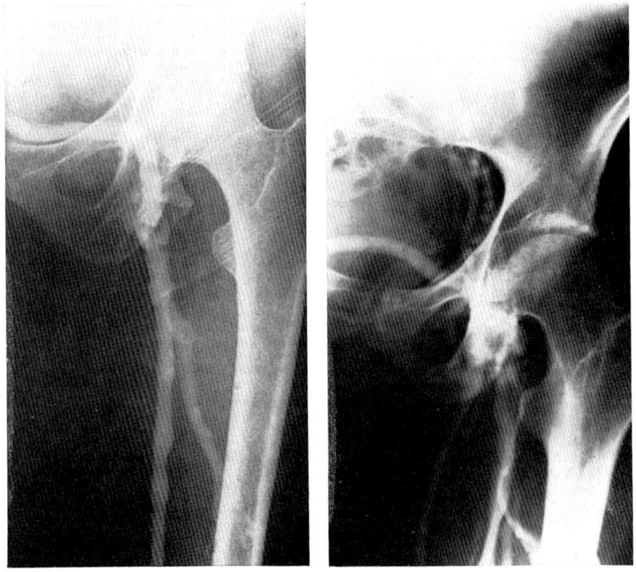

a b

Fig. 7.20. Sites of anastomosis in Palma's operation. The long saphenous is connected with the femoral vein (*a*); the long saphenous is connected with the saphenous vein (*b*).

Venous pressure measurements will yield this information (p. 161). The condition of the leg veins is also important, however.

If the thrombosis is mainly limited to the pelvic veins, and the leg veins are tolerably well preserved, much better results may be expected than when there are additional injuries to the leg veins. In these cases, we hesitate to perform this procedure and question whether the Palma operation should be performed at all. Additional peripheral stasis and failure of the calf muscle pump are a considerable burden.

Further Problems

There are decisive differences between arterial and venous anastomoses. When the clamps are removed, an arterial anastomosis remains open on its own, as soon as the flow is released, because the blood pressure ensures it. However, if there is a sudden drop in pressure during or after arterioplasty, the risk of thrombotic obstruction is real.

On the other hand, pressure in the vein is too low to ensure a patent anastomosis.

In addition, anyone who has dissected a subcutaneous vein knows that the vein is suspended in the surrounding tissues by fibrous strands. These stays must unfortunately be destroyed during operation.

The Palma operation, carried out on a healthy person, would probably cause thrombosis of the anastomosis, since there is no functional necessity for it. Also, the thrombotic process must have fully "burnt out." This obvious requirement is not always observed. Reconstructive interventions during florid or incompletely subsided thrombosis have been attempted in some cases. Thrombosis occurred in every one unless a temporary arteriovenous fistula was applied as well.

In most cases, occlusion of pelvic veins is due to thrombosis. Occasionally, old trauma or inflammation may be the cause. Dale (1966) showed that the Palma operation is indicated in these cases also.

We have not so far operated on pelvic veins occluded as a result of malignant processes. They are almost without exception inoperable and frequently are irradiated recurrences of gynecologic conditions. This type of obstruction is rather common, and patients are much distressed by the tensely swollen leg. Dale (1966) operated on some of these cases. He reported that the legs of patients were relieved and thus improved. This indication needs serious investigation, for even if the suffering of these patients could be alleviated for only a few months, much would have been achieved from a psychologic viewpoint. The patients were under the impression that their disease had improved. On review we were not convinced. Unfortunately, stagnation is only partly venous; it is chiefly caused by impaired lymph drainage. Pain in the leg is also due to growth of the tumor into nervous tissue. The decision whether to operate must be based on both phlebography *and* lymphography.

Bilateral occlusion remains a *contraindication*. We are still unable to provide relief in these cases. Bilateral bridging to the vena cava has not been attempted so far. Certainly, the worse side could be bridged with the vena cava, but our studies have not convinced us that this major intraperitoneal operation is justified.

It is especially important that the *patient be mobile* and be able to walk well. The leg also must be freely movable. Vigorous exercises in bed and early mobilization are essential for successful outcome.

If the *great saphenous* that is to be pulled through is *varicosed*, this operation should not be used since the risk of thrombosis is too great.

The primary requirement for success of the Palma operation is a notable drop in the pressure gradient.

For this reason, preoperative *venous pressure measurements* in the common femoral vein in the groin should be obtained, as described on page 161.

Venous pressure measurements are required for another reason. *We should be able to check our success objectively by a functional method of measurement* (Fig. 7.21). We require this for any operation on chronically changed deep veins, including leg veins, because only in this way can the inaccurate phrase "impression of clinical improvement" be eliminated. Disregard of this requirement leads to discussion of doubtful surgical methods for 10 years and longer. With arterial grafts, success and failure are immediately evident. With surgery on deep veins, patients are seen time and again to leave the hospital happy despite clear failure. Bed rest and the magic of surgical intervention have deceived them.

We should clarify what can be achieved in the most favorable case. Venous hypertension is eliminated. This is what causes the sensation of heaviness and, even more, the peculiar venous claudication typical of pelvic vein occlusion, pain on rapid walking. These complaints are easily influenced by subjective considerations. The swelling is only partly venous. Deep thrombosis of the leg veins does not cause obliteration of lymphatic vessels primarily, as was formerly believed. Lymphatic vessels are affected only when extensive secondary skin changes or leg ulcers are present. This is obvious since the

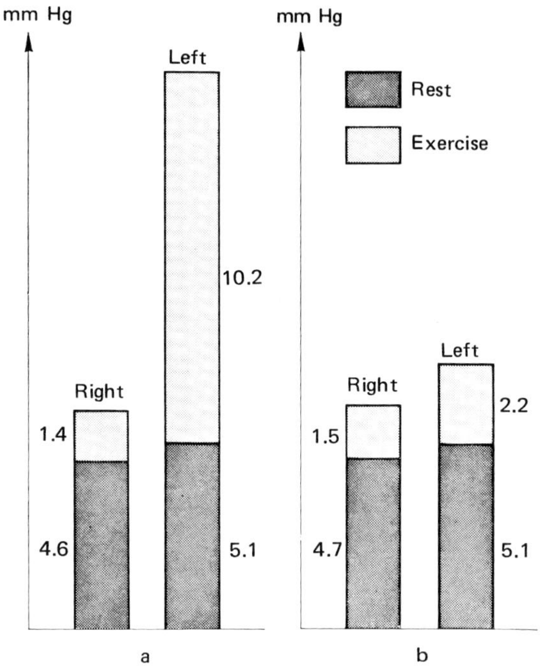

Fig. 7.21. Venous pressure measurements before (*a*) and after (*b*) the Palma operation on the left side.

lymphatics run along the long saphenous subcutaneously. There are no deep lymphatics connected with the femoral. The situation is different with the pelvic veins. The lymphatics course close to the large veins and may easily be affected by periphlebitis. Hence we stress again that isolated pelvic thrombosis is not accompanied by edema. If edema is present, it is lymphogenic, and even successful pelvic venoplasty will not relieve it. Or the edema may be due to concomitant injuries to the deep leg veins, and these are not at all affected by pelvic venoplasty.

We record the values obtained in venous pressure measurements in the form of columns in the patients' case sheets, since visual evidence is more striking than figures (Fig. 7.21).

Absolute values are of secondary importance in the examination of *post-thrombotic conditions*. We largely ignore them.

What *is* significant is

— the *difference in pressure values between the two sides at rest*, and
— the *degree of elevation of the values* on stress; the more marked the elevation following exercise, the greater the drainage block.

We should like to emphasize again that roentgen examination of the pelvic veins, especially when surgery is being considered, should always parallel venous pressure measurements during rest and exercise. Both investigations can be carried out in one session. The needle used for injection of the contrast medium into the femoral vein in the groin can be connected with the manometer. The values obtained complement the x-ray picture, which yields only a very limited indication of disturbed function. In addition, the values are an infallible indicator of the success of the operation from the point of view of function.

Results and Complications

We divided our results into two groups. In one group (14 cases) assessed three years ago, the *operation was successful in seven cases.*

This is a very poor result. It made us doubt whether the operation could be justified in the future. The fact that the results of other vascular surgeons were just as bad was small comfort.

The cause of failure is the *progressive stenosis of Kunlin*, which makes any venoplasty problematic. Unlike that in arteries, the flow velocity in veins is poor, too slow for successful vein-to-vein anastomosis. Hence, scarring occurs near the anastomosis which narrows the lumen progressively and finally closes it (p. 54). Every vein-to-vein anastomosis depends on the prevention of progressive stenosis.

There are several possible ways of avoiding *progressive stenosis.*

— *Suspended suture or mechanical suture.* Animal experiments indicate that use of Kunlin's ring suture improves results decisively. We have not yet decided to use it because of the risk, in the groin, of tilting of the rings and because of the likelihood, if a stabilizing rod is affixed to the ring to prevent tilting, of trauma to the vein on movement. Extreme bending occurs just at the site of anastomosis in the groin. Our fears may be unjustified. Other mechanical sutures with clips are unsuitable for end-to-side anastomosis, as are Nakayama's rings. Mechanical suture can be used only for anastomosis of the two long saphenous veins.

Since Nakayama rings proved useful in our hands for anastomosis of small arteries, we were particularly interested in his experiments (1962) to construct rings for veins. Unfortunately, technical difficulties of production have not yet been overcome (personal communication). Among the possibilities of mechanical anastomosis, the idea of Gottlob and Blümel (see p. 66) appears to us the best at the moment. After animal experiments yielded favorable results, first trials on patients are under way. We selected patients in whom the poor state of the deep veins did not permit anastomosis, so that anastomosis of the two great saphenous veins was the only practical possibility anyway. Unfortunately, this technique, too, requires implantation of a foreign body, but its shape and position exclude the risk of kinking or arrosion bleeding.

— *Extremely careful technique*. Jakobson and Katsumara (1965) showed in experiments that excellent results were obtained when the finest suture material and magnifying spectacles were used and delicate handling was observed. In a second series of studies in the last three years, we paid careful attention to these operative details: finest suture material, magnifying spectacles, avoidance of clamps, compression only with rubber catheters, elongated and oblique anastomosis, cautious handling of venous margins, strict avoidance of restitching the suture line, total heparinization and automatic intermittent suction drainage. In this series, the anastomosis remained patent in 16 of 22 cases. The future will show whether these results last or whether they need improving. Generally, we are under the impression that if a vessel is patent after one year, it will remain patent. We watch with greatest interest patients who have become pregnant.

Studies in three cases showed—fortunately—widening of the graft, *not* varicose change.

Otherwise there is only one other way to avoid progressive stenosis. Success is almost certain, but a double, much more difficult operation is required.

— *Temporary arteriovenous fistula*. Kunlin (1950) was the first to show by experiments (p. 48) that a temporary arteriovenous fistula will keep the anastomosis patent forever. Other authors confirmed this in numerous animal experiments. The protective hemodynamic action of the arteriovenous fistula was elucidated by Dost (1968) with careful measurements. It is not due to *augmentation of pressure*, as frequently supposed. The effective component is exclusively *elevation of blood flow velocity*. Obviously, the fistula must be distal to the venous anastomosis. Dost also determined how long an arteriovenous fistula must be maintained in order to guarantee success. For vascular prostheses, with their unfavorable prognosis, 4 to 6 weeks suffice. This is especially important, since in this length of time a serious retrograde effect on the heart is not anticipated. In fact, Dumanian (1968) reported excellent results with a Palma operation using this procedure. The method was systematically completed by Vollmar (1970), who, rather than anastomosing the femoral artery and vein, separated the long saphenous, inserting the proximal stump into the femoral artery like a bucket handle (Fig. 7.22). True, the method requires sacrifice of the long saphenous, a vessel important for collateral circulation. Recently, following a suggestion of Senn (1968), Vollmar has modified the procedure to spare the long saphenous and uses any suitable tributary. Elimination of the fistula, about 4 months later, is considerably easier if a black silk suture is loosely applied around it. On reoperation the suture is easily identified and the loosely applied loop needs only to be tightened. These apparently minor technical improvements are extraordinarily important, since formerly reoperation to close an arteriovenous fistula proved very difficult at times, and stenosis of the femoral artery

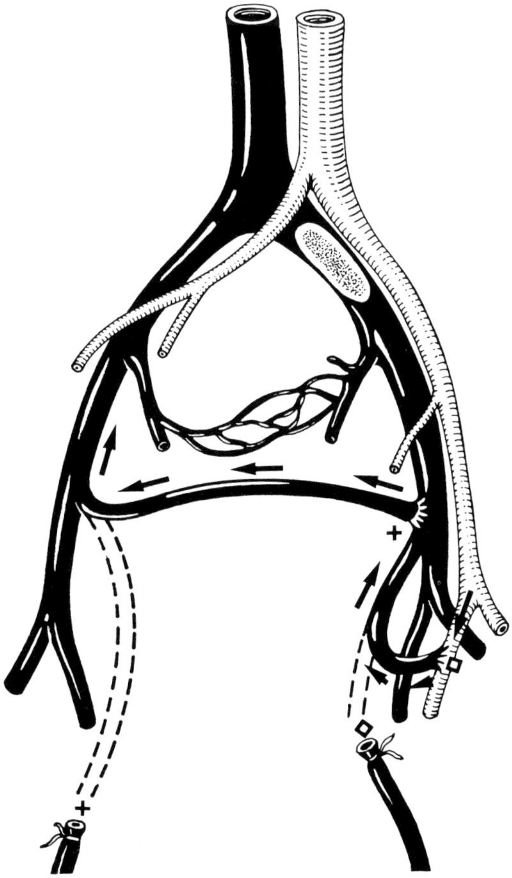

Fig. 7.22. Temporary arteriovenous fistula of Vollmar distal to the bypass of Palma. (From Vollmar, J.: Act. Chir. 5 (1970) 79.)

always was a possibility. It will be seen in the next few years whether improved technique alone suffices in order to achieve good results or whether a temporary arteriovenous fistula should be applied in all cases.

We noticed that the scars after the Palma operation were particularly ugly and bulging. The cause is unquestionably disordered scar formation owing to heparinization. We are designing an applicator for placement of thrombin into the wound. In the past, we have excised the scars after one year in cosmetically unacceptable cases and glued the wounds.

Temporary arteriovenous fistula is increasingly being used for all operations on deep veins in centers of any magnitude. It is applied not only to safeguard the Palma operation but also following removal of thrombi from pelvic veins. It has made possible intercalation of prostheses in caval defects, which before had almost always thrombosed.

The fistula is usually applied a handbreadth below the groin. The medial branch of the long saphenous, which is usually a few centimeters distal to its junction, is anastomosed with the femoral artery, and the anastomosis is marked by a loosely applied loop of black silk. Constructing the fistula at the ankle is also being discussed. For some indications, especially when using plastic prostheses, it will not be possible to dispense with the temporary arteriovenous fistula in the future. Experience in the next few years will show whether it is necessary after thrombectomy.

Temporary arteriovenous fistula during the Palma operation is at present the only method that guarantees a patent anastomosis in more than 90 per cent of cases. Nevertheless, we would like to be able to do without this aid. We hope to achieve patency of the anastomosis without arteriovenous fistula by careful selection of patients (venous pressure measurements), improved suturing techniques and suspension of the anastomosis (similar to Kunlin's ring procedure). This is of practical importance. Bridging venous defects with a graft or another vein would always remain rare, but considering the frequency of post-thrombotic states, the Palma operation, possibly improved, will become a routine procedure of the vascular surgeon. Apart from the fact that elimination of the fistula requires a second operation, it can be expected to increase complications that might present serious consequences for the artery under certain conditions.

Temporary Arteriovenous Fistula

Since this volume went to press, experience has yielded the following results:

Application of a temporary arteriovenous fistula during the Palma operation is currently the most suitable method of guaranteeing a patent graft. It should be also employed for thrombectomy of pelvic veins in all cases in which thrombosis is not very recent. Furthermore, Vollmar established the surprising findings that with an arteriovenous fistula even older venous thrombi (iliofemoral, axillary, that are about to become organized usually recanalize more rapidly—at a time when treatment with streptokinase is no longer effective. In other words, the spontaneous course of phlebothrombosis can be considerably influenced by a change in hemodynamics—increased flow velocity and flow minute volume. With venous thrombectomy, which is frequently incomplete, the temporary arteriovenous fistula produces a rapid "clearing effect"; that is, the lumen is fully restored, and persisting blockades of the central drainage can be corrected by a bypass operation (autologous vein graft) in a second session, with remarkable chance of success. Patency of the disobliterated segment should be tested and ascertained angiographically before the fistula is closed.

An arteriovenous fistula is probably not needed when the *femoral bypass of May* is used. However, if the femoral bypass is combined with the Palma operation, this protective measure should be employed, and it is best applied in the region of the medial malleolus between the posterior tibial artery and vein.

The temporary arteriovenous fistula represents a decisive tactical advance in reconstructive surgery of pelvic and caval veins (after trauma and resection of tumors). This procedure also secures a place again for caval prostheses. Alloplastic veins had a thrombosis rate of 50 to 60 per cent.

Site of fistula. For the Palma operation and after thrombectomy of pelvic veins, the fistula is applied about four fingerbreadths below the inguinal ligament. This site at the level of the adductor canal proved satisfactory in only a few cases and cannot be recommended as routine procedure.

Kunlin showed in Chapter 2, Experimental Venous Surgery, that an arteriovenous fistula is a reliable aid for keeping venous anastomoses open. But there was concern for routine application in man because of the reoperation, which is risky and by no means simple.

These drawbacks are avoided by the *technique of Ellis and Vollmar*, using a *bucket handle shunt*.

After the venous anastomosis is completed, the skin incision is extended by about 1 cm distally. The superficial femoral artery is dissected for

5 cm and loops are placed around it. The great saphenous is then exposed. A strong branch, if one is present, or even better, the end of the Palma graft should be used. We use magnifying spectacles and employ 6–0 sutures. The vein should form a loose sling, the anastomosis not exceeding a width of 4 to 5 mm. The anastomosis can be marked with a strong black metal suture, which is loosely tied. The suture should be long enough to lie subcutaneously at the lower angle of the wound but ought to be palpable through the skin. The length of the suture is measured and recorded. The wound is closed in layers. The patency of the fistula can be verified by stethoscope. Routine arteriographic evaluation is unnecessary. The fistula is left no longer than three months. A longer period is not required, and the leg would swell unnecessarily and reoperation would be more difficult.

Closure of the fistula. The skin scar is excised. The black suture is found and used as guideline to the fistula. Recently it has proved more efficient to look for the artery in the distal angle of the wound where it is not yet adherent. Dissection follows proximally along the artery and not along the vein.
The fistula is then closed. With a sterile stethoscope the surgeon checks to be sure the hum at the anastomosis has disappeared. Not until this is done is the operation completed.

Varicocele of the Female Pelvis

Varicosities of the uterovaginal plexus and in the broad ligament are fairly common. They are the basis for a series of vague complaints, including a sensation of heaviness in the true pelvis and dysmenorrhea. But just as often they are symptomless, and the patient is unaware of them. They often are a fortuitous finding on pelvic radiology following pelvic vein thrombosis. They are said to occur frequently in the absence of thrombosis, after inflammation in the small pelvis, salpingitis, and other infections, and to prevail in multiparas.

Follow-up study of the results of the Palma operation to the present time (1977).
1. The ideal indication for the operation obtains when the pressure in the femoral vein on the side of the occluded pelvic vein yields a pressure difference during exercise that is three times as great as that of the opposite side. The pressure difference at rest is of slight significance only (May, 1976).
2. The slow venous flow is only a secondary cause of early closure of the anastomosis following a Palma operation. According to the studies of Gottlob, the essential cause is endothelial damage of the vein during the operation. This can be demonstrated in animals and in man. The edges of the endothelial cells are stained with silver, and the degree of endothelial damage can thus be assessed. If the vein is carefully handled so that only those parts of the vein are touched with instruments that can be excised after establishing the anastomosis, and the suture applied is completely atraumatic, the endothelium will be preserved, and the anastomosis remains patent. This technique is now called by us "*atraumatic technique of Gottlob and May.*"
The endothelium regenerates within three weeks. If the anastomosis remains patent during the first three weeks, it remains open permanently. Later closure has not been observed by us.
With careful atraumatic technique and correct indication, i.e. considerable difference in venous pressure on movement, additional measures, e.g. temporary arteriovenous fistula, are not necessary. If the diameter of the long saphenous vein used for the anastomosis is less than 4 mm, we do not succeed in preserving the endothelium with absolute certainty at present.
In these cases, we advise either establishment of a temporary arteriovenous fistula or spreading the suture with a ring according to Kunlin—see p. 43 in Chapter 2, Experimental Surgery. Lately, oval, and not circular, rings have been used by us.
3. Checkups ten years later showed that varicose degeneration of the grafted long saphenous vein is minimal also following pregnancy.

Roentgenologic Findings

The method of roentgen demonstration was elaborated by Helander and Lindbom (1960). The contrast medium is injected into Seldinger catheters after bilateral percutaneous introduction into the femoral veins and pushed proximally up to the union of external and internal iliac veins. Simultaneous compression of the vena cava is recommended. The catheter may also be pushed further upward and the contrast medium injected into the left renal vein. The ovarian vein and the varicose plexus in the parametrium are thus filled retrogradely.
Detailed studies including a survey of the literature were published by Chidekel and Edlundh (1968) and by Helander and Lindbom (1960). Chidekel and Edlundh also reported an important comparative study, showing that injection of the contrast medium into the renal vein was markedly superior to transuterine phlebography.

Surgical Procedure

At present, the most successful operation is considered to be ligation of the left ovarian vein 10 to 15 cm distal to its union. It is stripped. Local coils are resected. Unfortunately, there is no means of postoperative x-ray evaluation. The symptoms are so vague that their disappearance presents only an uncertain measure of possible success.

The *varicose ovarian vein* merits special mention. It may assume the thickness of a lead pencil or even greater size. Recently thrombosis of the ovarian vein causing fatal pulmonary embolism has been observed. It may also enlarge greatly after interruption of the inferior vena cava and cause thrombosis or embolism, thus jeopardizing caval interruption. It should therefore be ligated prophylactically in these cases.

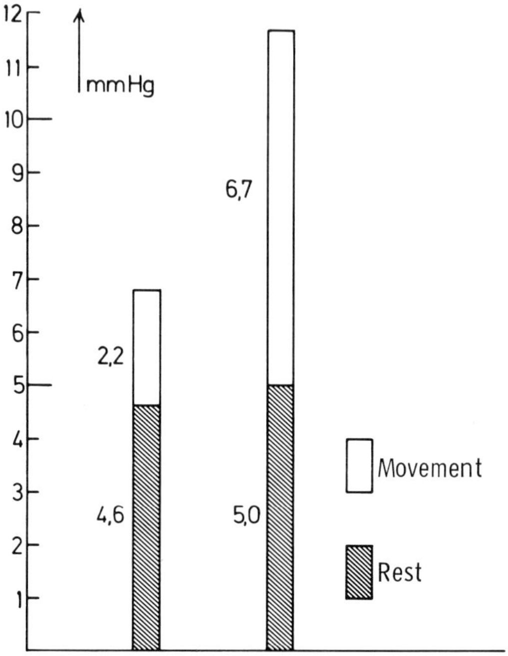

Fig. 7.23. Ideal indication for Palma operation. The pressure on movement, measured in the femoral vein on the side of the occluded pelvic vein, is three times that of the opposite side.

Interruption of the Inferior Vena Cava for Pulmonary Embolism

J. A. DeWeese

Historical Aspects

The first known ligations of the inferior vena cava below the renal veins were performed in the late 1800s. The ligations were performed accidentally or to control hemorrhage following injury, and they demonstrated that a patient could survive such a procedure. In 1906, Trendelenburg reported ligation of the inferior vena cava to prevent progression and pulmonary embolism of infected thrombi occurring in puerperal pyemia. In the early 1900s, there was increasing awareness of pulmonary embolism as a cause of death or morbidity following prolonged periods of bed rest or operations, as well as infection in the pelvic organs. Several studies based on autopsy findings demonstrated that thrombi in the veins of the lower extremities or pelvis were almost always the source of these pulmonary emboli (Rössle, 1973; Hunter et al., 1941; Ravdin and Kirby, 1951; Byrne and O'Neil, 1952; Short, 1952). On the basis of these observations, Homans and others advocated ligation of the femoral or common iliac veins, or in some instances the inferior vena cava, to prevent pulmonary embolism when deep venous thrombosis existed (Homans, 1941, 1947). During the same period, anticoagulants such as heparin or coumarin derivatives were used with increasing frequency to prevent the formation or propagation of venous thrombi. It became accepted practice to administer anticoagulants when the diagnosis of venous thrombosis or pulmonary embolism was made. If pulmonary embolism occurred despite adequate anticoagulation, it was felt that propagation of thrombi was not being prevented. Ligation of the inferior vena cava was then advised. It became a popular operation and several large series of cases were reported. It was noted, however, that ligation of the inferior vena cava occasionally resulted in catastrophe. Some patients went into shock and died at the time of ligation, presumably as a result of the sudden decrease in venous return from the lower extremity (Wheeler et al., 1966; Gazzaniga et al., 1967; Maraan and Taber, 1968). Other patients experienced distal progression of the venous thrombosis and developed the painful, blue, massively swollen extremities characteristic of phlegmasia cerulea dolens (Nabseth and Moran, 1965; Mozes et al., 1966). Most authors also noted a high incidence in these patients of edema, pain, recurrent phlebitis, dermatitis or ulceration. These postphlebitic or post-thrombotic changes were observed in up to 75 per cent of patients (Donaldson et al., 1961,

Mozes et al., 1966; Agrifoglio and Edwards, 1961; Bowers and Leb, 1955; Dale, 1962; Shea and Robertson, 1951).

In hopes of avoiding the adverse effects of ligation of the inferior vena cava and still preventing pulmonary embolism, several methods of partial interruption were advocated. M. S. DeWeese (DeWeese and Hunter, 1963) constructed a harp-grid filter across the inferior vena cava by placing mattress sutures through the occluded vein walls 3 to 4 mm apart and then tied the sutures when the vein was distended (Fig. 7.24*a*). Spencer et al. (1965) compartmentalized the vein by placing mattress sutures through the occluded vein a few millimeters apart and then tied the sutures snugly (Fig. 7.24*b*). Moretz (1965) applied a Teflon clip with two smooth edges (Fig. 7.24*c*). Miles used a clip with two serrated edges which was modified by Adams and DeWeese so that only one edge was serrated (Fig. 7.24*d*) (Miles, 1966; Adams and DeWeese, 1966). Experimentally, all these techniques were shown to prevent passage of significant emboli without obstructing blood flow (Adams and DeWeese, 1965). On the basis of these theoretical advantages and subsequent clinical experience, partial interruption of the vena cava as contrasted to ligation has become the procedure of choice of increasing numbers of surgeons.

Indications

Although nonoperative management is the treatment of choice, approximately 5 per cent of patients have occurrence or recurrence of pulmonary embolism during such treatment. In addition, anticoagulant therapy may be contraindicated in patients with active or potential bleeding problems in the gastrointestinal, genitourinary, or neurologic systems, or immediately following major injuries or operations.

Vena caval interruption is indicated in the following situations:

— second pulmonary embolism in a patient receiving adequate anticoagulant therapy for his previous pulmonary embolism;
— first pulmonary embolism in a patient being treated adequately with anticoagulants for deep venous thrombosis; and
— first pulmonary embolism in any patient who cannot receive anticoagulants.

Operation

Preparation

Patients receiving heparin are given protamine sulfate to return the clotting time to normal, and those receiving coumarin derivatives are given a vitamin K preparation to return the prothrombin time to normal.

Exposure of the Vena Cava

The vena cava can be approached retroperitoneally or transperitoneally. The main advantages of the retroperitoneal route are that it is associated

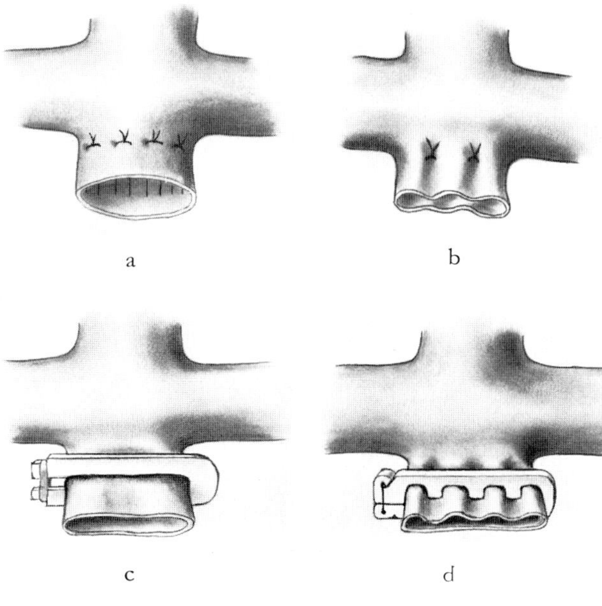

Fig. 7.24. Various methods of partial interruption of the vena cava. Filter method of DeWeese (*a*); compartmentalization technique of Spencer (*b*); Moretz clip (*c*); and Adams-DeWeese serrated clip (*d*).

with less mortality and it can be used on some very ill patients who would not survive the transperitoneal operation. The main disadvantage is that it is very difficult to expose the vena cava just distal to the renal veins retroperitoneally. *It is important that, whenever possible, interruptions be performed just distal to the renal vein*, since fatal emboli have been reported from thrombi forming in the cul-de-sac left distal

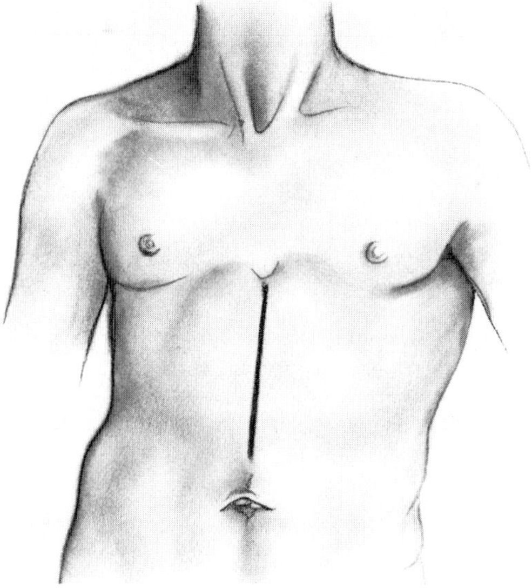

a

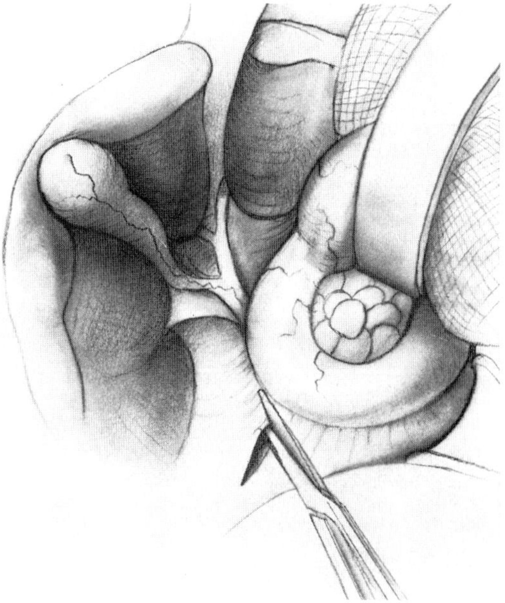

b

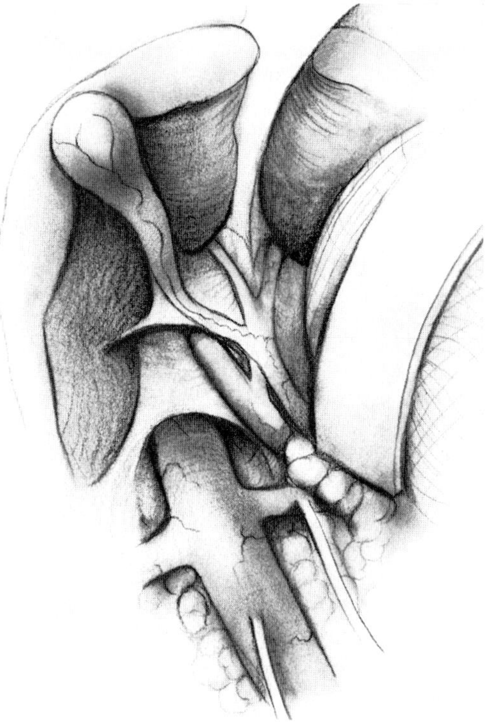

c

Fig. 7.25. Transperitoneal approach to the inferior vena cava. Midline incision (*a*); Kocher maneuver (*b*) and exposure of vena cava and spermatic or ovarian veins (*c*).

to the renal veins when interruption was too low (Crane, 1964; Nabseth and Moran, 1965). In addition, the left ovarian vein is difficult to expose retroperitoneally.

Transperitoneal Approach

This is the preferred method (Fig. 7.25). A midline incision is made from xiphoid to umbilicus. A Kocher maneuver is performed by dividing the right lateral duodenal attachments to reflect the duodenum medially. The renal veins and inferior vena cava are thus exposed. In addition, the right spermatic or ovarian vein, which usually enters the vena cava slightly below the right renal vein, can be seen. The left spermatic or ovarian vein, which usually enters the left renal vein, is also exposed and ligated.

Retroperitoneal Approach

This is used for very ill patients without pelvic vein thrombosis (Fig. 7.26). A transverse incision

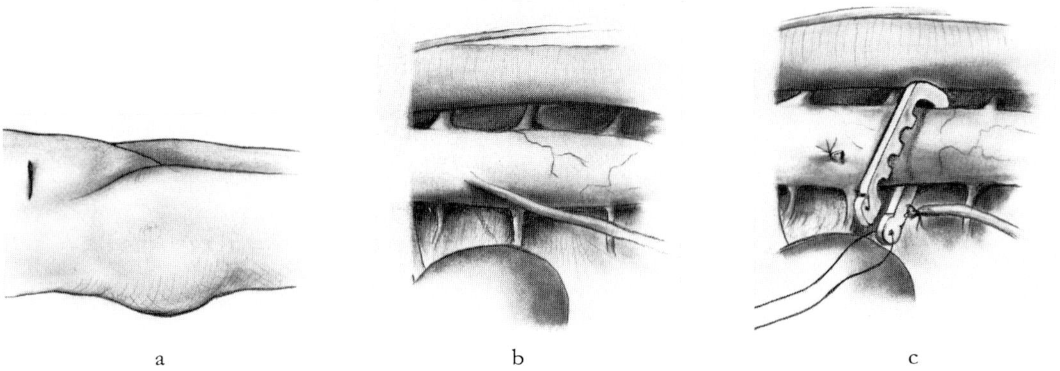

Fig. 7.26. Retroperitoneal approach to the inferior vena cava. Transverse incision to the right of the umbilicus (*a*); exposure of the vena cava (*b*); and application of the Adams-DeWeese clip just inferior to the major lumbar vein (*c*).

is made to the right of the umbilicus. The rectus muscle is divided and the external oblique, internal oblique and transversus abdominis muscles are split in the direction of their fibers. The peritoneum and underlying structures are retracted medially to expose the vena cava. The right spermatic or ovarian vein is ligated and divided.

Interruption of the Vena Cava

Ligation

Ligation is not desirable. If it is performed, the vena cava should be ligated just distal to the renal veins or to a large lumbar vein. One or two heavy silk ties are passed around the vena cava and tied to completely occlude it. Division is not necessary.

Partial Interruption

Although any of the techniques shown in Figure 7.24 is satisfactory for partially interrupting the vena cava, we prefer either the serrated clip or the production of a filter.

Application of an Adams-DeWeese clip (Figs. 7.24*d* and 7.26*c*). A suture is passed through the hole of the flat limb of the clip. A large right-angled clamp is passed around the vena cava just distal to the renal veins or large lumbar vein. The suture on the clip is grasped, the limbs are spread and the suture is used to pull the clip around the cava. The flat limb and serrated limb are then approximated and held in place with a heavy suture.

Creation of a filter. The cava is occluded with two vascular clamps about 1 cm apart. With atraumatic needles several sutures are passed through the occluded vessel as a mattress stitch with sutures separated 2 to 3 mm. The vascular clamps are removed and the cava is allowed to distend. The sutures are then tied so that all sutures are taut within the lumen and yet do not decrease the size of the lumen.

It is important that either filter or clip be placed just distal to the renal vein or a major lumbar vein to avoid leaving a cul-de-sac in which thrombi can form (Crane, 1964; Nabseth and Moran, 1965).

Early Postoperative Management

It is important to remember that vena caval interruption is performed only to prevent pulmonary embolism and does not treat the venous thrombosis from which the emboli arise. Therefore, bed rest and elevation of the legs are resumed for 7 to 10 days. In addition, anticoagulation is resumed 2 days following the operation if there is no evidence of bleeding. Heparin is administered for 7 days and coumarin derivatives for an additional 1 to 6 months.

Late Postoperative Management

Later management is directed toward preventing or minimizing a postphlebitic syndrome. The primary aim is prevention of edema, which can be accomplished in two ways:

Elevation of the legs. Elevation of the legs above the level of the heart is necessary for varying lengths of time during both day and night, depending on the severity of the venous thrombosis. Following femoral or iliofemoral venous thrombosis, it may require 3 to 6 months before sufficient collaterals form or recanalization reduces venous hypertension. During this time, the patient may have to spend several hours each day with the legs elevated. Eventually, most patients are able to lead normal lives. They are all advised, however, to lie down with their legs elevated, rather than sitting for prolonged periods.

Elastic stockings. Most patients require elastic support to prevent edema. Initially this means the use of heavy stockings. In time, lighter stockings may suffice. It should be reemphasized that the primary aim of therapy is to prevent edema. The amount of elevation and the strength of elastic support prescribed should be whatever is needed to prevent any swelling. If the edema can be prevented, then more disabling sequels, such as venous ulcers, can also be prevented.

Results

In order to give a better idea of the results of interruption of the vena cava and also to compare the results of ligation with partial interruption, the results of several large series are combined and summarized in Table 7.2.

Table 7.2 Comparative results of Ligation and Partial Interruption of the Vena Cava

	Ligation	*Partial Interruption*
Operations	600	309
Nonfatal emboli	3.2%	5.6%
Fatal emboli	1.0%	1.0%
Fatal shock	1.0%	—
Patent vena cava	—	71.0%

Six hundred ligations were reported by 13 different groups (Agrifoglio and Edwards, 1961; Bergan et al., 1965; Crane, 1964; Dale, 1962; Donaldson et al., 1961; Ferris et al., 1967; Gurewich et al., 1966; Krause et al., 1963; Mozes et al., 1966; Babseth and Moran, 1965; Schauble et al., 1962; Stevens et al., 1965; Wheeler et al., 1966).

Twelve different groups reported 309 partial interruptions (Bergan et al., 1964, 1965; Burget et al., 1967; DeWeese and Hunter, 1963; Leather et al., 1968; Miles, 1966; Moretz, 1965; Royster, 1967; Spencer et al., 1965; Taber et al., 1966; Wheeler et al., 1966; Whitcomb and Mostyn, 1965).

The primary purpose of caval interruption is to prevent pulmonary embolism. There was a 3.2 per cent incidence of small pulmonary emboli following ligation and a higher incidence, 5.6 per cent, following partial interruption. However, the 1 per cent incidence of fatal embolism was the same for the two groups.

In addition, there was a 1 per cent incidence of fatal shock secondary to sudden massive edema and distal progression of venous thrombosis following ligation, which was not seen following partial interruption. There were no reports of a patent vena cava following ligation even when the cava was ligated with catgut. In fact, it has been demonstrated that numerous large collaterals can form about the site of the ligation through which emboli can pass (Fig. 7.27) (Parrish et al., 1968). On the other hand, when

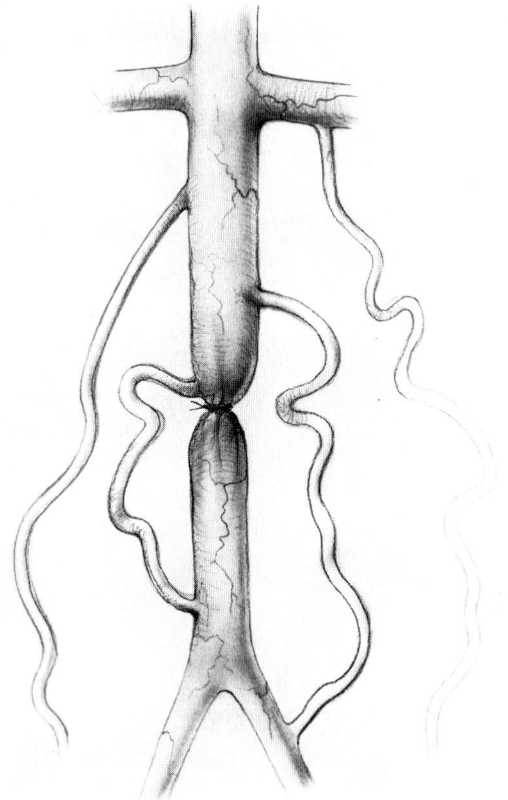

Fig. 7.27. Patterns of collaterals following caval ligation. Spermatic or ovarian vein collaterals to the vena cava on the right side and the renal vein on the left. Ascending lumbar collaterals illustrated on the left and lumbar-lumbar vein collaterals on the right side.

cavagrams were obtained from patients following partial interruption, patency above and below the site of interruption was found in 71 per cent (Fig. 7.28).

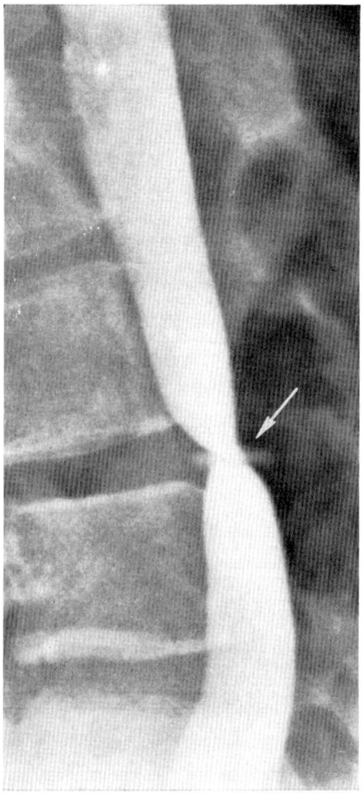

Fig. 7.28. Lateral cavagram of a patient in whom a serrated clip had been applied 6 months previously.

Meaningful comparisons cannot be made regarding the mortality rate because of nonthromboembolic complications. The mortality rate for either of the procedures is directly related to the number of elderly, poor-risk patients with significant cardiac disease. Their operative mortality rate may be as high as 55 per cent (Crane 1964). There have not been enough comparative long-term follow-up studies of the two groups to state definitively that the incidence of the postthrombotic syndrome is lower following partial interruption. Early follow-up indicates that this will be so. It is known that distal progression of a thrombus occurs more frequently following ligation than after partial interruption (Adams and DeWeese, 1965). It is venous thrombosis resulting in recanalized valveless veins or dilated valveless collaterals that produces late venous stasis. It seems logical, therefore, that there will be a lower incidence of sequelae, especially late sequelae, after partial interruption.

Caval Interruption by Preventive Filter Implantation

V. Schlosser

The filter implantation of Mobin-Uddin occupies an important place among methods of interruption of the inferior vena cava as surgical prophylaxis against pulmonary embolism.

While interruption of the inferior vena cava has two inherent disadvantages—the risks of an extraperitoneal abdominal operation and of acute reduction of the minute volume, application of the caval clips of Adams (1966), DeWeese and Hunter (1963), Miles (1966) and others has only the drawback of extraperitoneal exposure of the infrarenal vena cava.

The Mobin-Uddin filter implantation is practical, since the filter is introduced transvenously from a vein in the neck, and is a minor operation of prime effectiveness.

The right internal or external jugular is exposed under local or short general anesthesia. The filter is introduced folded by means of the applicator via the superior vena cava under television image-converter control. It passes the right atrium and is pushed as far as the infrarenal portion of the inferior vena cava. The site of application is the caudal margin of the third or the cranial margin of the fourth lumbar vertebra. In addition, the position of the renal pelves is marked by infusion pyelography so that the filter is secured distal to the junction of the renal veins. Once the applicator is in the correct position, the filter is pushed out of its casing, and it expands on its own because of its elasticity. A slight backward pull on the introducing catheter produces firm anchoring of

Table 7.3 Complications during and after Caval Interruption Following Mobin-Uddin Filter Implantation

	No.	%	No.
Total number of filter implantations (literature to March 1, 1974)	2267	100	—
Number of our own filter implantations (to April 1, 1975)			53
Filter migrating and displaced	33	1.5	2
Recent embolism	77	3.4	
(Fatal)	(19)	(0.8)	1
Marked postoperative edema of legs	116	5.1	5
Significant retroperitoneal hemorrhage	7	0.3	
Misplacement	35	1.5	1

the filter hooks in the wall of cava without perforating it. The applicator is then unscrewed without effort and removed from the venotomy. X-ray confirmation for documentation ends this brief intervention.

Later removal of the filter is not envisaged.

Possible complications (Table 7.3) are edema of the lower extremity, recurrent embolism, misplacement of filter and dislocation.

On questioning our 52 patients about the tendency to swelling after filter implantation, 10 per cent answered affirmatively (Table 7.4). Phlebographic evaluation of 25 of the 52 patients 1 to 2 years after implantation revealed eight with complete occlusion of the vena cava in the region of the filter with corresponding collateral circulation and moderate to marked swelling tendency of the lower extremity. In eight patients, an additional third, phlebography showed partial obstruction due to the filter with traces of collateral circulation but without swelling of the legs. In nine patients the vena cava was patent; the filter lay at the typical site and no collateral circulation had developed.

Table 7.4 Caval Filter Implantation for Prophylaxis against Pulmonary Embolism, 1971–1975. n=53. Postoperative Assessment

Questioned	50
Since died	2
Not available	4
Evaluable	44
Tendency to edema	14
Postoperatively	4
Pulmonary embolism	none
Anticoagulation	30 (60%)

We consider administration of anticoagulants necessary for 1 to 2 years after filter implantation. Recurrent emboli were observed with this method. They are due either to clots spreading from veins not reached (ovarian vein, collateral veins) or to clot formation proximal to the filter, which is being discussed. Misplacement of the filter can easily be corrected by reimplantation of a new filter.

The protective filter implantation of Mobin-Uddin as surgical prophylaxis against recurrent pulmonary embolism is distinguished by a high degree of certainty with a small operative risk. Hence, this procedure can be carried out almost without limitation on gravely ill patients with little surgical trauma and avoidance of general anesthesia.

The Eichelter catheter, which is applied through the saphenous vein only temporarily, has the drawback that it must be introduced via the pelvic veins, which may contain thrombi. The risk of infection is likewise increased by this method.

Mobin-Uddin filter implantation as prophylaxis against pulmonary embolism is indicated in the following conditions:

— after single threatening pulmonary embolism for prevention of recurrent, possibly fatal emboli;
— in recurrent multiple small emboli in the pulmonary arteries which might cause pulmonary hypertension (after lung scintigraphy or pulmonary angiography for demonstration of emboli if feasible); and
— with phlebographically proven fresh pelvic and leg thrombosis with floating thrombi immediately prior to major operations—orthopedic, traumatic, gynecologic or urologic—and generally postoperatively.

References

Adams, J. T., J. A. DeWeese: Experimental and clinical evaluation of partial vein interruption in the prevention of pulmonary emboli. Surgery 57 (1965) 82

Adams, J. T., J. A. DeWeese: Partial interruption of the inferior vena cava with a new plastic clip. Surg. Gynec. Obstet 123 (1966) 1087

Agrifoglio, G., E. A. Edwards: Venous stasis after ligation of femoral veins or inferior vena cava. J. Amer. med. Ass. 178 (1961) 1

Amador, E., T. K. Li, C. Crane: Ligation of inferior vena cava for thromboembolism: Clinical and autopsy correlations in 119 cases. J. Amer. med. Ass. 206 (1968) 1758

Antonopoulos, D.: Über die Beckenvenendarstellung von Knochenmark aus zum Studium der Tumoren des kleinen Beckens. Zbl. Gynäk. 77 (1955) 2048

Antonopoulos, D.: La phlébographie pelvienne chez la femme par la tuberosité ischiatique. Christon, Athènes 1959

Bales, Ch., J. A. DeWeese: Iliac vein stenosis. A case report and review of literature. Vasc. Dis. 3 (1966) 373

Bennek, J.: Die diagnostische Bedeutung des Kavogrammes bei retroperitonaealen Tumoren im Kindesalter. Z. Kinderchir. 3 (1966) 511

Bergan, J. J., H. A. Kaupp, O. H. Trippel: Critical evaluation of vena cava plication: Prevention of pulmonary embolism. Arch. Surg. 88 (1964) 1016

Bergan, J. J., D. W. Kinnaird, K. Koons, O. H. Trippel: Prevention of pulmonary embolism: Comparison of vena cava ligation, plication, and filter operations. Arch. Surg. 92 (1965) 605

Bowers, R. F., S. M. Leb: Late results of inferior vena cava ligation. Surgery 37 (1955) 622

Burget, D. E., Jr., J. H. Henzel, J. L. Smith, W. J. Pories: Inferior vena cava plication for prevention of pulmonary embolism: Results in 24 cases. Ann. Surg. 165 (1967) 437

Byrne, J. J., F. D. O'Neil: Fatal pulmonary emboli: A study of 130 autopsy-proven fatal emboli. Amer. J. Surg. 83 (1952) 47

Carey, L. C., R. D. Williams: Comparative effects of dicumarol, Tromexan, and heparin on thrombus propagation. Ann. Surg. 152 (1960) 919

Chidekel, N.: Female pelvic veins demonstrated by selective renal phlebography with particular reference to pelvic varicosities. Acta radiol. 7 (1968) 193
Chidekel, N., K.-O. Edlundh: Transuterine phlebography with particular reference to pelvic varicosities. Acta radiol. 7 (1968) 1
Cockett, F. B.: The role of lymphatic obstruction in the swollen leg of the post-phlebitic. In: Progrès cliniques et thérapeutiques dans le domaine de la phlébologie. Stenvert & Zoon, Apeldoorn 1970
Cockett, F. B., M. L. Thomas: The iliac compression syndrome. Brit. J. Surg. 52 (1965) 816
Coon, W. W., F. A. Coller: Clinicopathologic correlation in thromboembolism. Surg. Gynec. Obstet. 109 (1959) 259
Crane, C.: Femoral vs. caval interruption for venous thromboembolism. New Eng. J. Med. 270 (1964) 819
Dale, W. A.: Inferior vena caval ligation for venous thromboembolism. Rev. Surg. 19 (1962) 1
Dale, W. A.: Chronic iliofemoral venous occlusion including 7 cases of cross over vein grafting. Surgery 59 (1966) 117
Dale, W., H. W. Scott: Grafts of the venous system. Surgery 53 (1963) 52
DeWeese, M. S., D. C. Hunter: A vena cava filter for the prevention of pulmonary embolism. Arch. Surg. 86 (1963) 852
DeWeese, J. A., S. M. Rogoff: Phlebographic patterns of acute deep venous thrombosis of the leg. Surgery 53 (1963) 99
DeWeese, J. A., S. M. Rogoff, C. E., hr., Phillips, W. J. Pories: Deep venous thrombosis. Postgrad. Med. 29 (1961) 613
Dick, W.: Klinik und Therapie der Venensperre am Confluens der beiden gemeinsamen Iliacalvenen. Langenbecks Arch. klin. Chir. 301 (1962) 573
Donaldson, G. A., R. R. Linton, G. V. Rodkey: A twenty-year survey of thromboembolism at the Massachusetts General Hospital 1939–1959. New Eng. J. Med. 265 (1961) 208
Doppman, J.: Inferior vena caval compression. Amer. J. Roentgenol. Vol. C, (1967) 411
Dost, K.: Plastischer Ersatz der Vena cava inferior im Tierexperiment. Arch. Kreisl.-Forsch. 51 (1966) 191
Dost, K.: Druck- und Flußgeschwindigkeit in der Vene bei plastischem Venenersatz. Angiologica 5 (1968) 271
Dumanian, A. V.: Cross-over saphenous vein graft combined with a temporary femoral a. v. fistula. Vasc. Surg. 2 (1968) 116
Edlundh, K.-O.: Pelvic varicosities in women. Acta obstet. gynec. scand. 43 (1964) 399
Ferner, U., J. R. Gardham, A. Marston: Femoropopliteal saphenous vein bypass grafting. Br. J. Hosp. Med. (1975) 679
Ferris, E. J., F. J. Vittimberga, J. J. Byrne, D. C. Nabseth, J. H. Shapiro: The inferior vena cava after ligation and plication: A study of collateral routes. Radiology 89 (1967) 1
Gardner, A. M.: Partial inferior vena cava occlusion by clip. Proc. roy. Soc. Med. 67 (1974) 1185
Gazzaniga, A. B., J. L. Cahill, R. L. Replogle, N. L. Tilney: Changes in blood volume and renal function following ligation of the inferior vena cava. Surgery 62 (1967) 417
Gottlob, R.: Untersuchungen am Endothel arterialisierter Venen. Vasa 4, 243, (1975)
Gottlob, R., R. May: Der Frühverschluß der Palma-Operation. Vasa 1977 (in press)
Guilhem, P., R. Baux: La phébographie pelvienne. Masson, Paris 1954
Gullmo, A.: The strain obstruction syndrome of the femoral vein. Acta radiol. 47 (1957) 119
Gullmo, A.: Phlebographie als präoperatives Diagnosticum bei femoral- und Leistenhernien. In: Angiographie und ihre Leistungen. K. E. Loose (ed.). Thieme, Stuttgart 1968
Gumrich, H.: Therapie venöser Stauungen. Chirurg 40 (1969) 495–500
Gumrich, H., E. Kübler: Das phlebographische Bild der Beckenvenensperre und deren Ursachen. Fortschr. Röntgenstr. 82 (1955) 756
Gurewich, V., D. P. Thomas, K. R. Rabinov: Pulmonary embolism after ligation of the inferior vena cava. New Eng. J. Med. 274 (1966) 1350
Hardin, C. A.: Bypass saphenous grafts for the relief of venous obstruction of the extremity. Surg. Gynec. Obstet. 115 (1962) 709
Harris, J.: Cross leg venous graft for the relief of unilateral lower limb venous obstruction. Surg. Gynec. Obstet. 120 (1965) 1232
Helander, C. G., A. Lindbom: Varicocele of the broad ligament Acta radiol. 53 (1960) 97
Helander, C. G., A. Lindbom: Roentgen examination of the inferior vena cava in retroperitoneal expanding processes. Acta radiol. 45 (1956) 289
Henderson, R. R.: Pulmonary embolism and infarction. Med. Clin. N. Amer. 48 (1964) 1425
Holtz, S., W. E. Powers: Inferior vena cavagramms. Radiology 78 (1962) 583
Homans, J.: Exploration and division of the femoral and iliac veins in the treatment of thrombophlebitis of the leg. New Eng. J. Med. 224 (1941) 179
Homans, J.: Venous thrombosis and pulmonary embolism. New Eng. J. Med. 236 (1947) 196
Hunter, W. C., V. D. Sneeden, T. D. Robertson, G. A. C. Snyder: Thrombosis of the deep veins of the leg. Arch. intern. Med. 68 (1941) 1
Jackson, D. R.: Pseudoiliofemoral vein thrombosis secondary to aortic dacron bypass grafting. Vasc. Surg. 1 237 (1967)
Jacobson, J. H., T. Katsumura: Small vein reconstruction. J. cardiovasc. Surg. 6 (1965) 157
Kainberger, F.: Veränderungen der Beckenvenen nach Radikaloperation wegen Uteruscarcinom. Fortschr. Röntgenstr. 104 (1966) 157
Kainberger, F.: Vergleichende Untersuchung der postoperativen und der neoplastischen Venenveränderungen bei Uteruscarcinom am Beckenvenogramm. Fortschr. Röntgenstr. 106 (1967) 371
Krause, R. J., J. J. Cranley, M. A. S. Hallaba, E. S. Strasser, C. D. Hafner: Caval ligation in thromboembolic disease. Arch. Surg. 87 (1963) 184
Kunlin, J.: Le rétablissement de la circulation veineuse par greffe en cas d'oblitérative traumatique ou thrombophlébitique; greffe de 18 cm entre la veine saphène interne et la veine iliaque externe; thrombose après trois semaines de perméabilité. Mém. Acad. Chir. 79 (1950) 109
Leather, R. P., W. R. Clark, Jr., S. R. Powers, F. B. Parker, H. R. Bernard, C. Eckert: Five-year experience with the Moretz vena caval clip in 62 patients. Arch. Surg. 97 (1968) 357
Maraan, B. M., R. E. Taber: The effects of inferior vena caval ligation on cardiac output: An experimental study. Surgery 63 (1968) 966
May, R.: Die Diagnostik venöser Verschlüsse im Beckenbereich. 14th Intern. Congress I.C.S. 1964, Vienna. (Kongreßdruck)
May, R.: Die Problematik der Venenplastik. Zbl. Phleb. 4 (1965) 43
May, R.: Ormond'sche Erkrankung. Act. Chir. 3 (1968) 65
May, R.: Die Wiederherstellung der postthrombotisch geschädigten venösen Strombahn. Zbl. Phleb. 7 (1968) 24
May, R.: Die chirurgische Behandlung des postthrombotischen Syndroms. Hefte Unfallheilk. 107 (1971) 129
May, R.: Meßmethoden in der Venenchirurgie. Huber, Bern 1971
May, R.: Surgical management of chronic venous occlusion of the extremities. Intern. Europ. Congress Soc. Cardiovascular Surgery Belgrade 1–5 September, 1976
May, R., R. Nissl: Die Phlebographie der unteren Extremität. Thieme, Stuttgart 1959
May, R., J. Thurner: Ein Gefäßsporn in der v. iliaca com. sin. als wahrscheinliche Ursache der überwiegend linksseitigen Beckenvenenthrombose. Z. Kreisl.-Forsch. 45 (1956) 912
May, R., J. Thurner: The cause of the predominantly sinistral occurrence of thrombosis of the pelvic veins. Angiology 8 (1957) 419
Miles, R. M.: Prevention of pulmonary embolism by the use of a plastic vena caval clip. Ann. Surg. 163 (1966) 192
Moretz, W. H.: Discussion: cited in Spencer et al.
Mozes, M., H. Bogokowsky, E. Antebei, N. Tzur, S. Penchas: Inferior vena cava ligation for pulmonary embolism: Review of 118 cases. Surgery 60 (1966) 790
Nasbeth, D. C., J. M. Moran: Reassessment of the role of inferior-vena-cava ligation in venous thromboembolism. New Eng. J. Med. 273 (1965) 1250
Nakayama, K.: A simple new apparatus for small vessel anastomosis. Surgery 52 (1962) 918
Neistadt, A., S. I. Schwartz: Is venous blood in the left leg less than in the right? Arch. Surg. 93 (1966) 938
Negus, D.: The iliac veins in relation to lymphoedema. Brit. J. Surg. 56 (1969) 34
Negus, D., F. B. Cockett: Femoral vein pressures in postphlebitis iliac vein obstruction. Brit. J. Surg. 54 (1967) 522

Niedner, F. F.: Entstchung, Pathologie und Behandlung der Venenerkrankungen. Heilkunst 79 (1966) section 8

Nylander, G.: Haemodynamics of the pelvic veins in incompetençe of the femoral vein. Acta radiol. 56 (1961) 369

Palma, C. E., R. Esperon: Tratamiento del sindrome post-trombo-flebitico mediante transplante de safena interna. Angiologia 11 (1959) 87

Palma, C. E., R. Esperon: Vein transplants and grafts in the surgical treatment of the postphlebitic syndrome. J. cardiovasc. Surg. 1 (1960) 94

Palma, E. C., F. Riß, F. Del Campo, H. Tobler: cited in Palma and Esperon 1959

Parrish, E. H., J. T. Adams, W. J. Pories, D. E. Burget, J. A. DeWeese: Pulmonary emboli following vena caval ligation. Arch. Surg. 97 (1968) 899

Ravdin, I. S., C. K. Kirby: Experiences with ligation and heparin in thromboembolic disease. Surgery 29 (1951) 334

Rossle, R.: Über die Bedeutung und die Entstehung der Wadenvenenthrombosen. Virchows Arch. path. Anat. 300 (1937) 180

Royster, T. S.: Thrombophlebitis after vena caval clipping. Amer. J. Surg. 113 (1967) 754

Rubinson, R. M.: Inferior vena caval obstruction from increased intra-abdominal pressure. Arch. Surg. 95 (1967) 766

Schauble, J. F., D. L. Stickel, W. G. Anlyan: Vena caval ligation for thromboembolic disease. Arch. Surg. 84 (1962) 35

Senn, A.: Möglichkeiten und Grenzen der chirurgischen Therapie beim postthrombotischen Zustandsbild. In: Das postthrombotische Zustandsbild der Extremitäten. A. Kappert, R. May (eds.). Huber, Bern 1968 (p. 93)

Shea, P. C., jr., R. L. Robertson: Late sequelae of inferior vena cava ligation. Surg. Gynec. Obstet. 93 (1951) 153

Short, D. S.: A survey of pulmonary embolism in a general hospital. Brit. med. J. 1952/I, 790

Spencer, F. C., J. Jude, W. F. Rienhoff, III, G. Stonesifer: Plication of the inferior vena cava for pulmonary embolism: Long-term results in 39 cases. Ann. Surg. 161 (1965) 788

Stein, G. N., J. T. Chen, F. Goldstein, H. L. Israel, A. Finkelstein: The importance of chest roentgenography in the diagnosis of pulmonary embolism. Amer. J. Roentgen. 81 (1959) 255

Stevens, L. E., W. K. Fitzpatrick, G. K. Stewart, W. J. Burdette: Ligation of the inferior vena cava. Arch. Surg. 90 (1965) 578

Taber, R. E. E. Zikria, E. A. Hershey, C. R. Lam: Prevention of pulmonary emboli with a vena caval clip. J. Amer. med. Ass. 195 (196) 889

Trendelenburg, F.: A review of surgical progress. J. Amer. med. Ass. 47 (1906) 81

Vollmar, J.: Die Rekonstruktion unilateraler Beckenvenenverschlüsse. Act. Chir. 5 (1970) 79

Wacker, W. E. C., M. Rosenthal, P. J. Snodgrass, E. Amador: A triad for the diagnosis of pulmonary embolism and infarction. J. Amer. med. Ass. 178 (1961) 8

Wagner, H. N., D. C. Sabiston, Jr., J. G. McAfee, D. Tow, H. S. Stern: Diagnosis of massive pulmonary embolism in man by radioisotope scanning. New Eng. J. Med. 271 (1964) 377

Wanke, R.: Die operative Therapie der chron. Beckenvenensperre. Chirurg 26 (1955) 161

Wanke, R.: Chirurgie der großen Körpervenen. Thieme, Stuttgart 1956

Wanke, R., H. Gumrich: Chronische Beckenvenensperre. Zbl. Chir. 75 (1950) 1302

Wanke, R., H. Eufinger, L. Diethelm: Anatomie und Chirurgie der Vena iliaca communis sinistra. Dsch. med. Wschr. 85 (1960) 640

Wessler, S., L. E. Morris: Studies in intravascular coagulation. IV. The effect of heparin and dicumarol on serum-induced venous thrombosis. Circulation 12 (1955) 553

Wheeler, C. G., J. E. Thompson, D. J. Austin, R. D. Patman, R. L. Stockton: Interruption of the inferior vena cava for thromboembolism: Comparison of ligation and plication. Ann. Surg. 163 (1966) 199

Whitcomb, J. G., M. Mostyn: Experience with the vena cava sieve procedure for prevention of pulmonary emboli. Amer. J. Surg. 110 (1965) 767

8 Lymphovenous Surgery

F. B. Cockett

Recently, fresh interest has been focused on the anatomic abnormalities and compression syndromes of the vena caval bifurcation. These developmental abnormalities causing various degrees of obstruction and flow irregularities are now well documented (Ehrich and Krumbhaar, 1943; Wanke and Gumrich, 1950; May and Thurner, 1957; Cockett and Lea Thomas, 1965; Cockett et al., 1967). It is known that they are the basic lesions causing most cases of acute major iliofemoral thrombosis in *young* people. Improved techniques of serial iliac venography (Cockett and Lea Thomas, 1965; Lea Thomas and Fletcher, 1967; Cockett et al. 1967) have been of great use in visualizing these obstructions of the great veins (Fig. 8.1).

After iliofemoral thrombosis has occurred and the immediate swelling and pain have died away, the patient enters the chronic phase of the disease. In this period, which lasts for the rest of the patient's life, the post-thrombotic signs gradually accumulate. There are two distinct groups of signs.

— venous congestion and incompetent perforating veins (lead to some swelling, but particularly to deterioration of the skin of the

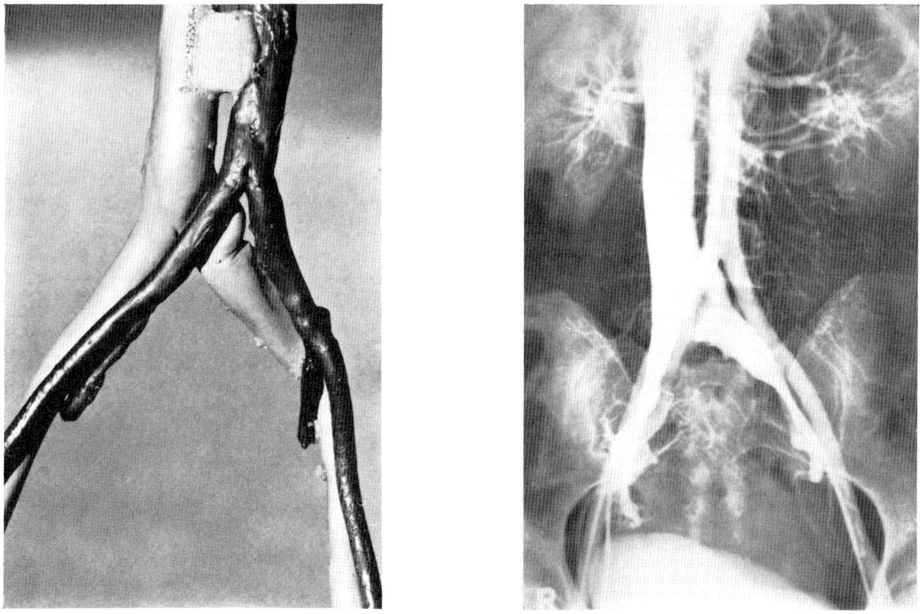

a b

Fig. 8.1. Iliac compression syndrome. Corrosion cast of the bifurcation of the aorta and vena cava in situ (*a*). The deep indentation and deformity of the left common iliac vein is immediately apparent. Simultaneous aortogram and venogram (*b*) from a patient who had a history of iliofemoral thrombosis, leaving him with a mildly swollen left leg. Note that in this case there is a marked compression defect both at the caval bifurcation and a little lower down on the left side where the left internal iliac artery crosses the vein. These are the two common sites where arterial compression of the great veins takes place; compression at both sites sometimes occurs in the same patient, as in this case.

periphery resulting eventually in ulceration); and
— generalized swelling of the limb.

These two sets of signs do not always go hand in hand, nor are they necessarily related to the extent and severity of the original thrombosis.

Some patients may have complete iliac vein obstruction only, with good collaterals and very little swelling.

Other patients may have a compensated iliac vein obstruction but extensive destruction of valves in the deep veins and incompetent distal perforating veins, with disastrous effects on the ankle skin (ulceration and fat necrosis) but surprisingly little general swelling.

Still other patients show increased swelling of the whole subcutaneous envelope of the limb, to such an extent that this swelling and sensation of heaviness are their main complaint.

These anomalies are explained when we consider the lymphatic drainage of the lower limb.

If iliac lymphangiograms and venograms are obtained simultaneously, it becomes apparent that the degree of swelling is *largely* dependent on the degree of obstruction in the iliac lymphatics.

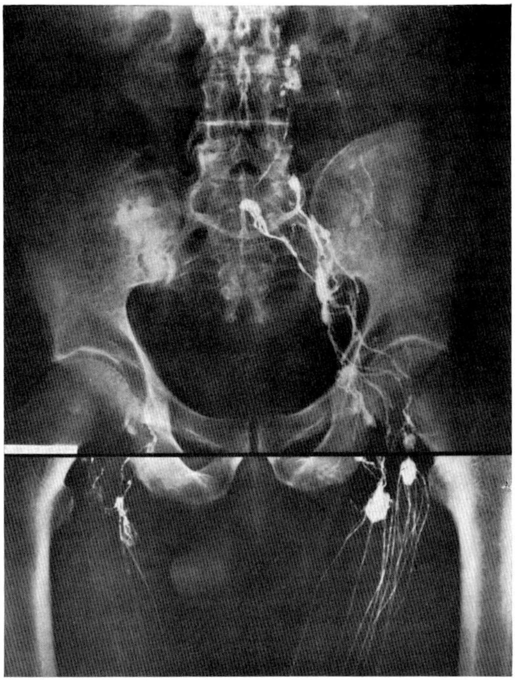

Fig. 8.2. Thigh and iliac lymphangiograms from a patient with gross swelling of the right leg (due to metastases from carcinoma of the prostate). Both legs were infused with Microlipiodol at the same time. The left side shows normal anatomy with the iliac lymph trunks closely applied to and following the course of the iliac veins to the caval bifurcation. The right side shows complete lack of filling of the iliac lymphatics, which persisted, indicating complete lymphatic obstruction.

Anatomy of Lymphatic Drainage

The lymphatics of the lower limb are essentially a superficial system of vessels running up to the groin, grouped more or less around the course of the internal saphenous vein. There is one deep lymphatic that runs with the posterior tibial vein, but these lymphatics deep to the deep fascia of the limb are extremely sparse, and it is doubtful that there are any deep to the deep fascia in the thigh. All these lymphatics (about 8 to 12 trunks normally) run up to the inguinal glands. The whole efferent system from the inguinal glands, draining the whole lower limb, continues as three to five large intercommunicating trunks closely applied around the external and common iliac veins to the caval bifurcation (Fig. 8.2).

Obstructed Lymphatic Drainage

It is apparent that these relatively few lymphatics grouped around the external and common iliac veins are very much exposed to possible obstruction associated with fibrosis and inflammatory reaction around a major iliac vein. At this point it is relatively easy for obstruction of the whole lymphatic outflow from the lower limb to occur. Iliac lymphangiograms obtained concurrently with venograms in cases of iliac vein thrombosis show that in those cases in which swelling is a major symptom, various degrees of obstruction of the iliac lymphatic trunks also exist.

Iliac Lymphatic Obstruction Coexisting with Iliac Venous Obstruction

If iliac lymphangiograms are done simultaneously with venograms in cases of iliac compression, patients can be divided roughly into three groups:

Patients with no or very little swelling. Lymphangiogram is normal.

Patients with moderate swelling. These patients show some degree of lymphatic obstruction in the iliac lymphatics. This can best be appreciated by doing the lymphangiogram with the aid of an image intensifier. On injection of the contrast material into the lymphatics in the foot, it is seen to ascend rapidly to the lymph glands in the groin on each side. There is then a considerable delay before small droplets of the Lipiodol infiltrate slowly into the iliac lymphatics, in marked contrast to the normal side, where ascent into the iliac lymphatics is normal (Fig. 8.3).

There is normally some holdup at the level of the inguinal ligament before filling of iliac lymphatics starts. Abnormal delay can be judged only if simultaneous lymphangiograms on both legs are done, and the times of filling of the iliac lymphatics on the two sides are carefully observed. It seems probable that this mild lymphatic obstruction is due to post-thrombotic fibrosis around the iliac veins, involving the lymphatics.

Patients with gross swelling. These patients show complete obstruction of the iliac lymphatics (see Fig. 8.2).

Conclusion. It is apparent, therefore, that the degree of swelling in the subcutaneous tissues in cases of post-thrombotic iliac vein obstruction is more directly related to the degree of accompanying lymphatic obstruction than to the venous obstruction itself.

Lymphedema without Obvious Iliac Vein Obstruction

It seems likely that many cases of primary lymphedema in young people originate in a primary lymphatic obstruction associated with or similar to the iliac compression syndrome.
These patients probably start with lymphatic obstruction in the region of the caval bifurcation; in the initial stages the swelling is only slight. However, as time goes on, stasis in the distended lymphatics leads to retrograde lymphatic thrombosis and obliteration. When most of the main lymphatic trunks of the limb have thus disappeared, the lymphedema becomes worse—solid and irreversible.
This sequence of events has been observed over the years by the author, in serial observations on a young girl, with very little abnormality at the caval bifurcation. All types of variants exist. At one end of the scale there are those with gross venous abnormalities at the bifurcation or in the pelvis, with relatively little in the way of lymphatic obstruction. At the other end of the scale are those with relatively little venous abnormality, but considerable lymphatic obstruction, the so-called *lymphedema praecox*.

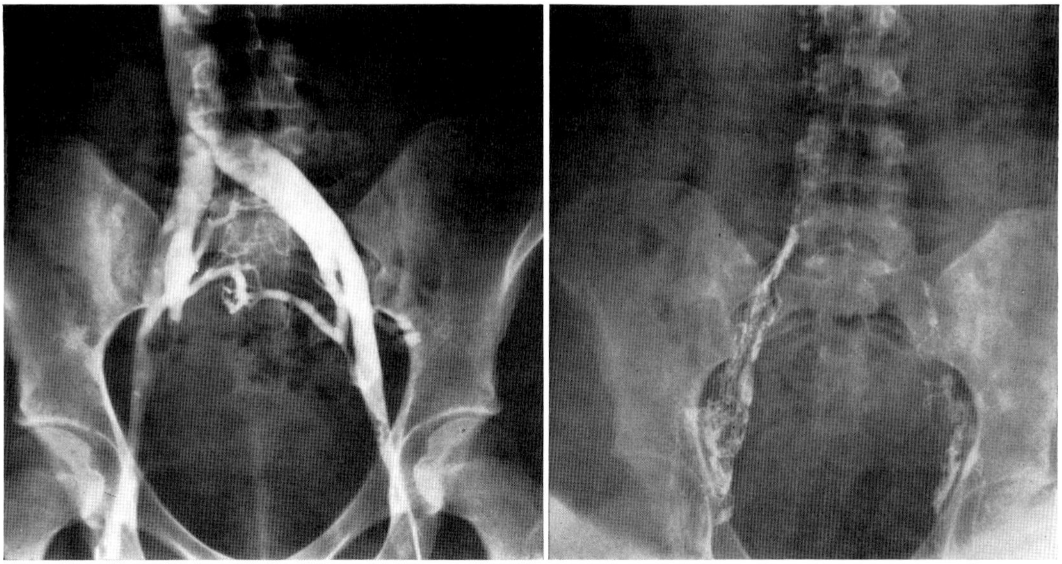

a b

Fig. 8.3. Venogram (*a*) and lymphangiogram (*b*) from a patient who had a history of possible iliofemoral thrombosis, with only a moderate degree of swelling. The venogram shows moderate compression of the left common iliac vein, with some collaterals. The lymphangiogram shows marked delay in filling of the iliac lymphatics on the left side.

Surgical Measures

In the *late stage* of lymphatic obstruction, when most of the lymphatic trunks have been obliterated by retrograde lymphatic thrombosis, only excisional surgery is possible. Among these methods *Thompson's operation* is probably the best. A long strip of subcutaneous tissue is removed on the inner aspect of the limb, from ankle to just above the knee. The anterior skin flap, from which the upper layer of the dermis containing hair follicles has been removed by dermatome, is sutured to the deep fascia, which has been incised close to the line of the posterior tibial vessels. The posterior flap is then stretched and folded over it. The procedure is shown in Figure 8.4.

In the early stages of lymphatic obstruction, before retrograde thrombosis and destruction of lymphatic trunks have occurred, it is possible to create a new lymphovenous anastomosis below the obstruction. This has been attempted in two ways:

— by transecting a lymph node with its afferent lymphatics intact and implanting this into the side of a major vein, for example, the external iliac or common femoral vein (Nielubowicz et al., 1968); and

— by direct implantation of one or more dilated lymphatics into a vein (Cockett 1968).

Implantation of Lymph Nodes into Veins

An anastomosis is established between a lymph node and a neighboring vein. If the lymph node is incised and sutured to the cut surface of the incised venous wall, subcapsular and medullary lymph sinuses remain patent and drain the lymph from the afferent lymphatics into the vein. Lymphostasis is thus eliminated.

Technique

The lymph nodes are exposed with care to spare the afferent lymphatics. A large lymph node is incised with a sharp scalpel. The capsule of the lymph node is sutured to the incised wall of the long saphenous, femoral or external iliac vein by continuous suture with 5-0 silk (Fig. 8.5)

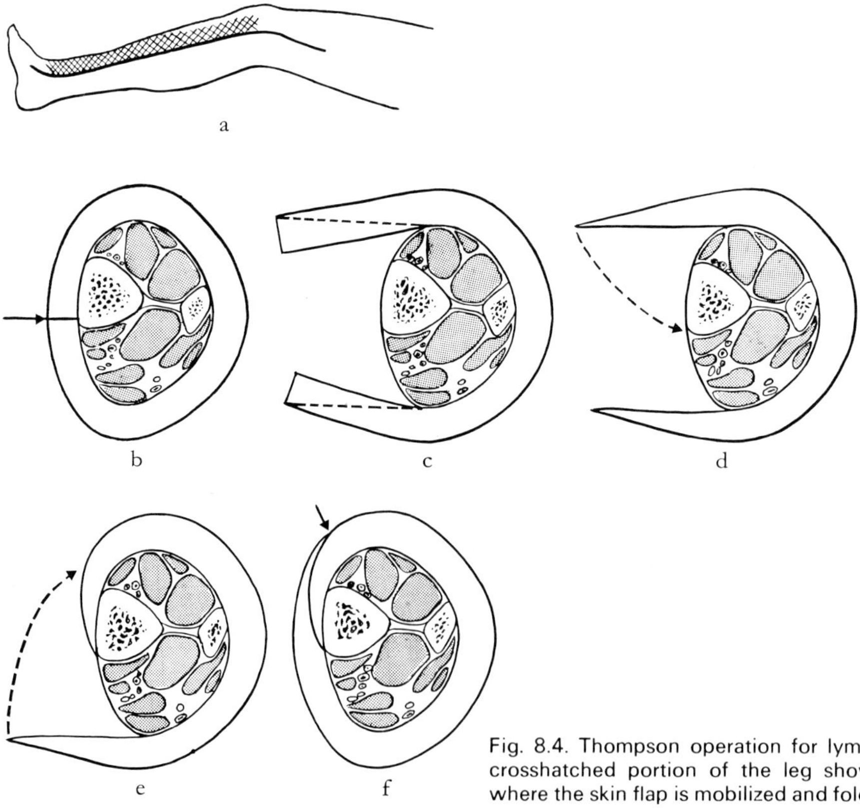

Fig. 8.4. Thompson operation for lymphedema. The crosshatched portion of the leg shows the region where the skin flap is mobilized and folded over (*a*).

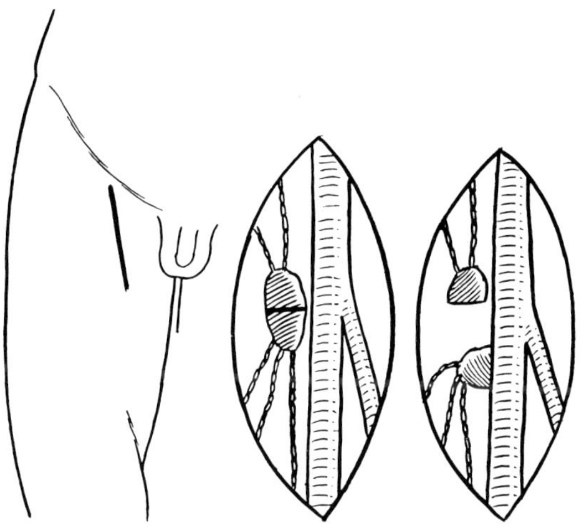

Fig. 8.5. Nielubowicz operation. Skin incision (*a*); lymph node incised (*b*) and implanted into the femoral vein (*c*).

Nielubowicz and Olszewski described their first cases: in 12 patients with secondary lymphedema, they anastomosed the inguinal lymph node four times with the long saphenous and six times with the femoral vein. Fibrotic nodes precluded anastomosis in two cases, which were used as controls.

In 17 cases of primary lymphedema, the inguinal lymph node was anastomosed with the long saphenous once, with the femoral ten times, and with femoral and long saphenous twice. The iliac lymph node was sutured to the external iliac once and into femoral and external iliac three times.

A subcutaneous drain was left after primary wound closure.

Postoperatively no pressure bandages or elastic stockings were prescribed, and the patients were checked every three months.

Prognosis

The results of the operation depend on careful suture technique and the state of the lymph node. The sutures must include only the capsule and should lie as far as possible away from the marginal sinus. Fibrotic, scarred lymph nodes are unsuitable.

If adequate nodes are available, a double anastomosis is preferred, namely, one anastomosis with the femoral and another with the external iliac.

Indications

Originally, the anastomoses were performed only in secondary lymphedema. For primary lymphedema, the operation is indicated only in selected cases when lymphography reveals much dilated lymphatics.

Postoperative Course

There were no serious complications. Oozing from the wound stopped between the third and fifth postoperative days. The patients were usually discharged after 10 days. Thromboembolic complications were not recorded.

The patients felt much improved on the fourth day after operation. Movement of knee and ankle joints was freer and tension in the leg declined. The circumference of the limb was noticeably reduced by the fourth postoperative day.

Results

It was shown in animal experiments that the anastomoses were still patent after 24 months.

The surgical results can be evaluated objectively only by measuring the circumference. These results vary according to time of day, external temperature and exercise of the patient; but a decrease in leg circumference of 1 cm means a diminution in volume of 200 ml.

Best results were seen in patients with secondary lymphedema. In them, reduction in circumference attained 9 cm. All patients reported disappearance of pain and easier movement of the limb. The average decrease of the calf circumference was 3.8 cm 3 to 9 months after operation. No final statements can be made about results after primary lymphedema. Evidently, satisfactory results are achieved only in selected cases. The average decrease in circumference was 1 cm. In two cases, the circumference increased by 0.5 cm.

The control patients, in whom only lymph node exposure was performed, showed increased edema.

Implantation of Lymphatics into Veins

This procedure was done by the author in a small number (ten) of selected cases by the technique shown in Figure 8.6.

In this method the dilated lymph trunk is implanted into the femoral vein by a nonsuture technique. The lymph trunk is first stained by patent blue injected subcutaneously into the web spaces of the toes (0.5 ml). It is then exposed by a

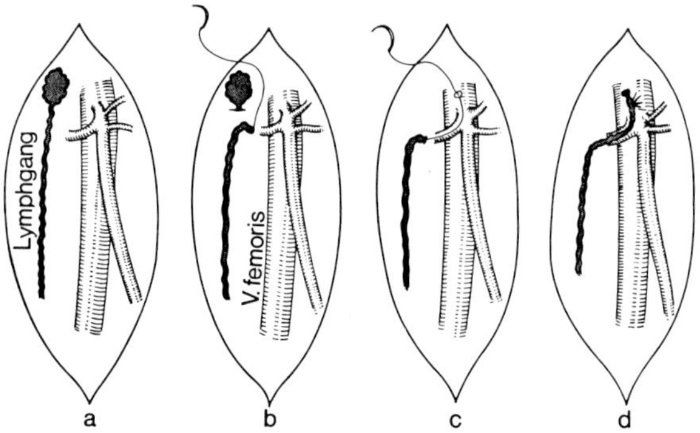

Fig. 8.6. Technique of implanting lymphatic trunks (*a–d*) by leading the trunk into the femoral vein through a side branch at the saphenofemoral junction.

large oblique groin incision. It is isolated, transected as high as possible and led to the inside of the femoral vein by introduction through a small side branch, as shown in Fig. 8.6. A side hole is cut in the lymphatic, from which it can empty its lymph into the lumen of the femoral vein. It is anchored to the inside of the femoral vein by the same fine silk suture that was used to pull it through.

It is advisable to heparinize the patients at a *low* dosage schedule for 24 hours after this operation, and then administer an oral anticoagulant for another 2 weeks, to discourage venous thrombosis.

The benefit of these operations is somewhat difficult to assess at times. In three patients, there was obvious reduction in swelling, and the patients reported that their subjective complaints of heaviness and bursting tightness of the limb, especially after exercise, were relieved.

The final proof that the operation works, however, must await the visual demonstration of the fistula by lymphangiography.

It must be emphasized that these attempts at creating lymphovenous anastomoses are as yet new and untried operations. It is not to be expected that they would produce dramatic cure of a lymphedema, but when they work they do provide some worthwhile improvement.

They are relatively minor operations, and not time-consuming. If they can be shown to halt the progress of lymphedema, they will be a useful addition to the equipment of a vascular surgeon.

References

Cockett, F. B.: A new technique for creating lymphovenous shunts. Boersma, Amsterdam 1968

Cockett, F. B., M. Lea Thomas: The iliac compression syndrome. Brit. J. Surg. 52 (1965) 816

Cockett, F. B., M. Lea Thomas, D. Negus: Iliac vein compression. Brit. med. J. 1967/II, 14

Ehrich, W. E., E. B. Krumbhaar: A frequent obstruction anomaly of the mouth of the left common iliac vein. Amer. Heart J. 26 (1943) 737

Kinmonth J. B. (1972) The Lymphatics, Arnold. London.

May, R., J. Thurner: Ein Gefäßsporn in der Vena iliaca communis sinistra als wahrscheinliche Ursache der überwiegend linksseitigen Beckenvenenthrombose. Kreisl.-Forsch. 45 (1956) 912

Nielubowicz, J., W. Olszewski: Surgical lymphaticovenous shunts in patients with secondary lymphedema. Brit. J. Surg. 55 (1968) 440

Nielubowicz, J., W. Olszewski, J. Sokolowski: Surgical lymphovenous shunts. J. cardiovasc. Surg. 9 (1968) 262

Thomas, M. L., E. W. I. Fletcher: The techniques of pelvic phlebography. Clin. Radiol. 18 (1967) 399

Thompson, N. (1962) Surgical Treatment of chronic lymphoedema of the lower limb. Brit. Med. J. ii p. 1566

Wanke, R., H. Gumrich: Chronische Beckenvenensperre. Zbl. Chir. 75 (1950) 1302

9 Venous Trauma

J. Vollmar

In vascular trauma that of the arteries has always occupied a predominant position. The risks of exsanguination and necrosis of limbs and organs were the obvious reasons. Most venous injuries are not so dramatic. They were therefore given little attention until a few years ago. Ligature of the veins was the prevailing therapeutic measure. Late sequelae of ligation of important main veins, especially manifest as post-thrombotic syndrome, have been clearly appreciated only in the last few years as a result of improved angiologic diagnosis (Shea and Robertson, 1951; Kappert and May, 1968), and more and more interest has focused on reconstructive procedures. Experience gained in reconstructive arterial surgery has been the guide.

Incidence

Precise statistics on injuries of large veins, i.e., those proximal to the knee and elbow joints, are not available as yet, for several reasons:

—Many blunt and penetrating venous injuries are concomitant with other trauma (fractures, organ ruptures, arterial damage and so forth). Care of the "main lesion" predominates; i.e., the venous trauma either is not recognized or is dismissed as unimportant and treated by ligation, and thus is not included in statistics.

—The sequelae of blunt venous trauma (post-traumatic thrombosis) are diagnosed only after the event; i.e., awareness of the relative and absolute frequency of traumatic venous lesions depends exclusively on the quality of intraoperative and postoperative diagnosis (cf. phlebographic evaluation after tibial fractures: in 43.6 per cent there was post-thrombotic venous damage—Hjelmsted and Bergvall, 1968).

In comparison, appreciation of arterial injuries is more reliable. since they are accompanied by clear-cut symptomatology. At the Heidelberg Clinic, arterial injuries in 168 patients were found to be associated with venous lesions in 111 (66 per cent). Because of greater vulnerability, the absolute frequency of isolated and combined venous injuries would be rather greater than that of arterial damage (the relative frequency of which is 0.3 to 0.5 per cent (Vollmar, 1967)). Conversely, if venous injuries are considered first, it is seen that 74 per cent of them are accompanied by arterial trauma (see Table 9.5). The close topographic relationship of artery and vein readily explains the extraordinary frequency of combined lesion.

Classification, Development and Clinical Signs

A classification of venous injuries is given in Table 9.1. This scheme is basically valid for both arterial and venous injuries, since the mechanism of insult is to a large extent the same.

Table 9.1 Classification of Venous Injuries

Direct injuries
Penetrating trauma
—cut, stab, shot
—iatrogenic (lesion during surgery, inadvertent ligation of a main vein)
Blunt trauma
—contusion
—compression (hematoma, fractures)
Indirect injuries
Tears due to stretching (usually with dislocations)
Acute and chronic sequelae
"Venous" embolism (air, foreign bodies, clots)
Post-thrombotic syndrome
Arteriovenous fistula

Like arterial injuries, most venous injuries—more than 90 per cent—are caused by direct impact (blunt or penetrating trauma). Indirect mechanisms of trauma (stretching, torsion or shearing of vessels) are seen very much less frequently. A third group comprises sequelae to accident—venous embolism, the post-thrombotic syndrome and arteriovenous fistula.

Direct Impact

Penetrating Trauma

The direction of a penetrating injury is from without inward, i.e., from adventitia toward intima. As with arteries, three grades of severity may be distinguished.

Grade I. Partial splitting of the wall without entrance into the lumen. Probably of no practical importance in venous injury.

Grade II. A slit or hole in the lumen of the vessel. This probably represents the most common type of injury. Clinically there is external or internal venous bleeding. The hemorrhage may stop spontaneously because of autotamponade, that is, compression of the vascular gap by the hematoma and surrounding tissues.

Grade III. Complete transection of the vein. This, when involving vessels of large caliber proximal to the elbow or knee joint, only rarely causes spontaneous closure of the bleeding vascular stump, which is observed time and again with corresponding arterial lesions because of retraction and involution of the intima. In the absence of adventitia (widely patent wound or opening of a neighboring body cavity), the blood loss may be followed by death in a short time.

Direct venous injuries of grades II and III, freely communicating externally or internally, are no less dangerous than arterial lesions. The life of the injured can in most cases be saved only by immediate surgical control of bleeding.

For instance, mortality in caval injury is about 50 per cent (Quast et al., 1965; Duke et al., 1965; Wood, 1966). Most injuries of large veins in body cavities are due to sharp penetrating trauma: 71 per cent by gunshot; 12 per cent by stab wounds; and 17 per cent by blunt trauma.

Practically all direct penetrating venous injuries cause strictly localized damage to the vessel which can usually be corrected directly by suture without a vascular substitute.

Blunt Trauma to Vessels

In blunt trauma, the intensity of the damage to the vessel wall runs from within outward; i.e., it decreases steadily from intima to adventitia. Depending on the intensity of the trauma, three grades of severity can be distinguished here, too.

Grade I represents a purely intimal lesion.

Grade II affects intima and media.

Grade III represents complete crushing of the vessel, the adventitia frequently being preserved as a mantle. Grades I and II may become the starting point of a secondary deep vein thrombosis.

The clinical picture is generally characteristic immediately after injury only in Grade III. Acute obstruction of a main drainage vein (proximal to elbow and knee joints) usually causes livid discoloration, soft tissue swelling and extreme filling of subcutaneous veins in the corresponding limb (Table 9.2). Collapse of the vein on elevation of the extremity does not occur.

Table 9.2 Diagnosis of Venous Lesions

1. *History*
   Penetrating foreign body?
   Blunt impact?
2. *Hemorrhage*
   Dark red, not pulsating
   Shock due to blood loss?
3. *Blockage of venous drainage*
   Livid swelling of soft tissues?
   Absence of venous collapse on raising the limb?
   Congestive hyperthermia?
4. *Venography*
5. *Exploratory exposure*

The nearer the obstruction of venous drainage to the vena cava, the more powerful are the hemodynamic reactions in the limb in general; this is the opposite of what happens in acute obstruction of the arterial stream. Acute interruptions of the superficial femoral vein or of one or two of the main veins of the leg may be clinically silent for a time, since there is usually an adequate collateral circulation in this type of localized stenosis. Signs of the post-thrombotic syndrome appear only some time after the accident, resulting from static strain. The same applies to blunt venous trauma of grades I and II, which may lead to blockage of deep veins via a traumatically induced deep phlebothrombosis.

Venous injuries due to blunt impact are only rarely accompanied by (internal or external) hemorrhage. There may be no external wound at all. Diagnosis is often difficult because of considerable secondary injury, especially fractures.

Thus, roughly one third of all fractures of the leg are accompanied by damage to the deep veins of the leg and a subsequent post-thrombotic syndrome (Hjelmstedt and Bergvall, 1968). Many of these unnoticed traumatic venous injuries are labeled "post-traumatic edema." This much used clinical term for post-traumatic swelling of the extremities is pathophysiologically not well founded. Precise angiologic examination almost

regularly reveals an unrecognized post-thrombotic syndrome or lymphatic blockage.
Unlike the case in penetrating vessel injuries, a more or less extended lesion of the vascular wall is seen in most cases after blunt venous trauma (and injuries due to indirect insult). Surgical correction by suture or simple thrombectomy is only rarely successful. The method of choice is vascular grafting, although application of these techniques in the deep venous system is limited at present.

Indirect Impact

Among indirect venous injuries, of particular importance is overstretching of the vessels due to luxation of large joints, e.g., of the axillary vein in dislocation of the humerus and of the cubital vein in dislocation of the forearm. In fractures with marked displacement, on the other hand, contusions as well as longitudinal distortions of neighboring veins may result. The mechanisms of injury just mentioned usually terminate in thrombosis, rarely in hemorrhage. As a rule, the skeletal injury dominates the clinical picture, so that the accompanying damage to the vein is frequently overlooked.*
A rare indirect lesion is tearing of the inferior vena cava at its point of emergence through the diaphragm, caused by blunt abdominal trauma with tearing of the diaphragm. These injuries usually lead to death in a few moments. Isfort (1967) managed to save one patient by direct transperitoneal caval suture.

Iatrogenic Lesions

Iatrogenic venous trauma occurs sometimes as an associated injury in surgical interventions, and sometimes is due to puncture or radiation (Table 9.3).
Among surgical injuries, penetrating lesions of the venous wall due to scalpel or scissors predominate. Less frequently blunt contusions of a main vein occur from pressure of a hook or as a result of unintended ligature (e.g., ligature of the common femoral vein instead of the great saphenous vein in operations for varicosities, and piercing or ligation of the external iliac vein during suturing in the Bassini operation. Among puncture injuries those of a mechanical-technical nature must be emphasized. Large perivenous hematomas may cause compression and thrombosis of a vein as a result of secondary bleeding from a puncture channel. This applies specifically in exploratory operations by introduction of catheters (e.g., cardiac catheterization). Wall dissection of large body veins produced by intramural injection is extremely rare. On the other hand, a relatively rigid catheter point or the mandrin may perforate large veins. Broken-off catheter points may embolize to the right heart or pulmonary arteries (Nissen-Druey, 1966; Wellmann, 1967; Pässler et al., 1972). A wrong injection—an error in site or mode or in quantity or concentration of the injected solution—is another possible cause of iatrogenic venous lesion (air or foreign-body embolism, chemicotoxic

*Recently, two important articles on venous injuries in fractures of the leg appeared (Spieler et al., 1972; Nylander and Semb, 1972). They show that this type of lesion is practically the rule, and hence post-traumatic thromboses are extremely common if preventive measures are not employed.

Table 9.3 Iatrogenic Vascular Damage (From Vollmar, J.: Rekonstruktive Chirurgie der Arterien. Thieme, Stuttgart, 1967)

Localization	Mechanism	Sequelae
Arterial	Operative injury to wall blunt (contusion, ligature) sharp (cut, stab, perforation)	1. Vascular occlusion (thrombosis, embolism), possibly ischemic tissue damage 2. Hemorrhage 3. Arteriovenous fistula
	Damage by puncture mechanical-technical mural dissection (intramural injection) injury to intima, detachment of arteriosclerotic plaques or mural thrombi	
Venous	Wrong injection (chemicotoxic or embolic) error of type, quantity, or concentration (air, mercury) error of site (intra-arterial instead of intravenous, intranervous or paranervous) Radiation damage	

damage of the intima with subsequent venous thrombosis). Thus, erroneous injection of an obliterating agent into the deep venous system or into an artery is usually followed by catastrophic consequences. Iatrogenic arteriovenous fistulas are due to combined damage of artery and accompanying vein, for example, by simultaneous ligation of arterial and venous stump on extirpation of an organ (nephrectomy, splenectomy, thyroidectomy) or by a combined penetrating lesion (arteriovenous fistula between terminal aorta and common iliac vein after surgery for intervertebral disk–Vollmar, 1968b).

An evaluation of 64 iatrogenic vascular lesions is shown in Table 9.4. Arterial injuries are numerically dominant, with 64 per cent. It is a fact worth noting that of 30 venous lesions requiring reconstruction, no less than seven, that is, almost one quarter, were iatrogenic (Table 9.5).

Table 9.4 Localization, Mechanism, and Sequelae of 64 Iatrogenic Vascular Injuries (From Vollmar, J.: Langenbecks Arch. klin. Chir. 322 (1968) 335)

Localization	Mechanism	Sequelae
Arterial 41	Operative injury of wall 48	Vascular stenosis 54
Venous 17	Injury due to puncture 12	Hemorrhage 8
Combined 6	Radiation damage 4	Arteriovenous fistula 2

Table 9.5 Injuries of Large Veins, Reconstructed (1960–1968)

Traumatic injuries	23*
Inferior vena cava	2
Common iliac vein	2
Brachiocephalic vein	1
Brachial vein	10
Axillary vein	1
Femoral vein	5
Popliteal vein	2
Iatrogenic injuries	**7**
Inferior vena cava (nephrectomy)	1
Inferior vena cava (aortoiliac plastic operation)	2
External iliac vein (ureterotomy)	1
External iliac vein (Bassini operation)	1
Common femoral vein (varicotomy)	1
Common iliac vein (broken intramural catheter)	1

*17 of them with arterial trauma (74 per cent).

Surgical Procedures

In the case of external bleeding of a limb, temporary hemostasis is obtained by application of pressure bandages (after aseptic dressing of the wound). The patient should be transported with the limb raised (to improve venous drainage after compression).

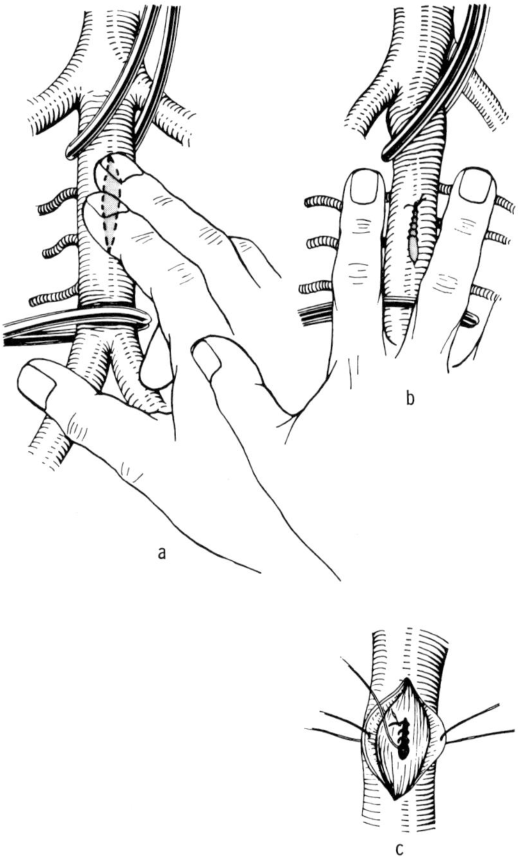

Fig. 9.1. Surgical procedure for inferior vena cava injury. Provisional hemostasis by digital pressure at the site of the lesion (best done by an assistant) (*a*). Meantime, preparatory isolation of the vena cava centrally and peripherally to the wall lesion is done. The vena cava is closed centrally and peripherally by hemostat, digital pressure is applied to the lateral inflowing lumbar veins (without isolating them) and the longitudinal tear is closed by continuous overhand sutures (suture material of 4–0 or 5–0) (*b*). For transluminal closure of a lesion at the posterior wall, the ventral opening in the vessel is enlarged by longitudinal incision and the posterior wall is closed by continuous suture (*c*). When there is great loss of lumen, the ventral gap of the cava is closed by marsupialization of a strip graft.

Attempts at provisional hemostasis at the place of accident by entering the wound and applying crushing forceps are contraindicated, since these maneuvers usually cause irreversible damage to vessel walls. Application of a *tourniquet*, using an Esmarch bandage or a sphygmomanometer cuff, runs the risk of producing too much pressure at the wound, so that venous backflow via collateral veins is impeded while arterial inflow is preserved. This results in excessive swelling of the limb and possibly increased bleeding.

If a lesion of a pelvic vein or the vena cava is suspected, the immediate measures are limited to replenishing the circulatory volume (blood transfusion, plasma expander). Because of the risk of exsanguination, transportation of the injured must be prompt and fast so that surgical control can be achieved as early as possible.

In injuries of the inferior vena cava, infusions should be given via the upper extremities, and in those of the superior vena cava, via the lower extremities; otherwise increased bleeding would result (Wood, 1966). If the patient does not respond to treatment of shock, exploratory thoracotomy or laparotomy must be performed immediately. In injuries of the superior vena cava, a preoperative full-size x-ray of the thorax is usually of diagnostic value (showing enlargement of the mediastinal shadow due to hematoma, hemothorax, an associated lesion of the lungs with pneumothorax, fractures of ribs and so forth). Contrast radiographs of the venae cavae usually only take time and are of limited diagnostic value. On surgical revision, digital pressure at the site of the venous lesion is the simplest and surest method of controlling bleeding (Fig. 9.1) (Starzl et al., 1962). Until hemostatic clamps have been applied atraumatically, preparation of the injured vein centrally and peripherally is carried out under digital control. Revision of large perivenous hematomas should in principle be performed only after the afferent and efferent main veins have been controlled, because of the possibility of instantaneous interruption of the bloodstream. Clearing the hematoma may otherwise trigger grave, profuse hemorrhage.

Choice of Surgical Procedure

Vascular Ligation

This is applied if the injury affects superficial subcutaneous veins and deep veins distal to the elbow and knee joints. Also, extended injuries in the knee and thigh or elbow and arm segments, whose restoration might require vascular grafting, should generally be tended by vascular ligation. Ligation in the pelvis (external and common iliac vein or inferior vena cava) is justifiable today only if severe associated injuries prohibit a protracted reconstructive vascular intervention.

With ligation of the inferior vena cava above the orifice of the renal veins there is a high risk of acute renal insufficiency, although with preservation of the left kidney, recovery of renal function is quite possible within a few days thanks to a rapidly established collateral circulation (review in Vollmar et al., 1973). Infrarenal ligation of the inferior vena cava is usually readily tolerated, but marked venous insufficiency of the lower extremities may result, the degree depending on the quality of the collateral circulation and supervention of a descending venous thrombosis (Shea and Robertson, 1951). Ligatures in the area of injured large visceral veins (lienal, renal and superior and inferior mesenteric veins) do not generally jeopardize survival of the corresponding organs since venous drainage is secured by collaterals in most cases. Ligation of the portal vein, however, is deleterious. It is generally accepted that ligatures in the area of the superior vena cava and its main branches are better tolerated than those of the inferior vena cava (because of absent or less hydrostatic pressure in the erect position, less flow minute volume and better chances of collateralization). Ligature of one internal jugular vein is easily tolerated; bilateral ligature usually has deleterious consequences.

If there is a prolonged interval between trauma and surgical intervention (more than 4 hours), thrombosis due to stagnation will very frequently follow in the venous system above and below the injury. The thrombus should first be removed completely, and from the vein being ligated as well (introduction of a Fogarty catheter or ring stripper and bandaging of the extremities centripetally with an Esmarch bandage—(Vollmar, 1966). This procedure considerably improves conditions for establishment of sufficient collateral circulation.

Another principle that requires attention when ligating injured veins is that the central (efferent) vein should be as far distal to the next lateral venous branch as possible. In this manner, "silent water zones" with formation of embolizing stagnation thrombi are avoided (Cook and Haller, 1962) (Fig. 9.2).

Thus, for example, in a lesion of the subclavian vein that cannot be reconstructed, it is best to ligate it directly before its junction with the internal jugular vein. In the area of the venae cavae, the points of reference are the junctions of the paired lumbar veins, and at the femoral, the junction with the deep femoral (ligation of the

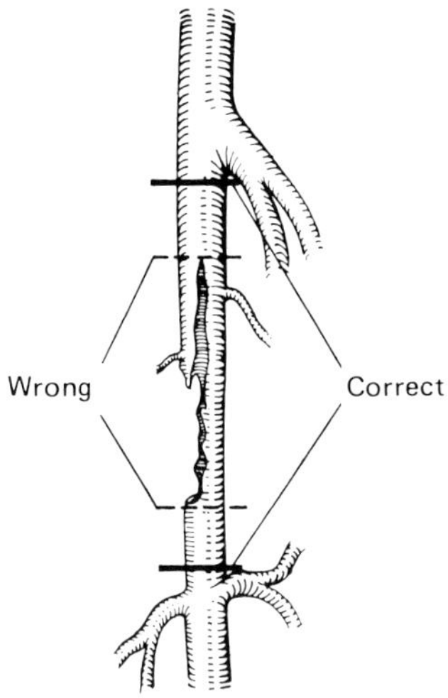

Fig. 9.2. Ligation of injured main veins when reconstruction of the flow path is impossible; to avoid "silent water zones," the ligature should be placed centrally and distally closely in front of or after junction with a large branch.

superficial femoral vein immediately distal to this vein). After each ligation of a main deep vein, strict compression treatment by elevation of the limb is required. The same therapeutic principles apply as for thrombectomy in deep vein thrombosis. If no concomitant lesions prohibit early mobilization, the patient should get out of bed with a pressure bandage on the second postoperative day to prevent propagation of an ascending or descending deep vein thrombus.

Reconstructive Surgery

Reconstructive surgery in trauma of large veins is indicated in all lesions of main veins proximal to the elbow and knee joints. This recent conception is considerably restricted, however. In the femoropopliteal segment, reconstructive interventions are at present justifiable only when there is a direct penetrating injury that can be reconstructed by immediate suture.* Otherwise, the main vein is ligated. In injuries of the superior and inferior vena cava, an attempt to maintain the venous blood flow should be made in any case.

For the success of surgical reconstruction three factors are of decisive importance:

—complete removal of thrombi from the venous afferent and efferent stream (free run-in and run-off);

—short time interval between injury and reconstruction (surgery within 4-hour limit when possible); and

—preferably autoplastic reconstruction under control of blood coagulation (systematic intravenous administration of heparin).

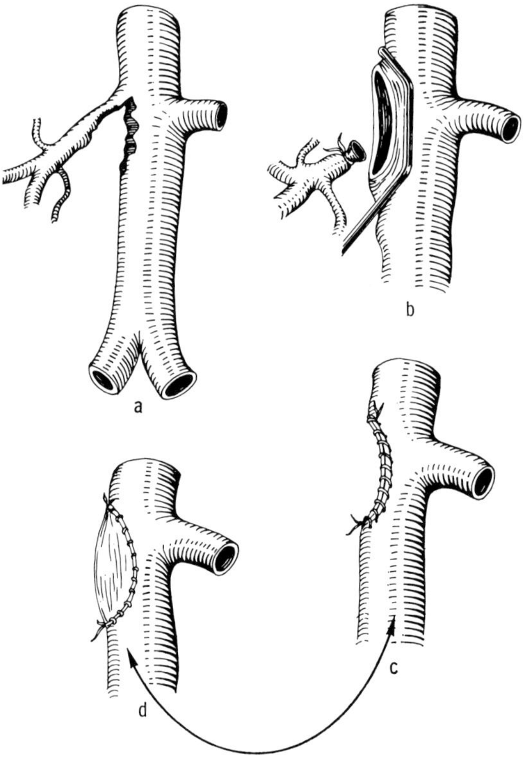

Fig. 9.3. Surgery of a caval defect with partial tear of the right renal vein: (*a*) Site of vessel. (*b*) Closure of the lateral caval defect by tangentially placed Satinski clamp; if the lesion is in close proximity to the vena cava, the renal vein can be ligated and the kidney preserved (sufficient venous drainage via testicular, ureteric, adrenal and capsular veins). (*c*) Surgery of the caval defect by means of lateral quilted sutures; narrowing of the lumen up to 50 per cent generally has no important hemodynamic effect. (*d*) Surgery of the caval defect by marsupialization of a venous strip graft (from the great saphenous vein).

*Brunner (1966): Direct end-to-end suture of the injured vein is not infrequently followed by suture thrombosis, which, however, remains limited segmentally, so that the normal vein connects distally and proximally with an elastic wall and sufficient valves. This localized suture thrombosis is usually recanalized in a few months so that in the end no loss of function results. Brunner furthermore advocates reconstruction of the functionally important common femoral vein.

The domain of reconstructive venous surgery includes penetrating and blunt injuries of the main veins of pelvis and venae cavae.

Direct suturing. Linear tears or sharp (partial or complete) divisions of large-caliber trunk veins can usually be repaired without difficulty by continuous atraumatic vessel suture (Mersilene, grade 4–0 or 5–0) in the majority of cases. An important requirement is perfect visibility, i.e., temporary interruption of the bloodstream (digital pressure by an assistant or application of artery forceps). The presence of thrombi in both inflow and outflow must be excluded by introduction of a balloon catheter or ring stripper from the site of the lesion both peripherally and centrally; if they are present, they are removed. In order to avoid air embolism the wound should be placed below the level of the right atrium (e.g., by raising the upper trunk in leg and pelvic injuries) and stopping respiration.

Lesions of the posterior wall of the vena cava may cause considerable technical difficulties, especially if tears of the dorsal lumbar veins are present simultaneously. Careful circular isolation of the cava, dissection of the lumbar veins and their ligation and division usually permit adequate rotation of the cava, so that the site of the lesion can safely be closed by atraumatic suture. Another solution is transluminal suture of the posterior caval wall (Field, 1965; Quast et al., 1965) (Fig. 9.1*c*).

In lateral defects of large-caliber main veins it is more useful to stop bleeding by means of lateral quilted sutures and to accept a relative stenosis than to perform a vessel graft, for instance (Fig. 9.3). Narrowing of the lumen to 50 per cent is of no practical importance hemodynamically (Wood, 1966). So far caval thromboses have not been observed when this method was used. An alternative is marsupialization of a strip graft.

In combined injuries of vein and artery, both vessels should, whenever feasible, be reconstructed if they are important main vessels proximal to the knee and elbow joints.* The prototype of this combined lesion is encountered in partial or complete severance of limbs. Experience in the last few years with reimplantation of limbs has underlined the great importance of venous suture for successful treatment.

Reimplantation is carried out in five surgical stages: (1) osteosynthesis, if practicable with shortening of the bone; (2) reconstruction of the venous path (direct end-to-end suture); (3) arterial suture; (4) joining of the nerve stumps; and finally (5) suture of the remaining soft tissues. It is important always to reconstruct the venous passages prior to arterial connection. Otherwise excessive edema usually results.

For technical details and results of treatment, the reader is referred to more specific publications (Vollmar, 1967; Malt, 1972).

In injuries of the superior and inferior vena cava, associated lesions of neighboring organs are almost regularly encountered (Quast et al., 1965; Wood, 1965). Below the diaphragm these are chiefly the duodenum, stomach, liver and pan-

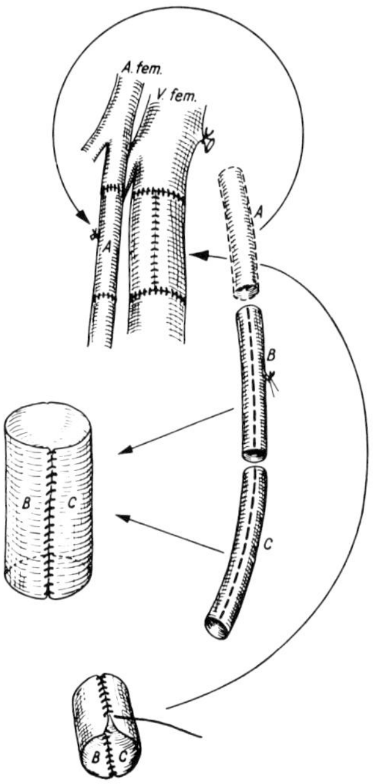

Fig. 9.4. Procedure in combined lesion of femoral artery and superficial femoral vein using autoplastic venous grafts from the ipsilateral long saphenous vein. (From Vollmar, J.: Rekonstruktive Chirurgie der Arterien. Thieme, Stuttgart, 1967.)

A, Segment of saphenous vein for interposition into the arterial stream.

B and *C*, Two venous segments are split longitudinally and sewn together along their longitudinal margins; a graft of double circumference results.

*The vast medical experience of the Vietnam war taught that in combined injuries of artery and vein in the extremities, reconstruction of both vessels is highly important. If, despite successful reconstruction of the popliteal artery, the leg had to be amputated, the reason was frequently nonrestoration of the popliteal vein (venous backflow not safeguarded). The procedure was either direct suture or autogenous venous graft. If the vein remains patent for at least 24 to 72 hours, collaterals may form. In addition, recanalization of the thrombosed vein or even of a venous graft is a common event. The leg was lost in some cases solely because of tearing of the popliteal vein, the popliteal artery being intact.

creas; in the thorax, the lungs, supra-aortic arteries and vertebral column with spinal cord (especially in bullet wounds). The prognosis as regards life depends decisively on recognition and proper attention to these accompanying lesions.

Reconstruction by grafts. For biologic reasons, autologous venous grafts occupy first place for reconstructive surgery of veins. Correction of partial defects of venous walls by venous strip grafts (patches) present no special problems (Fig. 9.3*d*). Considerably more complicated are the

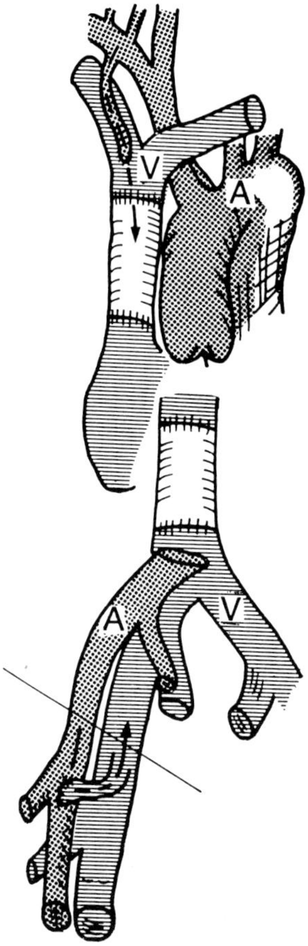

Fig. 9.5. Temporary arteriovenous fistula as a protective device in reconstructive intervention on large veins. For the inferior vena cava and pelvic veins, a flapped shunt is made below the inguinal ligament, using the great saphenous vein. For subclavian veins and the superior vena cava, the pedicled shunt of the mobilized internal thoracic artery and subclavian vein can be interrupted by simple ligation after 3 to 4 months. (From Vollmar, J.: Plastische Eingriffe an den tiefen Venen. In: Kappert, A., and May, R.: Das postthrombotische Zustandsbild der Extremitäten. Huber, Bern, 1968.)

conditions requiring complete substitution of wide-lumen veins, as for example the common iliac vein or inferior vena cava. No autologous vein graft of similar lumen size is available. Compound grafts from the long saphenous vein have proved useful, however (Fig. 9.4).

Synthetic grafts should be avoided whenever possible. Owing to the slight flow velocity and the low intravascular pressure, thrombosis of the graft occurs even in the caval and iliac segments (40 to 70 per cent of all cases). A new method of improving results with alloplastic veins, especially in the caval area, is creation of a temporary arteriovenous fistula (Bryant et al., 1958; Stansel, 1964; Vollmar et al., 1973) (Fig. 9.5). This increases flow velocity with only minor rise in venous pressure in the reconstructed vessel segment. It thus protects the graft to a certain degree. The arteriovenous fistula can be closed 3 months later.

In unilateral lesions of the pelvic venous system, a venovenous bypass should be considered in place of orthotopic vessel reconstruction. Because of its technical simplicity, the transverse femorofemoral in situ bypass (Palma and Esperon, 1950) is of great practical importance (Fig. 9.6). For protection of prolonged patency of this graft, we have recently been using a temporary arteriovenous fistula here also (bucket handle shunt between the central stump of the great saphenous vein on the injured side and the common femoral artery, with end-to-side connection—Vollmar, 1968a).

Correction of iatrogenic venous damage offers no particular problems to the vascular surgeon. Prompt recognition and prompt correction are decisive for success. This is especially true when the main vein in the thigh and pelvis has been inadvertently ligated.

After the site of the ligature is freed, the thread is cut and the vein in this area opened by longitudinal incision. Complete removal of stagnation thrombi from the inflow and outflow paths is essential. If the ligature has produced no marked damage to the wall, it is advisable to marsupialize an ovoid venous strip graft from the great saphenous vein into the venotomy.

The suspended suture recommended by Kunlin (1961), which relaxes tension of the vascular anastomosis, presents an interesting conception for improvement of results in reconstructive surgery of the veins. This technique of anastomosis appears to us to be of little importance in the care of venous trauma, however, since the vascular lesion is strictly localized and the risk of collapse of the anastomosis is extremely small with a free inflow and outflow. A rapid and atraumatic vascular reconstruction with strict

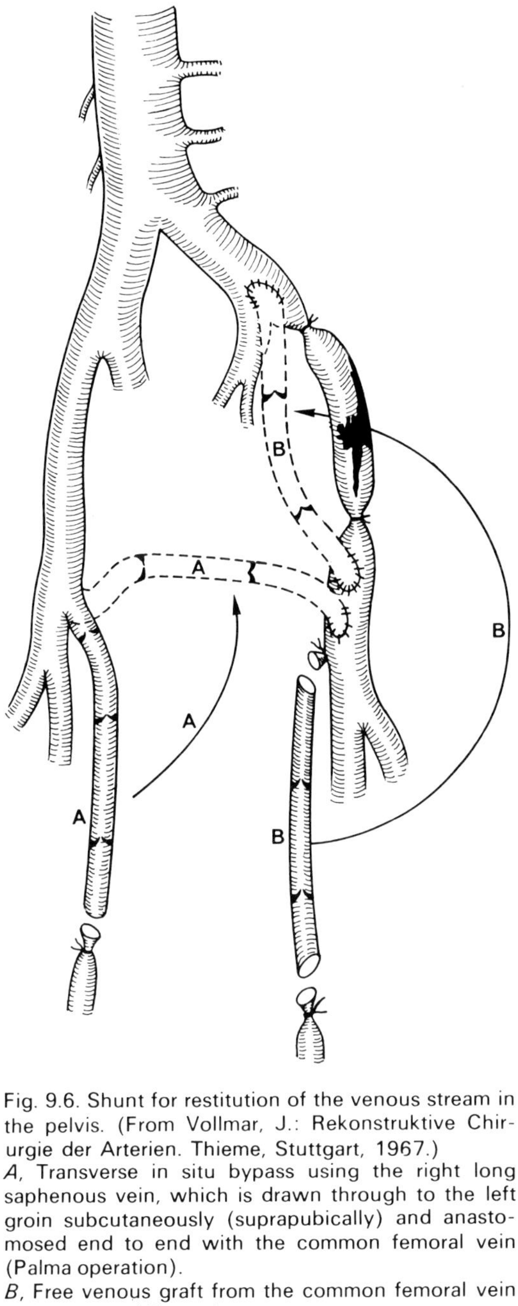

Fig. 9.6. Shunt for restitution of the venous stream in the pelvis. (From Vollmar, J.: Rekonstruktive Chirurgie der Arterien. Thieme, Stuttgart, 1967.)
A, Transverse in situ bypass using the right long saphenous vein, which is drawn through to the left groin subcutaneously (suprapubically) and anastomosed end to end with the common femoral vein (Palma operation).
B, Free venous graft from the common femoral vein to the external iliac vein.

control of clotting and restoration of a free run-in and run-off are the pivots of surgical success, in our experience.
Of 30 cases of venous injury requiring reconstructive intervention, lasting restoration of venous flow was achieved by direct suturing or grafting in 26. Best results were seen in those cases in which restitution by direct vascular suture was practicable.

Sequelae to Venous Injuries

A venous lesion may be followed by three important clinical conditions:
—venous embolism,
—post-thrombotic syndrome, and
—arteriovenous fistula.

An air embolism is usually an immediate or early complication; originating in the majority of cases from open or penetrating injuries of the superior vena cava or its great branches (jugular, subclavian or arm veins). Also, pneumothorax may be the cause of an air embolism in a simultaneous lesion of an intrathoracic vein, as Ellis and Brown (1964) observed; its occurrence depends on the combination of gaping wounds and intermittent negative pressure in the great thoracic veins. Intravenous infusions under pressure are the most frequent cause of iatrogenic air embolism.
Since introduction of intubation anesthesia with alternating pressure respiration, intraoperative air embolism due to opening of large veins, e.g., in surgery of the thyroid or intrathoracic organs, has become a great rarity. Still, though, open heart surgery with incomplete ventilation prior to release of the bloodstream is followed by air embolism usually of a cerebral artery. In addition, in surgery of venous injuries, especially of the cervical and caval veins, there is always danger of air embolism (for prophylaxis, see p. 197).
Thromboembolism after venous injuries originates from post-traumatic venous thrombosis. Unlike air embolism, thromboembolism appears several days after the injury. Stagnation thrombi may also embolize into the right heart and lung as a result of inexpert choice of the site of venous ligation (Cook and Haller, 1962). Overall, thromboembolic complications appear to be more common after lesions of the inferior vena cava and its branches than after lesions of the superior vena cava. Foreign body embolism after venous injury is extremely rare, apart from iatrogenic dispersion of broken venous catheters, guide wires, and the like. Popper (1966) reported a grotesque incident: on shaking down a clinical thermometer, a 19-year-old nursing student nicked a vein on the dorsum of her hand with the point of the thermometer. She died of disseminated mercury embolism in the small pulmonary arteries.
The sequelae of a post-traumatic venous occlu-

sion essentially depend on its localization and extent and on the quality of the collateral circulation.

The degree of spontaneous recanalization after post-traumatic venous occlusion has not yet been clarified. It may be assumed that the severity and extent of the primary damage of the vessel wall are decisive. According to clinical experience, after surgical ligation of an injured vein, spread of central and distal stagnation thrombosis depends entirely on hemodynamic conditions, i.e., on the distance to the next large venous branch that can act as a collateral vein.

The sequelae to ligation of important main veins at different vascular levels are discussed on page 194f.

Therapy of post-traumatic venous occlusion is basically the same as that for the post-thrombotic syndrome of other origin (p. 135ff).

Post-traumatic arteriovenous fistula is a matter of a combined vascular lesion of artery and vein. In most cases it follows a perforating injury by a small projectile or a sharp foreign body (such as a knife). The diagnosis is made only exceptionally in the stage of acute injury; usually it is discovered only after an interval of weeks or months. The aim of the therapy in each case is elimination of the arteriovenous short circuit as early as practicable, with preservation of artery and vein if possible, when large vessels proximal to the knee and elbow joints are involved (for surgical technique, see Vollmar, 1967).

Elimination of the arteriovenous shunt causes a drastic reduction of flow velocity and volume in the area of the venous branch of the vessel. Correspondingly, there is a postoperative risk of venous thrombosis, especially after closure of an arteriovenous fistula in the lower part of the body. Elevation of the limb on a splint, early mobilization and firm pressure bandages are routine measures of prevention.

References

Bolot, F., J. Germain, R. Ponson, J. Massotte: Bullet wound of the inferior vena cava above the renal pedicles: ligature of the vena cava. Mém. Acad. chir. 81 (1955) 393

Brunner, U.: Kasuistik zu den Problemen peripherer Venenverletzungen. Zbl. Phleb. 5 (1966) 121–130

Bryant, M. F., Jr. W. D. Lazenby, J. M. Howard: Experimental replacement of short segments of veins. Arch. Surg. 76 (1958) 289

Buckner, F., Ch. Lyons, R. Perkins: Management of lacerations of the great vessels of the upper thorax and base of the neck. Surg. Gynec. Obstet. 107 (1958) 135–142

Cook, F. W., J. A. Haller: Penetrating injuries of the subclavian vessels with associated venous complications. Ann. Surg. 155 (1962) 370

Duke, J. H., R. C. Jones, G. T. Shires: Management of injuries to the inferior vena cava. Amer. J. Surg. 110 (1965) 759–763

Ellis, G. R., J. R. Brown: Massive air embolism due to gunshot wound. J. Amer. med. Ass. 189 (1964) 953

Ellis, P. R., Jr.: Med. Trib. med. News 2 (1967) 2

Field, S. E., Jr.: Transluminal repair of penetrating injury of the inferior vena cava. Amer. Surg. 31 (1965) 6–8

Hjelmstedt, A., U. Bergvall: Incidence of thrombosis in patients with tibial fractures. Acta chir. scand. 134 (1968) 1

Hjelmstedt, A., U. Bergvall: Phlebographic study of the incidence of thrombosis in the injured and uninjured limb in 55 cases of tibial fracture. Acta chir. scand. 134 (1968) 229–234

Holle, F., W. Hart: Die Verletzungen venöser Gefäße und ihre Komplikationen unter besonderer Berücksichtigung der Begutachtung. Unfallheilk. 81 (1965) 74

Holt, M. H., F. J. Lewis: Experimental grafts of the superior vena cava with temporary arteriovenous shunts. J. thorac. cardiovasc. Surg. 49 (1965) 818

Isfort, A.: Isolierte Ruptur der Vena cava inferior zwischen Zwerchfell und Leber, eine seltene Folge nach stumpfem Thoraxtrauma. Thoraxchir. 14 (1967) 621

Kappert, A., R. May: Das postthrombotische Zustandsbild der Extremitäten. Huber, Bern 1968

Kunlin, J.: Techniques de la suture veineuse suspendue. Presse méd. 69 (1961) 1917

Malt, R. A., I. P. Remensnyder, W. H. Harris; Long-term utility of replanted arms. Ann. Surg. 176 (1972) 334

Nissen-Druey, C. Iatrogene Fremdkörperembolie. Münch. med. Wschr. 108 (1966) 788

Nylander, G., H. Semb: Veins of the lower part of the leg after tibial fractures. Surg. Gynec. Obstet. 134 (1972) 974–976

Pässler, H. H., H. Henkemeyer, C. Burri: Gefahren des Kava-Katheterismus. Helv. Chir. acta 39 (1967) 101

Palma, E. C., R. Esperon: Vein transplants and grafts in the surgical treatment of the postphlebitic syndrome. J. cardiovasc. Surg. 1 (1950) 94

Popper, L.: Tod nach Thermometerverletzung. Wien. med. Wschr. 116 (1966) 779

Quast, D. C., A. L. Shirkey, J. B. Fitzgerald, A. C. Beall Jr., M. E. De Bakey: Surgical correction of injuries of the vena cava: an analysis of sixty-one cases. J. Trauma 5 (1965) 3–10

10 Malformations of Leg and Pelvic Veins

J. Vollmar

Congenital anomalies of the venous system have attained increasing clinical importance since the development and general application of cardiovascular studies (angiocardiography, cardiac catheterization, venography). In this chapter, certain junctional and valvular anomalies, including structural changes in the venous wall and anomalies causing primary varicosis on a hereditary basis, will be excluded. The reader is referred to page 82ff for discussion of them. Knowledge of the development of the venous system is required for understanding of the vascular anomalies to be discussed.

Embryology

The primary venous system of the human embryo has a symmetric bilateral anlage in the fourth to fifth weeks (Fig. 10.1). Two cranial and two caudal cardinal veins drain the venous blood from the upper and lower parts of the body into the sinus venosus via two common collectors (right and left common cardinal veins). The omphalomesenteric veins join the confluence of the two cardinal veins in the midline. The omphalomesenteric veins are penetrated and surrounded by proliferating hepatic cords in the septum transversum. Thus, liver capillaries arise on the one hand, and liver veins as hepatic drainage to the right atrium on the other. This omphalomesenteric differentiation occurs simultaneously with development of the *subcardinal veins*, which form an extended venous plexus in the region of the mesonephron. Transverse vascular bridges are described as *intersubcardinal anastomoses*. The *pars hepatica* of the inferior vena cava originates from the right subcardinal vein; the *pars renalis* is made up of the intersubcardinal anastomoses. This metamorphosis in the median vascular zone is accompanied by involution of cardinal and remaining subcardinal veins, and by the appearance of a third, initially paired, venous system, the *supracardinal veins*, which later become the azygos system. The right supracardinal vein becomes the *pars infrarenalis* of the inferior vena cava.

It is significant that the development of the large body veins is closely connected with that of the heart. Cardiac asymmetry commences toward the end of the third embryonic week. Drainage of body and pulmonary veins is determined in the ensuing 4 weeks. Hence, determination of body veins is simultaneous with the basic phase of cardiac development, when torsion, looping and septation occur under the influence of the embryonal bloodstream (Goerttler, 1955, 1958, 1963). This explains why most anomalies of junction, course and anlage of the superior and inferior cava are associated with anomalies of the heart. Developmental disturbances of the cranial cardinal veins or the later superior vena cava are more frequent than those of the caudal cardinal veins (Goerttler, 1958; Anderson et al., 1961).

Anomalies of the Inferior Vena Cava

In contrast to anomalies of the superior vena cava, those of the inferior vena cava are much more infrequent. Solitary anomalies are a rarity. The commonest *combined malformations* are partial or total *visceral inversion* in thorax and

Table 10.1. Survey of the Most Important Congenital Malformations of Veins in the Lower Half of the Body

Inferior vena cava
Membranous stenosis and occlusion (pars diaphragmatica)
Aplasia of the pars hepatica (infrahepatic interruption with azygos continuation)
Duplication of or a left-ascending pars infrarenalis
Deep veins of the pelvis and legs
Aplasia or hypoplastic stenosis (in hemangiectatic hypertrophy = Klippel-Trenaunay syndrome)
Aplasia of valves (partial or complete)
Duplication and anomalous course and union of leg veins

abdomen, persistence of a left superior vena cava and various congenital anomalies of the heart (particularly septal defects, pulmonary stenosis, and transposition of the large vessels—Muelheims and Mudd, 1962; Bücheler et al., 1966. The most frequent malformations of the inferior vena cava are summarized in Table 10.1.

Congenital aneurysms of inferior vena cava and its tributaries have not been observed as far as we know. This type of venous aneurysm is restricted to the superior vena cava and jugular vein (Abbott, 1950; Abbott and Leigh, 1964; Kootstra, 1969). However, *acquired aneurysms* occur in the lower half of the body, most frequently along with excessive long-saphenous insufficiency, as a sequel to (acquired or congenital) *arteriovenous fistulas* (mural deficiency resulting from great flow volumes). A *congenital vascular bridge* between the left renal and lumbar veins (usually the left ascending) gains importance only in the pres-

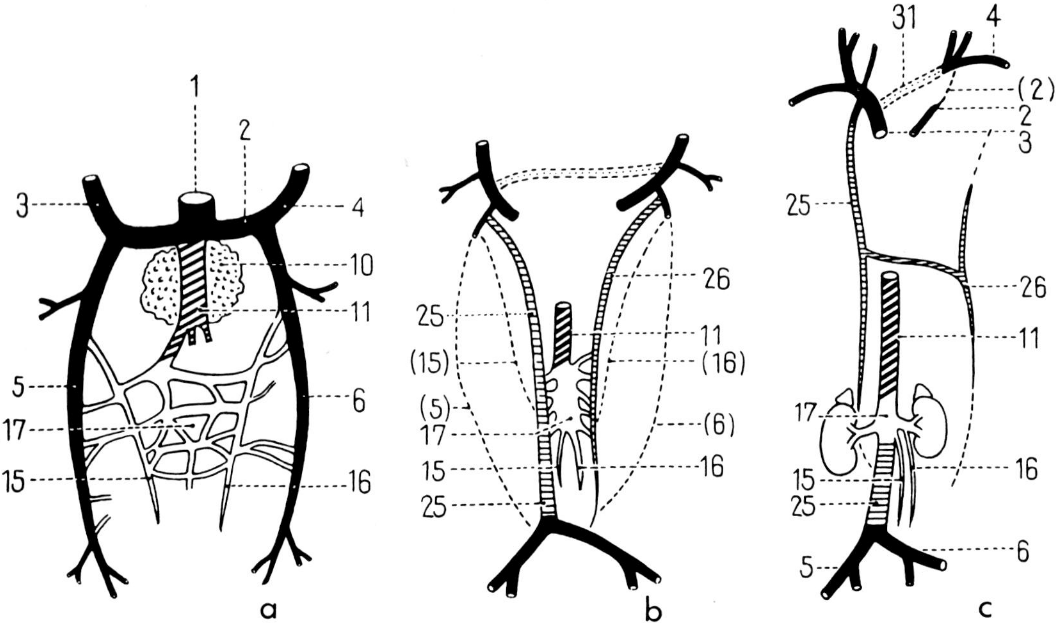

Fig. 10.1. Development of the venous system. Primary venous system (4 to 5 weeks), stage of largely morphologic symmetry (*a*). Secondary venous system (approximately 7 weeks), stage of increasing asymmetry, with predominant right supracardinal vein (*b*). Fully developed system of the large veins of the body (*c*). (From Elke, M., and H. Ludin: Fortschr. Röntgenstr. 103 (1965) 655.)

1 Sinus venosus
2 V. cardinalis communis sinistra (Ductus Cuvieri sinister) → Sinus coronarius
3 V. cardinalis cranialis dextra → V. cava superior, V. subclavia dextra, etc.
4 V. cardinalis cranialis sinistra → V. subclavia sinistra, V. jugularis sinistra, etc.
5 V. cardinalis caudalis dextra → Vv. iliacae dextrae
6 V. cardinalis caudalis sinistra → Vv. iliacae sinistrae
10 Rudimentary liver (venous tubes)
11 Venous sinuses of omphalomesenteric system and of right subcardial vein → Hepatic portion of inferior vena cava
15 V. subcardinalis dextra → V. ovarica or testicularis dextra
16 V. subcardinalis sinistra → V. ovarica or testicularis sinistra
17 Intersubcardinal anastomoses → Renal portion of inferior vena cava (the umbilical and omphalomesenteric veins flowing into the sinus venosus are omitted in the diagram)
25 Right supracardinal vein → Azygos (cranial portion) and right ascending lumbar vein → Caudal and subrenal portion of inferior vena cava
26 V. supracardinalis sinistra → V. hemiazygos, V. lumbalis ascendens sinistra
31 V. brachiocephalica (anonyma) sinistra
In parentheses: obliterating embryonic segments of veins

ence of pathologic conditions, namely, in obstruction of the left renal vein or inferior vena cava. This renolumbar venous anastomosis occurs in approximately every third person on the left and is only exceptionally seen on the right (Bücheler et al., 1968).

Membranous Stenosis and Occlusion in the Diaphragmatic Portion

These are partial or complete obstructions in the vena cava produced by valvular or septate membranes jutting into the lumen (Fig. 10.2). They are predominantly *situated* in the *pars diaphragmatica* (or pars hepatica), almost always proximal to the union with the *right* hepatic vein. The *left* hepatic vein was found to be occluded in most reports; its union lay above the membrane. In extreme cases, the caval lumen is totally interrupted by the membrane. Nevertheless,

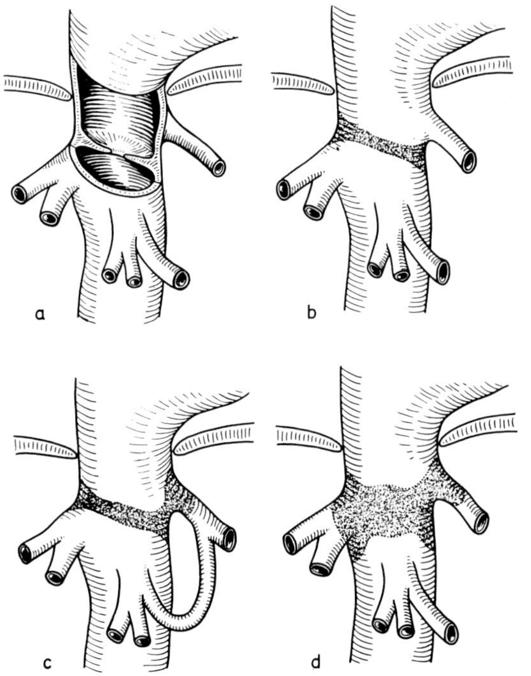

Fig. 10.2. Various forms of membranous stenosis of the inferior vena cava. Valvular stenosis (usually without hemodynamic significance) (*a*); complete membranous occlusion of the lumen (*b*), the left hepatic vein usually flowing into the free cranial, and the remainder into the caudal caval segment. Membranous occlusion includes the ostium of the left hepatic vein, which flows into the intermediate hepatic vein via a collateral (*c*); membranous occlusion with secondary thrombotic obstruction of the hepatic veins (*d*).

hemodynamic effects of drainage from the liver and lower half of the body are not serious because commonly a well developed collateral circulation has existed for many years.

Markedly dilated diaphragmatic veins reach the central caval portion as collaterals central to the membrane. Fibrotic obstruction of the left hepatic vein usually affects its junction. The distal portion of this vessel is frequently joined to the intermediate hepatic vein by a wide anastomotic arch running caudally and laterally (Fig. 10.2*c*).

Histologically, the membranes consist of connective tissue with an endothelial covering. They contain elastic but no muscle fibers (Kimura et al., 1963). The *liver* is usually much enlarged. Its surface is granular or nodular, and the thickened capsule adheres to the diaphragm. The liver is congested and cirrhotic.

Clinically, there is orthostatic edema and a marked collateral circulation visible on thorax and abdomen. Signs of *posthepatic block* (Budd-Chiari syndrome: hepatomegaly, splenomegaly, ascites and esophageal varices) are fully developed only when the hepatic veins have become occluded as well (Erlik et al., 1962; O'Hara et al., 1963; Eguchi et al., 1966).

These signs become *manifest* in the third decade as a rule. The course is eminently chronic. Remissions alternate with acute exacerbations. In the six observations of Kimura et al. (1963), the signs persisted for 2 to 10 years until operation or death. *Prognosis* depends on cardiac state, liver damage, possible thrombosis and the quality of the collateral circulation, in addition to the site and severity of the vascular block. Without surgery, death will occur sooner or later, usually from *hepatic coma* or *hemorrhage from esophageal varices.* Less common causes of death are intercurrent infection, thromboembolism and progressive cachexia.

The *first description* was presented by Bennett (1950). Up to 1970, 205 cases were observed and reported (Hirooka and Kimura, 1970). Only sporadic cases have appeared in the European and Anglo-American literature, however (Bennett, 1950; Boutelier and Couinaud, 1962; Watkins and Fortin, 1964).

The *causal* and *formal* genesis of membranous stenosis has not been elucidated. The proponents of the congenital hypothesis assume an inhibitory malformation of the venae revehentes, whereas others consider the membranes due to regression of the ductus venosus (Arantii). Extended obliteration of this fetal blood system, which joins the left hepatic vein, is supposed not only to occlude its junction but also to cause membranous constriction of the cava.

Kimura et al. (1963) compared this process with the development of aortic coarctation at the junction with the ductus arteriosus (Botalli). In fact, occasionally an externally visible, fusiform constriction of the inferior vena cava is found in addition to the membranous stenosis. Accordingly, Watkins and Fortin (1964) called the membranous stenosis *congenital coarctation of the vena cava*. The localization of this process and the common findings of valvular formations speak in favor of a congenital genesis. The relatively late manifestation of the stenosis is not a definite contradiction to this assumption, since undoubtedly, especially in the late stage, secondary thrombotic deposits increase it and may lead to complete obliteration of caval and hepatic veins. Bücheler et al. (1966) pointed out that the type of collateral circulation favors *acquired caval blockade* in the majority of cases; i.e., the almost regular persistence of embryonic veins seen in congenital caval interruption is absent. The geographic aspect also indicates this. Membranous stenosis has so far been observed almost exclusively in East Asiatics.

Indication for surgery. Surgery is indicated only when membranous stenosis of the vena cava clinically impairs drainage, i.e., when the Budd-Chiari syndrome is present or venous flow from the lower extremities is insufficient. Otherwise, surgical intervention is contraindicated in progressive cases with severe cirrhosis of the liver and cachexia.

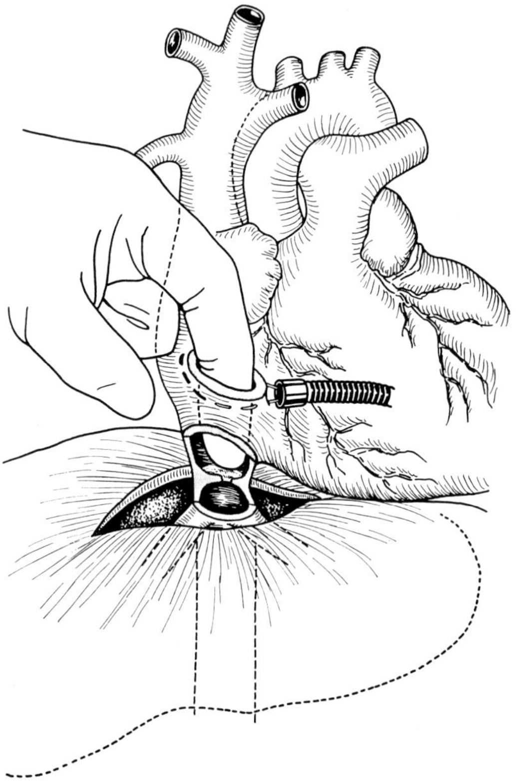

Fig. 10.3. Digital rupture of a membranous stenosis from the right atrium. Access by anterolateral thoracotomy (seventh or eighth right intercostal space); in addition, the diaphragm is split radially at the foramen of the vena cava in order to dilate the vein.

Surgical Procedure

In principle, two *methods* are available for correction of occlusion or stenosis of the inferior vena cava due to membranes:

Membranotomy and extirpation of membranes

—*half-closed, transcardial*, digital or instrumental rupture (Kimura et al., 1962b, 1963; Lamm et al., 1965; Hirooka and Kimura, 1970),

—*open direct method* (membrane extirpation under direct vision) (Watkins and Fortin, 1967).

Bypass operation (Ohara et al., 1963; Eguchi et al., 1966).

Indirect membranotomy (digital or instrumental, from the right atrium or right auricle) is the simplest and most commonly used procedure (Fig. 10.3), but it is suitable only when the membrane is thin. It precludes simultaneous correction of the hepatic vein ostia. Incomplete opening of the lumen and the risk of embolization are significant factors of uncertainty. These disadvantages are largely avoided by *open, direct membrane extirpation*, which, furthermore, permits exact revision of the hepatic vein ostia and should be considered first for cases in which secondary thrombosis is involved. The *bypass operation* requires operation on two cavities. The abdominal cavity may be avoided by using an extraperitoneal approach in cases of risk. The bypass operation precludes simultaneous correction of the hepatic vein ostia.

Open, Direct Membrane Extirpation

For this method (Fig. 10.4), the best approach to the upper portion of the inferior vena cava is by right *anterolateral* thoracotomy (seventh or eighth intercostal space). Additional laparotomy is required only exceptionally. The diaphragm is radially incised at the passage of the vena cava, with care to spare the phrenic nerve, and the inferior vena cava is circularly isolated at its junction with the right atrium and tightened. After the fixed portion is freed and the liver is folded back

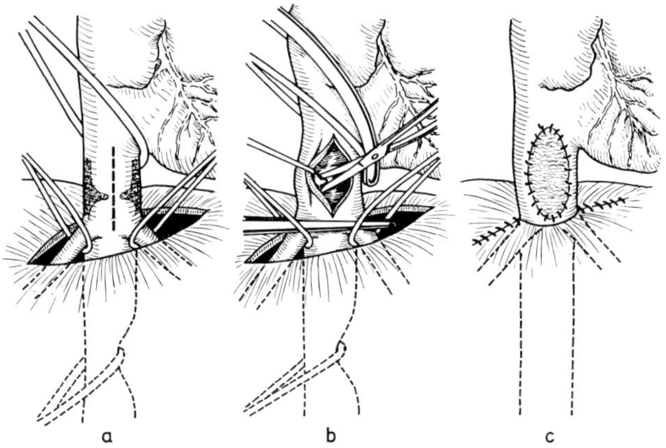

Fig. 10.4. Correction of membranous stenosis of the inferior vena cava by open excision. Exposure of the inferior cava transthoracically from the right (seventh or eighth intercostal space), radial splitting of the diaphragm at the foramen venae cavae, dissection of the junction with the hepatic veins (*a*); opening of vena cava longitudinally after total stoppage of blood flow, and excision of stenosing membrane under direct vision (*b*); closure of the cavotomy by implanting an oval patch graft and closure of the diaphragm (*c*).

around the cava, the union of the two or three hepatic veins is easily exposed. *Caval clamping* for the usual time of 10 to 15 minutes requires no particular protective measures. However, if prolonged interruption of the blood flow is anticipated, it is advisable to create a *venovenous shunt* from the common femoral to the right atrium or external jugular. A marked rise in pressure in the inferior vena cava and the portal system is thus avoided. Systemic (intravenous) administration of heparin is recommended for prevention of clot formation. Continuous recording of venous and arterial pressure is urged.

The vena cava is suitably exposed by *longitudinal incision*. Clear revision of the lumen and the junction of hepatic veins is thus ensured. The stenosing membrane is excised from the caval lumen, in conjunction with thrombectomy of the hepatic veins, if necessary. The venotomy is closed by continuous overhand suture (e.g. 4–0 Mersilene) or, with small-caliber vessels, by grafting a venous strip. The thoracotomy wound is closed by the usual technique with suction drainage for 24 hours.

Cavoatrial Bypass

This operation (Fig. 10.5), which is technically relatively easy, is justified only when the junctions of the hepatic veins are not involved in the occlusion. A *plastic prosthesis* (Dacron or Teflon) with a diameter of 14 to 16 mm is used as a graft. It is anastomosed caudally end to side with the infrahepatic portion of the inferior vena cava, the central insertion being end to side in the right atrium or auricle.

The inferior vena cava is exposed either by an incision in the right flank *extraperitoneally* or *transperitoneally* from in front (incision along the costal margin or transrectal or pararectal incision on the right). Exposure of the right atrium is best done by *anterolateral thoracotomy* (seventh or eighth right intercostal space). The operation begins with the caudal end-to-side anastomosis, with the vena cava clamped tangentially (with a Satinski clamp). The prosthesis is then drawn retroperitoneally to the right pleural cavity, preferably to the right of the cava, by means of dressing forceps pushed cranially against the diaphragm. An oval opening, large enough for the prosthesis to pass, is made in the diaphragm over the tip of the dressing forceps. The prosthesis is inserted only after it has

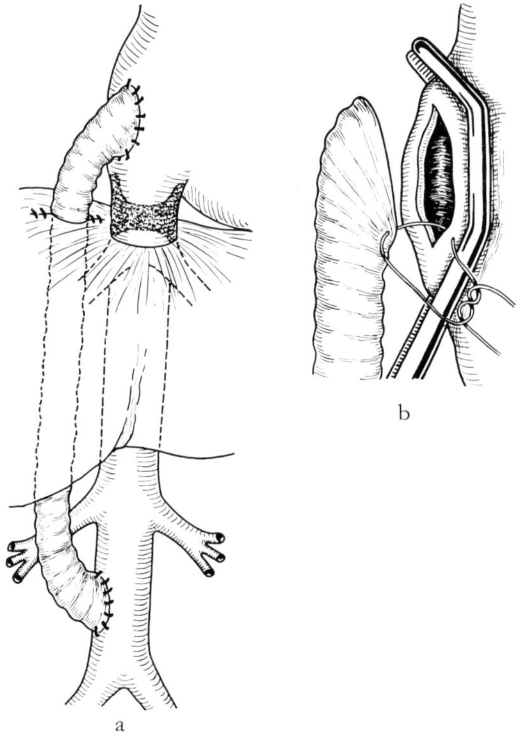

Fig. 10.5. Correction of membranous occlusion of the inferior vena cava by cavoatrial bypass. Dacron prosthesis (*a*) inserted retroperitoneally and transdiaphragmatically as a bypass graft. End-to-end anastomosis during partial clamping of atrial or caval wall with a Satinski clamp (*b*).

been sealed by preclotting with autologous blood. The operation is completed by end-to-side anastomosis of the central end of the prosthesis with the right atrium or the resected auricle or the terminal segment of the cava. Reliable, bloodless operating is safeguarded by partial exclusion of the atrial wall by means of an atraumatic Satinski clamp.

Complications

The chief danger of all reconstructive operations of the vena cava is intraoperative *air embolism*. In the first place, it occurs with inadvertent injuries of the cava during exposure. Adequate removal of air from the clamped segment of the vessel must be ensured before the bloodstream is released. *Thromboembolic complications* are to be feared especially when clamping is prolonged and clotting is insufficient because of heparin administration.

Aplasia of the Hepatic Portion

(infrahepatic interruption with azygos continuation)

In this congenital anomaly, the hepatic portion is absent; i.e., the renal segment of the inferior vena cava does not directly continue to the right atrium or the junction with the hepatic veins. Almost always there is the compensating malformation of persistence of the right, or occasionally the left, supracardinal vein. This means that the renal segment of the cava continues on the right directly into the azygos vein and flows into the superior vena cava by this vessel, which is compensatingly much dilated, in a ventromedial arch, the so-called azygos continuation (Anderson et al., 1955) (Fig. 10.6).

If the left supracardinal vein also persists, the cava on the left is continued by the dilated hemiazygos, which joins either the azygos in typical fashion or a persisting left-sided superior vena cava. The hepatic veins flow individually or as a common trunk into the right, or rarely into the left, atrium (Anderson et al., 1955; Muelheims and Mudd, 1962).

The azygos and hemiazygos replace the suprarenal cava in this anomaly, and also receive the portal vein in rare cases (Gould, 1953). The terminal segment of the azygos may contain aneurysms (Walker, 1963). If the renal and subrenal inferior caval segments are included in this developmental inhibition, the two persisting supracardinal veins may appear as large-caliber drains, ascending parallel with the vertebral column, and may mimic *duplication* of the whole cava (Fig. 10.7) (Elke and Ludin, 1965). In this case, the renal veins flow into the corresponding supracardinal vein.

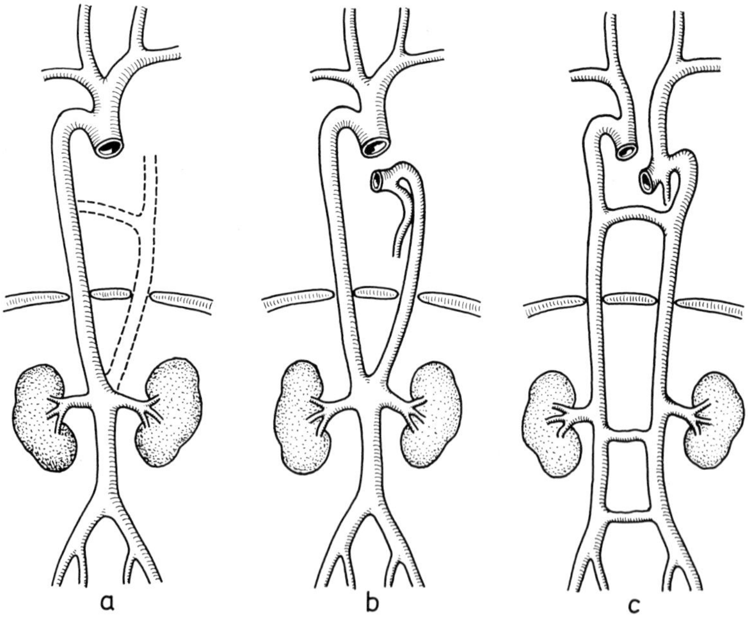

Fig. 10.6. Different forms of aplasia of the hepatic portion (so-called infrahepatic caval interruption with azygos continuation). Persistence of the right supracardinal vein, i.e., continuation of the renal cava segment into the compensatingly dilated right azygos (dashed line: additional persistence of the left supracardinal vein, i.e., caval continuation into hemiazygos ascending on the left and typical union with the terminal segment of the azygos) (*a*). Continuation of the cava into the azygos and hemiazygos, the latter flowing into the sinus venosus of the heart (*b*). Total duplication of inferior and superior cava; transverse bridges may persist in the lumbar and the thoracic portions between both main veins; separate junction of renal veins into the left or right substitute cava. The hemiazygos flows into the persisting left superior cava, entering the right atrium (or left atrium) via the sinus venosus (*c*).

Infrahepatic interruption of the inferior vena cava with azygos or hemiazygos continuation is the most common type of caval aplasia. It was first described by Stark in 1835 (in mammals), and first diagnosed angiographically in the living by Stackelberg et al. in 1952. Approximately 70 cases had been reported in the world literature by the end of 1968. Anderson et al. (1961) estimate the incidence of the anomaly without other cardiac defects to be less than 0.3 per cent; in combination with congenital heart disease the incidence is about 0.6 per cent. But it must be remembered that these data refer to selected patients (incidental diagnosis during cardiac catheterization).

Clinically, congenital anlage anomalies of the inferior vena cava are usually silent, unless they are associated with malformations of the heart or other organs (defects of the interventricular and interatrial septa, transposition of the large vessels, situs inversus or absence of the spleen). Venous drainage of the lower half of the body is only minimally affected, if at all.

The *diagnosis* can occasionally be guessed if there is a prominent azygos shadow (on a standard x-ray film of thorax) combined with increased venous markings of the anterior trunk and abdomen. Proof is obtained by *cavography*. The contrast medium flows from the inferior vena cava paravertebrally via the markedly dilated azygos, or the hemiazygos on the left, describing in its terminal section an arch similar to that of the aorta, the so-called candy cane phenomenon (Anderson et al., 1955, 1961). Also typical are difficulties in introducing the cardiac catheter from the long saphenous (the tip stops in the terminal azygos, and enters the right atrium in a cranioconvex arch via the superior vena cava). Most cases reported are incidental phlebographic or autopsy findings in patients with congenital heart disease.

The anomaly gains practical importance in *cardiac diagnosis* and *surgery* (absence of caval drainage). Inadvertent ligature of the azygos may cause death in these cases (Effler et al., 1951).

Surgical correction is hardly ever indicated since this venous anomaly is almost always associated with embryonically determined spontaneous correction. Exceptions are those cases in which the "substitute cava," ascending on the left, flows into the left atrium, producing a more or less marked degree of cyanosis. A left-sided inferior vena cava flowing into the left atrium may occasionally be encountered also without caval interruption (Loogen and Kreuzer, 1962).

Differential diagnosis. This anomaly must be distinguished from other forms of right-to-left shunts. Correction consists of transposing the caval junction into the right atrium (Gardner and Cole, 1955; Gautam, 1968).

Duplication and Left-Ascending Infrarenal Portion

Doubling and ascending on the left of the caudal caval segment reveal many morphologic variants

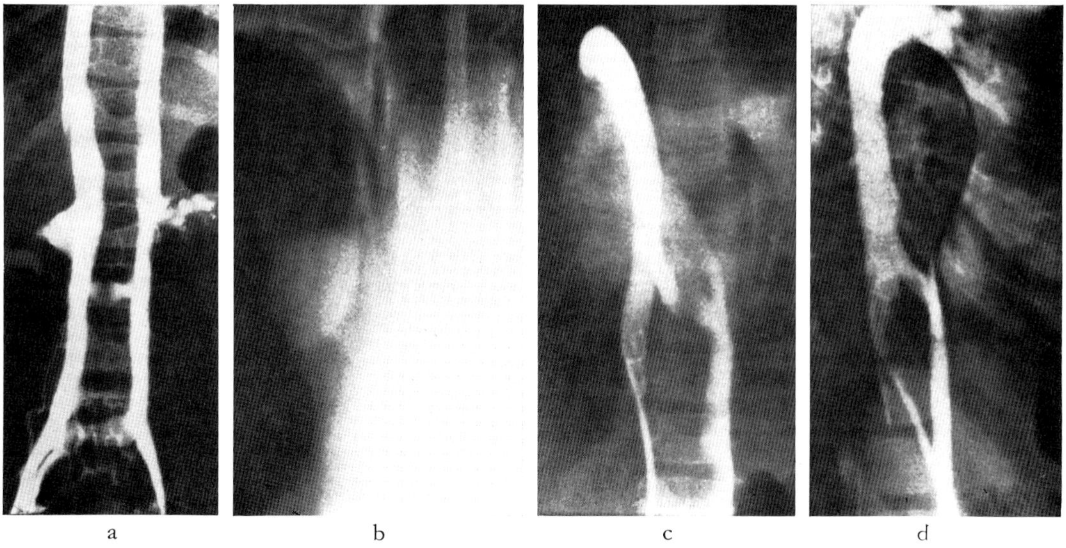

Fig. 10.7. Early embryologic disturbance of the inferior vena cava. Persistent supracardinal veins, which reveal several distinct transverse connections at the level of L5, L3 and T10. The renal veins flow into the supracardinal trunks (*a*). Tomogram of much dilated azygos with prominent vascular shadows on the right (*b*). Union of persisting supracardinal veins (azygos with hemiazygos above the diaphragm), and common junction with the superior vena cava via the markedly dilated azygos arch (candy cane phenomenon) (*c, d*). (From: Elke, M., and H. Ludin: Fortschr. Röntgenstr. 103 (1965) 665.)

with assorted unions. Both morphologic varieties are based on the same ontogenetic errors.

Developmentally, the infrarenal portion of the inferior vena cava arises from the right supracardinal vein and the pelvic veins from the initial segment of the posterior cardinal veins. Differential regression or persistence and abnormal anastomoses between the central portions of the cardinal veins and left and right supracardinal vein are responsible for the development of numerous morphologic variants. Details of the embryology are given by McClure and Butler (1925), Eufinger et al. (1961) and Sarma (1966).

Incidence. Reis and Esenther (1959) found duplication or left-sided inferior vena cava 11 times among 500 autopsies. This means an incidence of 2.2 per cent for the former and of 0.2 per cent for the latter type. Seib (1934) found doubling of the inferior cava in approximately 3 per cent, and left-sided position alone in approximately 0.5 per cent of cases. Adachi (1937) encountered no instances of this anomaly in 1055 autopsies.

Morphologically, Sarma (1966) distinguished two main types, but with varying transitions (Fig. 10.8).

Type I. An additional inferior vena cava is found on the left, distal to the renal vein. The inferior venae cavae may have the same or different calibers. Three subgroups are distinguished depending on predominance of the left or right vessel:

Doubling of the inferior vena cava (caliber approximately identical), *accessory left inferior cava* (the right predominating), and *left-sided inferior vena cava* with accessory right cava (right vessel hypoplastic, transition to type II).

When the *caval veins* are *duplicated*, both vessels usually arise from a normal confluence of the common iliac veins. An oval ring results. Much less common is a left-ascending inferior vena cava as a continuation of the left external and internal iliac vein, and a right cava as a continuation of the right external and internal iliac. The latter variety can be described, if less correctly, as high confluence of the common iliac veins. The union of internal and external iliac veins also occupies varied sites. Thus Eufinger et al. (1961) described the junction of the left internal iliac with the confluence of the common iliac veins, that is, complete absence of the left common iliac vein.

Duplication of the vena cava may be associated with a *retrocaval ureter*. A cava ascending on the left may in rare cases flow into the left atrium.

Clinically, the inferior caval and pelvic vein anomalies mentioned do not usually cause any symptoms, but awareness of them is important to the surgeon, since they may be injured during operations on the terminal aorta, ureter and sympathetic trunk. Billroth is alleged to have inadvertently ligated an anomalous inferior vena cava (with fatal results) during a nephrectomy (cited by Sarma, 1966). In the differential diagnosis, distinction of caval anomalies from total situs inversus is important.

Type II. Transposition of the infrarenal portion of the inferior vena cava in the *absence* of visceral inversion is complete. The pelvic veins join to the left of the bifurcation of the aorta. The cava courses abruptly to the right, crossing the aorta ventrally, closely caudal to the branching of the superior mesenteric artery, and receiving the left renal vein. The cava then runs cranially in normal fashion. The right common iliac vein is crossed by the left common iliac artery; this produces worse drainage conditions than are found on the left (unlike the normal situation).

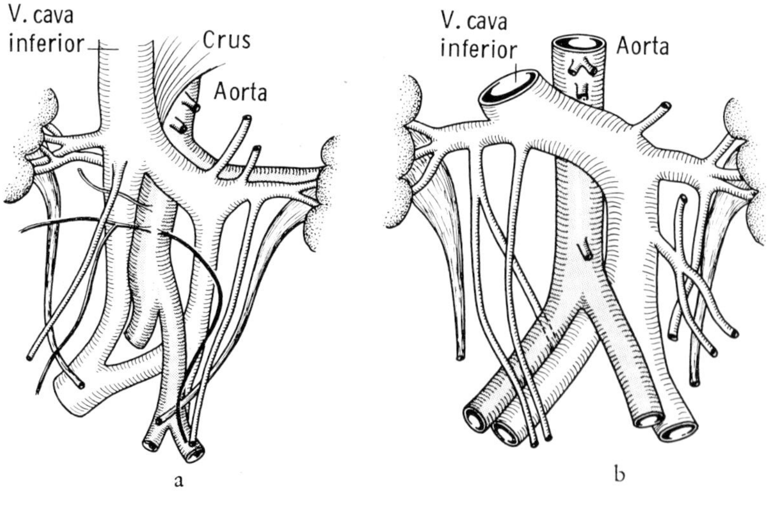

Fig. 10.8. Main types of anomalies of the infrarenal portion of the inferior vena cava. Duplication of the inferior vena cava, the most common form of type I anomaly (*a*); transposition or left-ascending inferior cava (type II anomaly) (*b*). Persistence of the vena cava and two testicular veins on the right. (From Sarma, K. P.: Brit. J. Surg. 53 (1966) 600.)

Anomalies of the Deep Pelvic and Leg Veins

Aplasia and Hypoplastic Stenosis

These are malformations comprising defects for short or, less frequently, longer distances, or hypoplastic stenoses of the deep veins (popliteal, femoral and external and common iliac). These venous anomalies were found regularly associated with hemangiectatic hypertrophy, of the Klippel-Trenaunay type.

Combination of the Klippel-Trenaunay syndrome with this aplasia of deep veins appears to be extraordinarily rare. For instance, Servelle (1949) encountered it only three times among 110 cases, but he saw compression of the veins by scarring. In the first place, the popliteal, femoral or external iliac vein is supposed to be affected by the aplasia. Olivier (1955) reported one case with an extended defect from popliteal to inferior vena cava. In the case of Langeron et al. (1963), drainage of the limb occurred via superficial veins, and an atypical deep collecting vein, which coursed from the lateral aspect of the thigh, crossed the common femoral ventrally and disappeared in the groin to flow directly into the external iliac vein. The superficial femoral and popliteal could not be found on exploration. The observation of Lindauer (1965) of aplasia of the deep veins on phlebograms of 11 patients with the Klippel-Trenaunay syndrome (confirmed by surgery in two patients) needs to be verified.

Presumably these malformations, hypertrophy and hypoplasia or aplasia of the deep venous system, are coordinated and not subordinated. This means that it is highly improbable that the resulting venous flow insufficiency would stimulate increased length and circumference of the extremity. Evidence in favor of this hypothesis is the fact that at most 1 to 2 per cent of patients with the Klippel-Trenaunay syndrome are affected by deep vein anomalies, and it is supported by the clinical observation that the post-thrombotic syndrome during childhood does not influence disunited epiphyseal cartilages.

The forms of hypertrophy of the limb concomitant with aplasia of the deep veins usually show the *clinical* picture of venous decompensation with a tendency to swelling, formation of secondary varices and occasionally recurrent leg ulcers. The combination with more or less extensive dermal angiomas or telangiectasia is typical, and at times lymphomas and lipomas are also present. The extremity assumes the ugly features of elephantiasis. In contrast, *Weber's syndrome* (macrosomia with congenital arteriovenous fistulas) usually reveals *proportioned* hypertrophy (Table 10.2) (Vollmar, 1967).

Table 10.2. Special Forms of Hypertrophy of the Extremities

	Klippel-Trenaunay (1900)	Weber's Syndrome (1907–1918)
Gigantism	disproportionate, elephantiasis	proportionate
Vascular nevi or hemangiomas, lymphangiomas	almost the rule	rare
Arteriovenous fistulas	absent	present (usually near epiphyses, intraosseous)
Anomalies of deep veins (aplasia, stenosis)	rare	absent
Prognosis	good, largely stationary	doubtful, tends to deteriorate

Recognition of hypoplastic stenosis or aplasia of deep leg and pelvic veins is practical only by angiography (ascending and descending phlebography). Perfect *phlebographic technique* is essential. Only too often, absence of deep veins on ascending phlebography of a "patchy" limb is evaluated by the inexperienced as proof of aplasia. In three patients admitted with this diagnosis, repeat phlebograms of good quality revealed a normal and patent deep venous system. The increased volume of the limb makes it extremely difficult to direct the contrast medium into the deep venous system (the tourniquet above the ankle must be tightened).

Surgical correction of congenital aplasia of deep veins can be considered in principle only for short defective segments of the pelvic system (*free venous grafting* or *transverse in situ bypass* of Palma). For reconstruction in the knee and thigh, a saphenous in situ bypass safeguarded by an arteriovenous fistula is the most suitable. In the presence of leg ulcers symptomatic relief may be provided by ligation of incompetent perforators or elimination of valve-deficient subcutaneous veins. In the presence of aplasia of the deep drainage system, collateral function of the subcutaneous veins should be tested phlebographically and clinically before sclerosation or extirpation of subcutaneous veins. If this is

omitted, their interruption may aggravate venous blood flow (Forster and Kirtley, 1959).
As far as we know, no report is available of successful reconstruction of the deep venous system in a patient with the Klippel-Trenaunay syndrome.

Aplasia of Venous Valves

Congenital absence of the valves in body veins, both complete and incomplete, is extraordinarily rare. Only about 20 cases had been reported by the end of 1968. This anomaly is as insignificant clinically as it is interesting for pathophysiologic studies (Basmajian, 1952; Lodin, 1961).
Clinically, orthostatic edema is the first sign, usually occurring in the second decade. *Varicosities* are secondary. The sign of "transport insufficiency" in the deep venous system is present, just as in the post-thrombotic syndrome. Venous return is much less affected than in the latter, however, since flow resistance is normal or reduced, unlike the case in the post-thrombotic syndrome, and the lymphatic system is evidently able to compensate for many years (Kappert and May, 1968).
Diagnosis is mainly based on venography. In typical cases, both subcutaneous and deep veins of the upper and lower extremities reveal complete absence of valves. The veins are widely placed and of smooth outline, and venous drainage is more or less retarded.
In the *differential diagnosis*, a post-thrombotic syndrome with extensive destruction of the valves must be excluded.
Surgical correction of partial or total absence of valves is *not* feasible. Treatment must remain conservative (pressure bandages and elastic stockings).

Duplication and Anomalies of Course and Union of Leg Veins

Numerical anomalies, particularly *duplication*, are not so rare, either in the deep veins of the femoropopliteal segment or in the subcutaneous veins (especially the long saphenous). The same applies to the numerous variations of the *saphenofemoral junction* and *communicating veins* between the small and great saphenous system. For their morphology, see pages 9 and 11.
The *clinical importance* of these anomalies is small. They are of no hemodynamic significance, but it is important to know of them in undertaking surgery of varicosities, understanding so-called recurrent varices and obtaining venous grafts.

Addendum to the Therapy of Congenital Angiodysplasias

Hypertrophy with Connatal Arteriovenous Fistulas (Weber Type)

The multiplicity and topographic extent of connatal arteriovenous fistulas preclude definite surgical correction in the majority of cases. Nevertheless, in view of the *tendency to progression, active surgical intervention* is indicated as early as the first or second decade if hemodynamically relevant arteriovenous shunts become apparent (ectasia of an afferent artery, positive Nicoladoni-Branham phenomenon or systolic-diastolic machinery murmur).
In planning and execution of plastic surgery, a technically faultless *arteriogram* is imperative (for localization of arteriovenous fistulas or recognition of the most important collateral afferent and efferent paths).

Direct arteriovenous fistulas between main vessels of the extremities (type I) can be *directly* operated on and ligated (separation method). Such a radical operation is not practicable for the far more common generalized form (type II, multiple transverse shunts in soft tissues and skeleton). The so-called *skeletization operation* (ligature of all afferent and efferent branches of main arterial and venous trunks) has proved useful. The occasional sacrifice of the limb that formerly was incurred because of deleterious remote action on the heart and large vessels can thus largely be avoided, in our experience.
Proximal ligature of the main artery must be strictly warned against: in type II, it has no notable effect on shunt volume and risks necrosis of the limb. Operative removal of *secondary varices* is just as objectionable, as long as the venous shunts are not definitely excluded. Sclerosing therapy is also senseless; the veins are recanalized under the influence of arterial recrudescence in a short time.

Correction of linear extension: for that up to 3 cm, by raising the heel of the shoe; if it is more than 4 cm, a shortening osteotomy should be considered after termination of epiphyseal growth.

All *other methods* (epiphysiodesis or removal or irradiation of the epiphyseal cartilage) are of little use.

Klippel-Trenaunay Type

This prognostically more favorable vascular variant of hypertrophy becomes *stationary* with completion of epiphyseal growth. The problem of extreme elephantiasis is cosmetic rather than medical. *Therapeutically, expectant conservatism* takes first place (tight pressure bandages and elastic hose).

There are two main indications for *surgery*:

1. In the presence of *dyplastic varices* of trunks (frequently valveless with atypical course, e.g., as "ventral or dorsal garland" on leg and thigh). Venographic exclusion of hypoplasia or aplasia of the deep venous system is essential prior to intended extirpation with ligature of incompetent perforators.
2. *Reducing operations* (eliminating elephantiasis by extirpation of lymphangiomas or hemangiomas or fibrous, indurated subcutaneous tissues in the "lymphostatic form").

If the limb volume is mainly of lymphatic origin, particularly at the margins of the foot and toes, hyperkeratosis with rhagades develops occasionally, which may be starting point of recurrent erysipelas or cutaneous fistulas.

Lymphangiographically, aplasia or marked hypoplasia of the efferent lymphatics can usually be demonstrated. *Local excision* (wedging with direct wound closure) of the hyperkeratotic margins is practical. Caution is necessary with free skin grafts. The poor healing tendency and keloid formation must be kept in mind in these operations.

The commonly present *nevus flammeus* is of barely any consequence in comparison with the enormous volume of the limb. Radiation is senseless, and surgical correction almost never justified. Regarding equalization of length of the limb, the principles are the same as those for the Weber type.

Note: The use of expert angiologic diagnosis and clinical checkups in the last few years have made it obvious that the two vascular variants of this hypertrophy can be clearly differentiated in most cases, particularly as regards their therapeutic consequences. To consider the Klippel-Trenaunay-Weber syndrome a single unit is not justifiable, either historically or clinically. Both syndromes are special forms of macrosomia, considerably distinguished by their clinical manifestations, prognosis and therapy.

References

Abbot, O. A.: Congenital Aneurysm of the Superior Vena Cava. Ann. Surg. 131 (1950) 259

Abbot, O. A., T. F. Leigh: Aneurysmal dilations of the superior vena caval system. Ann. Surg. 159 (1964) 858

Abrams, H. L.: The Relationship of Systemic Venous Anomalies to the Paravertebral Veins. Amer. J. Roentgenol. 80 (1958) 414

Adachi., B.: Cited in Sarma

Albert, H. M., R. L. Fowler, B. A. Glass, Yu. Shu-Kuen: Cardiac anomalies and splenic agenesis. Amer. Surg. 34 (1968) 94

Anderson, R. C., P. Adams Jr., B. Burke: Anomalous inferior vena cava with azygos-continuation (infrahepatic interruption of the inferior vena cava). J. Pediat. 59 (1961) 370

Anderson, R. C., W. Heilig, R. Novick, C. Jarvis: Anomalous inferior vena cava with azygos drainage: so-called absence of the inferior vena cava. Amer. Heart J. 49 (1955) 318

Bartel, J., L. Wierny: Zur Agenesie der V. cava caudalis. Fortschr. Röntgenstr. 99 (1963) 467

Basmajian, J. V.: The distribution of valves in the femoral, external iliac, and common iliac veins and their relationship to varicose veins. Surg. Gynec. Obstet. 95 (1952) 537

Bennet, I. L., Jr.: A unique case of obstruction of the inferior vena cava. Bull. Johns Hopkins Hosp. 87 (1950) 290

Berk, R. N.: Dilatation of the left superior intercostal vein in the plain-film diagnosis of chronic superior vena caval obstruction. Radiology 83 (1964) 419–423

Boenig, H.: Leitfaden der Entwicklungsgeschichte des Menschen. Thieme, Leipzig 1944

Boutelier, P., C. Couinaud: Les Anomalies dites "Primitives" de la veine cava inférieure. J. Chir. (Paris) 83 (1962) 199

Brunner, U.: Gemischte kongenitale Angiodysplasien: Chirurgische Maßnahmen im Rahmen des Syndroms von Klippel-Trenaunay-Weber. Zbl. Phleb. 9 (1970) 230

Bücheler, E., A. Düx, A. Sobbe: Die renolumbale Anastomose im direkten retroperitonealen Veno- und selektiven Azygogramm. Fortschr. Röntgenstr. 109 (1968) 713

Bücheler, E., A. Düx, P. Thurn: Membranöser Verschluß und Agenesie der Vena cava inferior. Fortschr. Röntgenstr. 105 (1966) 806

Capdevila, J. M., J. Farre, F. Bongera, J. M. Curria, E. Samaniego: Situación anómala de la vena cava inferior a propósito de tres observaciones personales. Angiologia 20 (1968) 11

Derra, L., F. Loogen, P. Satter: Anomalien der unteren Hohlvene. Dtsch. med. Wschr. 90 (1965) 689, 701

Effler, D. B., A. E. Greer, E. C. Sifers: Anomaly of the vena cava inferior; report of fatality after ligation. J. Amer. med. Ass. 146 (1951) 1321

Eguchi, S., S. Endo, A. Yamaguchi, K. Asano: Inferior caval occlusion associated with the BUDD-CHIARI-Syndrome: treatment with bypass operation. J. cardiovasc. Surg. 7 (1966) 490

Elke, M., H. Ludin: Drainage der unteren Körperhälfte bei Agenesie und erworbenem Verschluß der Vena caudalis. Fortschr. Röntgenstr. 103 (1965) 665

Erlik, D., A. Shramek, S. Brandstaetter, H. Bassan: Cure of hepatic vein occlusion by side-to-side portacaval shunt. Surg. Gynec. Obstet. 114 (1962) 368

Eufinger, H., L. Diethelm, E. May: Röntgenologische und Operationsbefunde bei chronischer Beckenvenensperre und ihre Bedeutung für die Operationsindikation. Bruns' Beitr. klin. Chir. 203 (1961) 152

Forster, F. H., J. A. Kirtley: Unilateral lower extremity hypertrophy. Surg. Gynec. Obstet. 108 (1959) 35

Gallucci, V., P. W. Sanger, F. Robicsek, H. K. Daugherty: Aneurysm of the superior caval vein. Vasc. Surg. 1 (1967) 158–161

Gardner, D. L., L. Cole: Long survival with interferior vena cava draining into left atrium. Brit. Heart J. 17 (1955) 93

Gautam, H. P.: Left atrial inferior vena cava with atrial septal defect. I. Thorac. cardiovasc. Surg. 55 (1968) 827

Goerttler, K.: Über Blutstromwirkung als Gestaltungsfaktor für die Entwicklung des Herzens. Beitr. path. Anat. 115 (1955) 33

Goerttler, K.: Normale und pathologische Entwicklung des menschlichen Herzens. In: Zwanglose Abhandlungen aus dem Gebiet der normalen und pathologischen Anatomie. Section 3. W. Bargmann, W. Doerr (eds.). Thieme, Stuttgart 1958 (p. 96)

Goerttler, K.: Entwicklungsgeschichte des Herzens. In: Das Herz des Menschen. Vol. 1. W. Bargmann, W. Doerr (eds.). Thieme, Stuttgart 1963 (p. 512, 522)

Gould, S. E.: Pathology of the Heart. Thomas, Springfield Ill. 1953

Hirooka, M., C. Kimura: Membranous obstruction of the hepatic portion of the inferior vena cava. Arch. Surg. 100 (1970) 656

Kappert, A., R. May: Das postthrombotische Zustandsbild der Extremitäten. Huber, Bern 1968

Kimura, T., K. Joya, H. Hirooka, M. Torada, K. Iwahashi, S. Maeya: Clinical and embryological findings in case of membranous obstruction of the hepatic inferior vena cava associated with Chiari's disease. Presented before the General Meeting of the 62nd Japan Surgical Society, Tokyo, 1962

Kimura, C., H. Shirotani, M. Hirooka, M. Torado, K. Iwahashi, S. Maetani: Membranous obliteration of the inferior vena cava in the hepatic portion. J. cardiovasc. Surg. 4 (1963) 87
Kimura, C., H. Shirotani, T. Kuma, M. Hirooka, K. Havashi, K. Tsunekawa, S. Matsuda: Transcardiac membranotomy for obliteration of the inferior vena cava in the hepatic portion. J. cardiovasc. Surg. 3 (1962) 393
Klippel, M., P. Trenaunay: Du naevus variqueux ostéohypertrophique. Arch. gén. méd. 3 (1900) 641
Kootstra, D. G.: Ectasieen van halsvenen. Ned. T. Geneesk. 113 (1969) 2233
Krestinov, G., D. Arnaudov: The diagnosis and treatment of the congenital aneurysm of the internal jugular vein. Vestn. Chir. (Mosk.) 94 (1965) 96–98
Lam, C. R., E. Green, H. Gale: Transcardiac membranotomy for obstruction of the hepatic portion of the inferior Vena cava. Circulation, Suppl. 31 (1965) 188
Langeron, P., B. Delecour, R. Vogel: Syndrome de Klippel-Trenaunay avec importante agénésie veineuse—relativité de la notion angiographique de retour veineuse précoce. Angéiologie 15 (1963) 5
de La Riega, E., E. Kuhn: Alleinige persistierende linke obere Hohlvene. 2. Kreisl.-Forsch. 54 (1965) 734–738
Lindauer, S. M.: The Klippel-Trenaunay-Syndrome: Varicosity, Hypertrophy and Hemangioma with no arteriovenous fistula. Amer. Surg. 162 (1965) 303
Lindvall, N., A. Lodin: Congenital absence of valves in the deep veins of the leg. Acta derm. venereol. Suppl. 45 (1961)
Lodin, A.: Congenital absence of valves in the deep veins of the leg. Acta derm. venereol. Suppl. 45 (1961)
Loogen, F., H. Kreuzer: Einmündung der unteren Hohlvene in den linken Vorhof als isolierte Anomalie. Z. Kreisl.-Forsch. 51 (1962) 1033
Loogen, F., R. Rippert: Anomalien der großen Körper- und Lungenvenen. Z. Kreisl.-Forsch. 47 (1958) 677
Lucas, R. V., H. N. Neufeld, R. C. Lester, J. E. Edwards: The symmetrical liver as a roentgen sign of asplenia. Circulation 25 (1962) 973
McClure, C. F. W., E. G. Butler: The development of the vena cava inferior in man. Amer. J. Anat. 35 (1925) 331
Martorell, F., J. Monserrot: Atresic iliac vein and Klippel-Trenaunay syndrome. Angiology 13 (1962) 265
Muelheims, G. H., J. G. Mudd: Anomalous inferior vena cava. Amer. J. Cardiol. 9 (1962) 945
Nißl, R.: Röntgenstudien zur Anatomie der Beinvenen. In: Angiographie. K. E. Loose (ed.). Thieme, Stuttgart 1966
Ohara, I., H. Ouchi, K. Takahashi: A bypass operation for occlusion of the hepatic inferior vena cava. Surg. Gynec. Obstet. 117 (1963) 151
Olivier, C.: Les varices symptomatiques de malformations vasculaires. Presse méd. 66 (1955) 1822
Palma, E. C., R. Esperón: Vein transplants and grafts in the surgical treatment of the postphlebitic syndrome. J. cardiovasc. Surg. 1 (1960) 94
Portsmann, W., S. Platzek: Obliteration der V. cava sup. et inf bei einem 19jähr. Patienten. Fortschr. Röntgenstr. 101 (1964) 90
Reis, R. H., G. Esenther: Cited in Sarma
Sarma, K. P.: Anomalous inferior vena cava—anatomical and clinical. Brit. J. Surg. 53 (1966) 600
Seib, G. A.: The azygos system of veins in American whites and American negroes, including observations on the inferior caval venous system. Amer. J. Phys. Anthropol. 19 (1934) 39
Servelle, M.: La veinographie va-t-elle nous permettre de démembrer le syndrome de Klippel-Trenaunay. Presse méd. 26 (1945) 363
Servelle, M.: Des malformations veineuses congénitales. Arch. Mal. Coeur 40 (1947) 125
Servelle, M.: Les malformations congénitales des veines. Rev. Chir. 68 (1949) 88
Stackelberg, Brita, J. Lind, C. Wegelius: Absence of inferior vena cava diagnosed by angiocardiography. Cardiologia 21 (1952) 583
Stark, C. G.: Commentatio anatomico-physiologica de venae azygos natura, atque munere. Breitkopfii Haertel, Lipsiae 1835
Swart, B.: Azygoserweiterung bei fehlender V. cava inferior und Situs inversus mit Laevocardie. Fortschr. Röntgenstr. 97 (1962) 523
Taussig, H. B.: Congenital Malformations of the Heart, Vol. II. The Commonwealth Fund, Cambridge 1960 (p. 948)
Vollmar, J.: Rekonstruktive Chirurgie der Arterien. Thieme, Stuttgart (2nd ed.) 1975
Walker, W. A.: Aneurysm of the azygos vein, etiology undetermined. Amer. J. Roentgenol. 90 (1963) 575
Watkins, E., jr., C. L. Fortin: Surgical correction of a congenital coarctation of the inferior vena cava. Ann. Surg. 159 (1964) 536

Index